Modern Radiotherapy
& Oncology

CENTRAL NERVOUS SYSTEM TUMOURS

Modern Radiotherapy & Oncology

CENTRAL NERVOUS SYSTEM TUMOURS

Edited by

THOMAS J. DEELEY

M.B., Ch.B., F.F.R., D.M.R.T.

Director, South Wales and Monmouthshire Radiotherapy Service, Velindre Hospital, University Hospital of Wales, Cardiff; Lecturer, Welsh National School of Medicine, Cardiff

BUTTERWORTHS

ENGLAND: BUTTERWORTH & CO. (PUBLISHERS) LTD.
                LONDON: 88 Kingsway, WC2B 6AB
AUSTRALIA: BUTTERWORTHS PTY. LTD.
                SYDNEY: 586 Pacific Highway 2067
                MELBOURNE: 343 Little Collins Street, 3000
                BRISBANE: 240 Queen Street, 4000
CANADA: BUTTERWORTH & CO. (CANADA) LTD.
                TORONTO: 14 Curity Avenue, 374
NEW ZEALAND: BUTTERWORTHS OF NEW ZEALAND LTD
                WELLINGTON: 26–28 Waring Taylor Street, 1
SOUTH AFRICA: BUTTERWORTH & CO. (SOUTH AFRICA) (PTY.) LTD.
                DURBAN: 152–154 Gale Street

Suggested U.D.C. Number: 615·849 : 616·83–006

ISBN 0 407 27590 8

Printed in Great Britain by
Western Printing Services Ltd., Bristol

Contents

Contributors

A. S. BLIGH, M.B., B.S., F.F.R., D.M.R.D.
Consultant Radiologist, University Hospital of Wales, Heath Park, Cardiff

G. DU BOULAY, M.B., F.R.C.P., F.F.R.
Consultant Radiologist, Lysholm Radiological Department, The National Hospital, Queen Square, London; Radiologist in Charge of the X-ray Department, Nuffield Institute of Comparative Medicine, The Zoological Society of London, Regent's Park, London

THOMAS J. DEELEY, M.B., Ch.B., F.F.R., D.M.R.T.
Director, South Wales and Monmouthshire Radiotherapy Service, Velindre Hospital, University Hospital of Wales, Cardiff; Lecturer, Welsh National School of Medicine, Cardiff

J. M. RICE EDWARDS, F.R.C.S.
Senior Registrar, The National Hospital, Queen Square, London

DOUGLAS GORDON, M.B., Ch.B., D.M.R., D.M.R.D.
Consultant Radiologist, Moorfields Eye Hospital (High Holborn); Consultant Ultrasonic Radiologist, Willesden General Hospital, London

J. M. HENK, M.A., M.B., B.Chir., F.F.R., D.M.R.T.
Consultant Radiotherapist, Welsh Hospital Board; Clinical Teacher, Welsh National School of Medicine, Cardiff

TAKAO HOSHINO, M.D., D.M.Sc.
Assistant Professor of Neurosurgery, University of Tokyo; Assistant Professor in Residence, Department of Neurological Surgery, University of California Medical Center, San Francisco, California

FAZLUR R. KHAN, M.D.
Chairman of the Department of Radiation Therapy, Weiss Memorial Hospital, Chicago, Illinois

SIMON KRAMER, M.D.
Professor and Chairman, Department of Radiation Therapy, Thomas Jefferson University Hospital, Philadelphia, Pennsylvania

J. G. LEOPOLD, M.B., B.Ch., M.R.C.Path.
Senior Lecturer in Pathology, Welsh National School of Medicine, Cardiff; Honorary Consultant Histopathologist, University Hospital of Wales, Heath Park, Cardiff

MARTIN B. LEVENE, M.D.
Deputy Director of the Joint Center for Radiation Therapy, Boston, Massachusetts; Associate Professor of Radiation Therapy, Harvard Medical School

HARRY NEWMAN, M.D.
Department of Radiology, University of California at San Francisco, California

C. PALLIS, D.M., F.R.C.P.
Reader in Neurology, Royal Postgraduate Medical School, London

THEODORE L. PHILLIPS, M.D.
Department of Radiology, University of California at San Francisco, California

J. JACKSON RICHMOND, F.R.C.S., F.F.R.
Honorary Consulting Radiotherapist, St. George's Hospital, London; Formerly Medical Director, Radiotherapy Centre, St. Luke's Hospital, Guildford, Surrey

WILLIAM R. SHAPIRO, M.D.
Associate Professor of Neurology, Cornell University Medical College, New York; Associate Attending Physician (Neurologist), Memorial Hospital for Cancer and Allied Diseases, New York

ANTERO VOUTILAINEN, M.D.
Professor of Radiotherapy, University Central Hospital of Turku, Finland

I. M. S. WILKINSON, B.Sc., M.D., M.R.C.P.
Consultant Neurologist, Addenbrooke's Hospital, Cambridge

Preface

The *Modern Radiotherapy & Oncology* series is designed to cover aspects of malignant disease at certain sites in the body. This volume is devoted to the central nervous system. The radiotherapist, concerned as he is with malignant disease, must have up-to-date knowledge not only of how to improve his techniques of treatment but of all aspects of the disease. Currently we apply the term *oncology* to this concept. The subjects of the chapters of this volume have been chosen with the hope that the radiotherapist treating malignant diseases at this site will benefit from this wide experience; with this in mind contributions have been invited from workers in other specialties. I hope that the resulting work will be of benefit to other clinicians as well as radiotherapists.

Diseases of the brain have always involved a feeling of apprehension because they strike at the body's most important organ; the results of treatment leave no room for complacency. Improvements in treatment demand considerable research on the part of many associated workers, all working together and fully aware of the problems not only in their own particular field but in associated disciplines. The contributors have described the advances that have already been made and have pointed out the paths which future developments may take. I am particularly grateful to all these authors for the willingness with which they have produced their chapters.

Miss J. M. Williams and Mrs J. James have given invaluable secretarial assistance and I am grateful to the Tenovus Cancer Information Centre, Cardiff, for their help. As usual, it has been a pleasure to work with the Editorial Staff of the Publishers.

T.J.D.

1—Introduction

J. Jackson Richmond

Since the earlier years of this century great advance has been made in the management of patients suffering from intracranial tumours. This has been due to improved surgical technique aided by modern methods of anaesthesia, more precise radiological localization of tumours and more sophisticated radiotherapy.

Harvey Cushing in America concentrated upon meticulous care in dissection of the tumour, watertight closure of the wounds and maintenance of a bloodless field in contrast to other surgeons of his era who relied on speed with an associated high operative mortality (McKissock, 1952). Later Olivecrona of Stockholm, using Cushing's gentle handling of tissues and replacement of the osteoplastic flap, devised methods whereby the operation time was reduced greatly. His technique has been adopted in many neurosurgical clinics today.

Despite these advances very few infiltrating gliomas can be totally excised by the surgeon without causing irreparable damage to normal brain tissue. Because of these limitations an increasing number of patients have been referred for radiotherapy. The results were extremely disappointing and no improvement in the mortality rate occurred until the dawn of a more realistic appraisal of the limited tolerance of the brain to irradiation. In some radiotherapy centres electromagnetic has been replaced by corpuscular irradiation in the form of high energy electron therapy. It is probable that neutrons will be employed to an increasing extent with the development of equipment more suitable for general practical use.

Chemotherapy by both the intra-arterial and systemic routes has a place in the treatment of the more anaplastic tumours. However, so far this is essentially a palliative method. With the advent of more selective and less toxic chemical agents this form of therapy may well be used more extensively.

This preamble leads to the important discussion of team work.

1

TEAM WORK IN SUCCESSFUL MANAGEMENT OF PATIENTS

Close co-operation between the following 'specialist team' should lead to more favourable results and achieve the maximum benefit to the patient.

Neurologist

The neurologist will in most cases make the provisional clinical diagnosis and refer the patient for radiological examination.

Neuroradiologist

The neuroradiologist uses straight and contrast radiographic studies and also isotope encephalography. It is remarkable to what extent valuable information may be deduced by expert radiologists from a study of plain radiographic views of the skull. How vividly I recall watching that great radiological teacher, the late Merrill Sosman, demonstrating to his students at his clinic in Boston, Mass. During the past decade radioactive isotopes have been employed to a progressively increasing extent in an attempt to gain more precise information regarding the localization of intracranial tumours. Ventriculography, formerly a standard procedure, has largely been replaced except in the investigation of pituitary adenomas. It is frequently possible to predict the pathology by studying the topography of tumours demonstrated by photo scanning (Bull, 1966). Furthermore in combination with angiography it is sometimes possible to estimate the degree of malignancy of a glioma, by the visual pattern of distorted normal blood vessels and the formation of new venous channels in the tumour.

Neurosurgeon

It is often possible to excise totally intracranial meningiomas and vascular tumours, in which case post-operative radiotherapy will not be indicated. Unfortunately this rarely applies when dealing with malignant gliomas. However, incomplete removal of these tumours can be of considerable value as a preliminary to a full course of radiotherapy. Also it is most important to have material available for histological study by the pathologist.

Pathologist

Very extensive experience is essential in the field of neuropathology before expressing a reliable opinion concerning the type and classification of a glioma. Even so there may be narrow differences in the assessment of experts concerning the degree of malignancy of individual tumours. Nevertheless the neuropathologist has made it possible for the relatively complex cytological features to be standardized. This forms a useful basis for comparison of results and estimation of prognosis in particular cases.

Radiotherapist

Supplied with comprehensive information resulting from the foregoing investigations, the therapist should be in the position to weigh the indications for radiotherapy. Of course, in practice many patients will fall into groups where a predetermined policy of combined surgery and irradiation has been decided upon.

Clinical Physicist

In planning the treatment design the services of the clinical physicist will be invaluable when working in collaboration with the radiotherapist. Individual cases will present problems in ensuring the optimum distribution of irradiation combined with protection of vital structures. Again the physicist will be involved with the operation of isotope scanning techniques.

Finally, this review would be incomplete without mentioning the important role played by the general practitioner. The patient's immediate medical adviser must be fully informed concerning the results of investigations and treatment and receive subsequent practical interval progress reports with suggestions regarding ancillary medical treatment.

FACTORS INFLUENCING CLINICAL RESPONSE TO RADIOTHERAPY

There are both *limiting* and *favourable* factors to be considered when contemplating the employment of irradiation in the treatment of tumours of the central nervous system. In the *first* group we must consider the following three items.

Vulnerability of Normal Tissues of the Central Nervous System to Irradiation

At an earlier stage in the history of radiotherapy it was generally believed that these normal tissues were relatively tolerant to ionizing irradiations. Subsequent experience has led to the opposing view. As more powerful therapy equipment became available there was a tendency to increase the tumour dose delivered to intracranial gliomas in an attempt to sterilize these relatively radio-resistant neoplasms. The dosage level was controlled by the tissues of the calvarium rather than those of the normal brain. However, there was no significant improvement in the appalling survival rate of patients. Indeed it was thought by many that radiotherapy was of little value in the treatment of gliomas, except perhaps in the case of the most highly sensitive tumours, e.g. medulloblastoma.

Subsequent careful microscopic studies of irradiated brain tissue removed at autopsy revealed evidence of post-irradiation changes of varying degrees, but in some cases no sign of active tumour. Supported by clinical and experimental evidence it is now well known that the normal tissues of the central nervous system are definitely vulnerable to dosages of irradiation little in excess of those frequently prescribed in the practice of radiotherapy. Experience has led to the acceptance of a 'maximum safe dosage level' under certain conditions. It is of the utmost importance that this principle in dosage prescription is adhered to even when dealing with tumours which are in immediate anatomical relation to but not actively invading the brain or spinal cord. Included in this category would be meningiomas, vascular tumours and pituitary tumours. Regions of the brain of major importance from the point of view of irradiation damage are the brain stem, mesencephalon, with particular stress on the hypothalamus.

Difficulty in Precise Localization of Gliomas

The glioma is a highly invasive tumour and it is difficult to define the limits of brain tissue to which the neoplasm is confined. Radiographic studies with contrast media are of great use to the surgeon in making the pre-operative diagnosis, but rarely give an accurate assessment of the full extent of the tumour. Bull and Rovit (1957) illustrated the point by comparing both air and arteriographic studies with autopsy brain specimens in a series of highly malignant gliomas with extremely short survival periods. While crude tumour localization could be obtained in a high percentage of cases by the two different contrast methods, in less than one half of all the cases studied could precise definition of the tumour outline be demonstrated. Although the common use of gamma encephalography (Howieson and Bull, 1966) has greatly improved the degree of localization of malignant gliomas it is not possible to delimit entirely the peripheral ramifications of the tumour in brain tissue.

Changing Order of Malignancy

There is evidence to indicate that the glioma is not a static tumour and the change is invariably to a higher order of malignancy. In an extreme case a relatively differentiated astrocytoma grade I may over a period of years revert to the highly anaplastic grade IV tumour. Again microscopic examination of samples taken from different sections of the same glioma may reveal dissimilar degrees of malignancy. This of course makes precise histological grading somewhat of a problem, but it is prudent to classify the glioma in the grade relating to the highest order of anaplasia detected in the complete specimen. The same process can at times occur in other primary intracranial tumours including meningiomas and haemangiomas which may change from the essentially benign to the locally invasive state.

The more *favourable factors* may be enumerated as follows.

(1) Malignant gliomas do not metastasize outside the central nervous system. This knowledge is of course of tremendous advantage in planning radical radiotherapy when compared with the position relating to malignant disease occurring at other sites in the body, e.g. breast, bronchus, etc. Looked at in essentially physical terms the entire supratentorial compartment is of very limited volume.

(2) Young age of patients. The patients for the most part are in early life. An average age of approximately 35 years would be a common finding in large groups of patients admitted to radiotherapy units with primary intracranial neoplasms. In cases where radical treatment is justified one hopes to effect a cure extending over many years of useful life.

(3) Usually the tumours are radio-responsive. The more anaplastic gliomas including the medulloblastoma are highly radio-sensitive. The haemangioblastoma and cellular meningioma are usually sensitive and the pituitary adenomata are by no means radio-resistant as a group.

(4) The tissues of the calvarium are relatively tolerant to irradiation. Even when employing orthovoltage multiple field systems there may be permanent epilation of hair, but there should be no other macroscopic evidence of skin atrophy if the prescribed tumour dosage has been kept within safe limits.

(5) Constitutional effects of the irradiation are minimal. Interruption of the course of therapy due to the onset of leukopenia or other untoward tolerance effects is most unusual except when extensive zones of the spine are being irradiated.

GENERAL PRINCIPLES OF TREATMENT PLAN IN PRIMARY INTRACRANIAL TUMOURS

Glioma Series

This group includes (*a*) astrocytoma, (*b*) oligodendroglioma, (*c*) ependymoma, and (*d*) medulloblastoma. These tumours are graded I to IV in ascending order of malignancy according to the classification first described by Kernohan and colleagues (1949). In this system the well-known label 'glioblastoma multiforme' is replaced by astrocytoma grade III or IV. These tumours are highly anaplastic, associated with a relatively short clinical history and carry a poor prognosis. Jefferson (1948) aptly described them as agents which 'in a few weeks can reduce a healthy man or woman to an aphasic, hemiplegic, incontinent caricature of humanity'. Nevertheless these tumours can be radio-sensitive and on occasions long-term regression can be achieved. It is difficult to select the patients most suitable for radiotherapy and one must expect a proportion to succumb, during the weeks and months following the completion of therapy, or even during the actual treatment period. Fortunately patients with the most advanced physical and mental deterioration in this group are those surviving for such a relatively brief period. In reviewing a personal series of 165 unselected cases of confirmed astrocytoma grades III and IV I found a mortality of 48 per cent during the first year after commencement of radiotherapy, and a five-year survival rate of 18 per cent (Richmond, 1959). From a statistical viewpoint these results depict the most depressing side of the picture and fortunately one can hope for a much more favourable outcome when treating other tumours in the glioma series.

There are two cardinal principles which should be obeyed when planning such treatment:

(1) The treated volume of brain should be sufficiently large to incorporate the probable extent of the tumour.

(2) The maximum tumour dosage should not exceed a level likely to lead to irreversible irradiation damage to normal brain tissue.

With these factors to the forefront it is possible to establish a series of standard regional multifield treatment plans. The volume of brain tissue irradiated will be extensive and include the ramifications of the glioma in the supratentorial compartment.

An adequate dosage distribution may be attained by two pairs of directly opposed orthovoltage x-ray fields 10 cm square disposed at right angles in antero-posterior and lateral planes (Richmond, 1952). Although there may not be complete uniformity of dosage it is reasonable to assume that the central zones of the glioma where the oxygenation may be reduced will require a higher dosage level to promote tumour sterilization. On the other hand the much smaller collections of tumour cells infiltrating brain tissue at the periphery of the irradiated volume may respond to a reduced dosage level.

The dosage prescription is all important. With orthovoltage x-ray therapy a tumour dose of 4,000 rads in four weeks at the 120 per cent isodose zone gives a maximum level of 4,500 rads. All four fields should be treated daily for a total number of 20 treatments given in an overall period of four weeks. The bone absorption factor may be disregarded for practical purposes when dealing with the relatively thin membranous bone of the calvarium. When using electromagnetic irradiation of higher energy levels, say 2–6 MeV, then the prescribed tumour dosage should not be increased by a factor of more than 10 per cent fractionated over the same time period. With high energy electron therapy (20–35 MeV) the dosage will correspond to that indicated for the standard cobalt unit and linear accelerator.

Medulloblastoma

For convenience this tumour will be considered in the glioma series, but there are special features relating to the pathological behaviour which will influence the design of treatment. These tumours occur exclusively in the infratentorial region in children and may spread by implantation along the cerebrospinal fluid pathways. Occasionally the ependymoblastoma may 'seed' in the same manner. Complete surgical excision of an actively growing medulloblastoma invading the cerebellum and brain stem of a child is virtually impossible. Accordingly, radiotherapy plays a dominant role in the treatment of this radio-sensitive tumour. If the therapy is to be planned on a rational basis then both the primary tumour and the possible paths of spread should be included in the zone of irradiation. There remains the problem of deciding whether the intracranial region and the spinal neuraxis should be treated by a combined technique or separately. In my view it is wise to adopt the latter plan, unless there is definite clinical or isotopic confirmation that the tumour has already disseminated in the spinal axis. Otherwise it is desirable to concentrate on the known extent of the disease in an attempt to promote early regression of the tumour and relieve the child's ataxia as early as possible. In practice the combined method is not very suitable for very young subjects up to two years of age. Again it is unusual for the intracranial treatment to be interrupted due to untoward constitutional effects including leukopenia. However, this complication may well occur when long lengths of the spine are included in the field of irradiation. This in turn would upset the rhythm of the treatment to the primary infratentorial tumour. Despite this, Paterson (1953) reported most encouraging results of over 40 per cent five-year survival rate using the combined technique. Care must be taken to ensure that the histological classification is precise. The true medulloblastoma is a rare tumour which does not metastasize outside the tissues of the central nervous system. Occasionally

7

the cytological features can closely resemble those found in the more common neuroblastoma.

Prescribed Irradiation Dosage for Children

It may be thought that gliomas of similar histological type should receive comparable minimum dosages irrespective of the age of the patient. However, the tissues of a baby just will not tolerate the quantity of ionizing irradiation which may be delivered with safety to an adult. For practical purposes the following guide can be useful.

With patients of 12 years and over a minimum dosage of 4,000 rads delivered in 20 equal fractions over a period of one month may be regarded as the adult standard. For a baby of one year 50 per cent of the adult dose is given over the same period. At five years 75 per cent is prescribed. For children of intervening ages the dosages are assessed on a *pro rata* basis (Richmond, 1953).

When using supervoltage x-rays or high energy electrons these dosages may be increased by a factor of 10 per cent.

Special attention should be given to the care of the child during the course of radiotherapy. Close co-operation between radiographers and nurses is required. Apprehension and restlessness can often be allayed if the child is accompanied by young friends of similar age from the ward to the treatment room. Frequently it is profitable to spend a few days in giving 'trial treatments' including the adjustment of the treatment moulds before the actual irradiation begins. Sedatives should be used sparingly. When the spinal axis is treated blood counts should be taken at least at weekly intervals. In the event of paresis of limbs or ataxia physiotherapy must be readily available to assist the promotion of muscle re-education as early as possible.

When dealing with highly radio-sensitive tumours in the posterior fossa it is important to precede the formal course of irradiation with two or three daily exposures at a conservative dosage level. Béclère (1926) first described the practical hazard of setting up a 'pressure cone' owing to the rapid regression of the tumour mass. This sudden change in the intracranial hydrostatics could lead to a fatal issue.

Unconfirmed Gliomas

Before leaving the 'glioma series' it is well worth while discussing briefly a group of tumours which after clinical and radiological investigation have been diagnosed as 'malignant gliomas', but lack histological confirmation. It may be that the clinical course was so rapid with marked deterioration in the condition of the patient that the neurosurgeon considered exploratory craniotomy unjustifiable. On the other hand biopsy may have failed in the case of a deeply situated tumour which in any case would be inoperable. In a large proportion of such a group there may be strong supportive evidence from the angiographic and isotope studies leading to the diagnosis of glioblastoma multiforme. Occasionally autopsy leads to confirmation should the patient die in hospital. On first consideration this group would appear to be most unpromising from the treatment point of view. However, unless the patient is 'in extremis' radiotherapy may lead to satisfactory palliation or even complete arrest of the progress of the disease over a period of years. If the general condition of the patient permits then the course of therapy should be prescribed as indicated above for a classified confirmed intracranial glioma. The dosage–time relationship should not be changed because the general prognosis may be considered unfavourable.

Meningiomas

It is in this group of tumours as opposed to the 'glioma series' that the surgical results are so outstandingly good. The tumour may advance to a very large volume compressing rather than infiltrating the neighbouring brain tissue. It is not surprising that the presenting sign or symptom is 'focal' rather than the classical triad of headache, vomiting and papilloedema occurring so frequently in the presence of a rapidly progressing glioma. Radiotherapy will be indicated only in cases where total removal cannot be accomplished. It may be that the tumour is attached to a dural sinus or perhaps invading bone in the sphenoidal region. The degree of radio-sensitivity varies considerably and appears to be related to the cellularity of the tumour. The cytological features differ from the typical 'whorls' of the psammoma to the highly cellular invasive neoplasm known to the older pathologists as the 'meningeal sarcoma'. Obviously the radiotherapeutic technique cannot be standardized and is tailored to conditions in individual patients. Thus the treatment zone may be limited to the site of attachment to a dural sinus following subtotal removal of the meningioma. On the other hand there may be an extensive basal tumour situated too deeply for excision. Fortunately photoscanning and angiography are of great value in determining the precise localization. As in the case of gliomas the irradiation dosage will be controlled by the tolerance of the neighbouring brain tissue. High energy electron therapy has a particular application in the treatment of these tumours. With the useful facility of being able to change the energy level the distribution of the high dosage zone can be confined conveniently to the required depth with a sharp irradiation 'fall off' in the normal tissues. Also it is possible in many situations to simplify the technique by using a single treatment field only.

9

Vascular Tumours

Radiotherapy has a limited although important part in this group of tumours. A distinction must be made between vascular malformations and true neoplasms. In the main the haemangiomata present a problem for the neurosurgeon, but on occasions the tumour may be situated too deeply or otherwise inaccessible to allow total excision. The true vascular neoplasms show a widely variable rate of progression and degree of radio-sensitivity. The haemangioma frequently has a delayed response to irradiation and slow tumour regression may occur over a period of many months. Therefore, unless there is definite evidence of extension or intracranial haemorrhage an assessment of the response to irradiation should not be made too early. At the other end of the scale the haemangioblastoma may advance relatively rapidly and is frankly malignant. These tumours may prove very radio-responsive with complete tumour regression following a full course of irradiation.

Again the treatment cannot be standardized and the technique will require individual planning as in the case of the meningiomata.

Pituitary Tumours

Radiotherapy may be indicated for each of the following types.

Chromophobe Adenoma

Usually a visual field defect or impairment of visual acuity leads to clinical investigation before any endocrine disturbance is detected. In studying the case histories of 78 female patients it was found that no less than 41 had an early menopause. Yet the average interval from the time of cessation of menstruation until confirmation of the diagnosis was 7·5 years (Richmond, 1958). In women with unexplained amenorrhoea even a simple lateral radiograph of the skull may lead to the correct diagnosis before vision is threatened.

The most satisfactory treatment plan is a combination of surgery and radiotherapy. Henderson (1939), when reviewing Harvey Cushing's large series of cases, pointed out that patients receiving post-operative x-ray therapy showed a significant percentage increase in the five-year recurrence-free period. With the advent of higher voltage x-ray equipment and the knowledge that chromophobe adenomas were in most cases relatively radio-sensitive, there was a general tendency for therapists to increase the prescribed tumour dosage substantially. This led to a high morbidity and indeed mortality rate usually during the first or second year after the completion of the irradiation. It is now more generally accepted that however impeccable the treatment technique the maximum tumour dosage must be controlled by the limited tolerance to irradiation of the hypothalamus which is in immediate anatomical relationship to the pituitary. In some neurosurgical centres, particularly in the United States of America (Horrax and colleagues, 1955), patients are referred for radiotherapy in the first instance and excision of the tumour is performed only in cases which do not respond to the irradiation. However, the operative mortality is low in the hands of experienced neurosurgeons and the case for partial excision of the adenoma followed by carefully controlled radiotherapy can be supported by the following arguments:

(1) Usually there is already visual impairment with the ever-present threat of permanent blindness. Decompression of the visual pathways can forestall this tragedy should the adenoma prove relatively radioresistant.

(2) Many of these tumours are of surprisingly large volume and removal of the greater part of the friable tissue will allow the subsequent irradiation to be standardized to a smaller volume.

(3) Histological verification and classification of the adenoma may be obtained. Several other conditions may stimulate the 'pituitary syndrome'. An infratentorial tumour, a solitary intracranial metastasis, a meningioma, an aneurysm of the circle of Willis, or a glioma of the optic nerve could possibly lead to confusion in the preoperative diagnosis.

In my own view there may be a case for confining the treatment to surgery or radiotherapy alone in patients over 50 years of age when the vascular compensation in the operative field is to some extent more precarious than in the younger subject.

The irradiation technique will consist of multiple small fields directed by radiographic control to give a uniform dosage zone in the target area.

With orthovoltage x-ray therapy this tumour dosage should be 3,500 rads delivered in 20 equal fractions over a total period of 28 days. In most radiotherapy units orthovoltage has been replaced by supervoltage equipment when the tumour dosage will be 3,850 rads with the same fractionation. This dosage level may be regarded as 'safe' and as a benign tumour is the object of attack the prescription will be appreciably more conservative than in the presence of frank malignancy.

This combined surgical and radiotherapeutic method should give a five-year recurrence-free result of at least 80 per cent.

The post-treatment care of the patient is of great importance. Clinical examination including perimetry is advised when possible at quarterly intervals during the first year and thereafter at six-monthly or yearly periods according to progress.

The patient's endocrine status should be checked and the adequacy of replacement therapy assessed clinically (Nabarro, 1972).

Eosinophil Adenoma

These actively secretory tumours are less common than the chromophobe adenoma and are associated with gigantism in adolescence and acromegaly in the adult. The tumour can progress slowly over a number of years without necessarily causing visual impairment. The response to radiotherapy is somewhat variable in individual cases but can be of considerable value in arresting the advance of the acromegalic changes in face, hands and feet. The tissues are rarely restored to normal texture and appearance. Also the onset of visual defects may be prevented or delayed. The treatment technique and prescribed irradiation dosage will correspond closely with that relating to the chromophobe tumour.

Basophil Adenoma

This adenoma is rare but of considerable interest, being associated with the typical Cushing syndrome resembling that seen with hyperplasia or adenoma of the adrenal cortex. Unlike the other types of pituitary adenoma these tumours are extremely small and do not expand the sella. Consequently there is no associated impairment of vision. The irradiation should be accurately localized to a small volume. The results are variable but occasionally the clinical improvement is quite dramatic, indicating a high degree of radiosensitivity.

Craniopharyngioma

These tumours are predominantly suprasellar and tend to cause a lower quadrantic defect from pressure on the optic pathway from above. Formerly they were considered to be radio-resistant as a class, but this certainly is not the case. Fortunately the response to irradiation is most encouraging in a considerable proportion of patients which is helpful as the tumour may be adherent to neighbouring vital structures and render surgical excision a difficult procedure.

Pituitary Carcinoma

This is uncommon but probably the incidence is higher than generally suspected. Carcinoma may occur as a malignant transition from a highly cellular invasive chromophobe adenoma or less commonly as frank carcinoma developing in normal pituitary tissue. These tumours may metastasize intracranially. The prognosis is of course more serious than in the case of the benign adenoma, but radiotherapy can be effective in some patients. It is justifiable to increase the prescribed tumour dosage to that recommended for intracranial gliomas.

Primary Spinal Tumours

Primary spinal tumours are not very common, particularly when compared with the relatively high incidence of spinal metastases causing spinal cord compression. These primary tumours may for convenience be divided into intramedullary and extramedullary according to the site of origin. All members of the glioma series may arise in the spinal cord although they advance less rapidly than their intracranial counterparts. Frequently these intrinsic tumours are not histologically classified, owing to the inadvisability of taking biopsy material when the tumour is exposed at laminectomy. As expected there is a wide range of radio-sensitivity, but radiotherapy is always worth a trial as these intramedullary gliomas are necessarily inoperable.

In the extramedullary group such tumours as haemangiomas, meningiomas, primary sarcomas, neurofibromas and Hodgkin's lymphadenoma may be encountered. Treatment is planned to meet individual cases according to the extent of the neoplasm assessed by radiographic contrast studies or surgical exposure. The use of supervoltage therapy greatly facilitates the treatment technique from the point of view of planning uniform dosage at a depth, avoiding heavy skin reactions and reducing the problem of bone absorption of irradiation.

Particular care is required in the management of patients while the treatment is in progress and during the immediate post-therapy period. There may be the added complication of paraplegia and the skin needs constant attention to prevent bedsores, more particularly when there are extensive areas of skin anaesthesia. The care of the bladder is important where there is interference with nervous control. Instrumentation should be avoided if possible when retention of urine occurs. Antibiotics will be required for associated cystitis. Expert and regular physiotherapy should be instituted to deal with paralysed limbs. A careful check on the blood count is necessary because a profound leukopenia may be induced when extensive areas of the spine are irradiated. Rehabilitation is of great importance to the permanently disabled and much can be done to help the patient's readjustment to life.

13

Intracranial Metastases

Palliative radiotherapy can be of great benefit to the patient despite the limited span of life remaining. However, the indications for this form of therapy should be carefully weighed in each individual case. Although metastases may develop from many primary neoplasms, the commonest sites of origin are the bronchus and breast.

Photoscanning will often reveal the presence of multiple secondary intracranial tumours when a solitary neoplasm is suspected on clinical examination. Of course the general condition of the patient will be an important factor when contemplating palliative irradiation. For instance, cerebral metastases rendering a patient in a semistuperose state may be a blessing in disguise in the presence of advanced bronchial carcinoma. At least the burden of distressing respiratory symptoms is relieved and it would be a disservice to destroy this degree of symptomatic relief during the patient's terminal illness.

In my view the application of palliative radiotherapy for cerebral metastases, although of value at times, should be restricted. The chief indications are: (*a*) persistent uncontrolled headache, and (*b*) impending blindness.

SUMMARY AND CONCLUSIONS

An attempt has been made to review the value, hazards and indications for the employment of radiotherapy in the management of patients suffering from tumours related to the central nervous system.

Stress has been laid on the importance of the radiotherapist working as a member of a team of specialists in the field.

Guiding principles have been suggested for the development of suitable methods of treating groups of tumours commonly encountered in practice.

Precise details of radiotherapeutic techniques will be discussed by colleagues in subsequent chapters.

I have underlined the importance of respecting the proved vulnerability of the normal tissues of the central nervous system to ionizing irradiations.

Some of the suggestions which I have made regarding the management of patients may be controversial, but are based for the most part on my own experience in this particular field.

Neuroradiotherapy represents an interesting but challenging branch of medicine: too often fraught with disappointment, but frequently most rewarding.

REFERENCES

Béclère, A. (1926). 'Les Dangers à éviter dans la Radiothérapie des Tumeurs de la Cavité Cranio-radulenne.' *J. Radiol. Électrol.*, **10**, 556.

Bull, J. W. D. (1966). 'Topographical criteria for pathological diagnosis of intracranial masses by means of gamma encephalography.' *Acta radiol.*, **5**, 754.

— and Rovit, R. L. (1957). 'The radiographic localization of intracerebral gliomata.' *J. Fac. Radiol. Lond.*, **8**, 147.

Henderson, W. R. (1939). 'The pituitary adenomata. A follow-up study of the surgical results in 338 cases (Dr Harvey Cushing's series).' *Br. J. Surg.*, **26**, 811.

Horrax, G., Smedal, M. I., Trump, J. G., Granke, R. G. and Wright K. A. (1955). 'Present day treatment of pituitary adenomas.' *New Engl. J. Med.*, **252**, 524.

Howieson, J. and Bull, J. W. D. (1966). 'Radiologic detection of astrocytoma involving the corpus callosum.' *Am. J. Roentgenol.*, **98**, 575.

Jefferson, G. (1948). 'Clinical preamble on the brain.' In *The Treatment of Malignant Diseases by Radium and X-rays*, Ed. by Ralston Paterson, Chap. 28, pp. 455–63. London; Edward Arnold.

Kernohan, J. W., Mabon, R. F., Svien, T. T. and Adson, A. W. (1949). 'A simplified classification of the gliomas.' *Proc. Mayo Clin.*, **24**, 71.

McKissock, W. (1952). 'Intracranial tumours. Part II.' In *Malignant Disease and its Treatment by Radium*, Ed. by Sir Stanford Cade, Vol. IV, pp. 461–486. Bristol; John Wright.

Nabarro, J. D. N. (1972). 'Pituitary tumours and hypopituitarism.' *Br. med. J.*, **1**, 492.

Paterson, Edith (1953). 'Treatment of cerebral tumours in children by irradiation.' *J. Fac. Radiol. Lond.*, **4**, 175.

Richmond, J. Jackson (1952). 'Intracranial tumours. Part III.' In *Malignant Disease and its Treatment by Radium*, Ed. by Sir Stanford Cade, Vol. IV, pp. 486–519. Bristol; John Wright.

— (1953). 'Radiotherapy of intracranial tumours in children.' *J. Fac. Radiol. Lond.*, **4**, 180.

— (1958). 'Pituitary tumours: the role of radiotherapy.' *Proc. R. Soc. Med.*, **51**, 911.

— (1959). 'Malignant tumours of the central nervous system.' In *Cancer*, Ed. by R. W. Raven, Vol. 5, pp. 375–389. London; Butterworths.

2—Neuroectodermal Tumours of the Brain

J. G. Leopold

INTRODUCTION

Both neurones and neural support tissue, the true glia, are products of the neuroectoderm. On the other hand, the phagocytic glial cells, usually known as the microglia or Hortega cells, are of mesodermal derivation and the representative in the brain of the ubiquitous reticulo-endothelial tissue. The majority of primary brain tumours arise from glia. Microglial tumours are rare. So are neuronal tumours, except in infancy. The differentiated cells of the true glia are the astrocytes, the oligodendroglia and the ependymal cells, and each can give rise to its own type of glioma.

A common feature of the glial and the neuronal cells is the possession of abundant cell processes. It is these that make up the background feltwork between cell nuclei, which is apparent in routine haematoxylin and eosin stained sections of brain cut from paraffin blocks. In such preparations the processes of the individual cells are not identifiable; sometimes they are a little clearer in sections cut by freezing techniques. A general assessment of the presence and extent of glial fibre production in tumours is obtained from sections stained with phosphotungstic haematoxylin. However, the fact that the cell types have distinctive processes is of no diagnostic help. Proper demonstration of the processes requires metallic impregnations which can be notoriously capricious to perform. They often require special fixatives which must be available at the time of biopsy and, even when impregnation is successful, the results are not always easy to interpret.

In practice the major part of diagnostic brain tumour pathology is done on paraffin-prepared sections stained by conventional methods.

16

In these the various elements in the glia are recognized by their nuclear characteristics, by the arrangement of the cells and, sometimes, even by artefacts to which certain populations of cells are prone.

INCIDENCE

The incidence of primary neuroectodermal tumours, and their various types, is difficult information to obtain. Hospitals differ in the factors which determine, sometimes selectively, the admission of patients suffering from disease.

The London Hospital figures for gliomas identified at autopsy show that, prior to the development of a neurosurgical centre there in 1928, the incidence was 0·8 per cent. The figures for the years following rose to 2 per cent of the autopsy population (Russell and Rubenstein, 1971).

The same source gives a breakdown for the incidence of different types of glioma and neuroectodermal tumours. However, since the analysis is by autopsy record it might be expected to overscore the anaplastic tumours relative to the differentiated, because the former are more likely to die in the hospital where they received their primary treatment.

The figures for other centres are equally open to criticism and for this reason any figures provided can only be regarded as approximate. The London Hospital figures for the various tumour types have been inserted in Table 1.

CLASSIFICATION AND GRADING

Difficulty of classification, as always, arises not with the more differentiated tumours but in respect of the anaplastic examples. The latter span the range between examples showing minor deviation from the picture of well-differentiated tumours and tumours composed entirely of anaplastic cells. However, amongst neoplasms whose anaplasia is such that they show little resemblance to any one type of differentiated glial cell, group similarities may often be apparent. The existence of group similarities in the range of anaplastic tumours explains why there has been the adoption of special names, e.g. glioblastoma multiforme, spongioblastoma. The construction of these well-used titles and of some other less well-used titles in the field of neural oncology, indicates opinions, variously well substantiated, that the constituent anaplastic elements are the counterparts of cells arising during the maturation of embryonic glia (Bailey and

Cushing, 1926). However, the alternative possibility has to be acknowledged that these cells are not throwbacks to stages of development but are entirely pathological cells with no normal, be it developmental, representative. Fortunately, from the point of view of prognosis and treatment, the different interpretations and the choice of names that spring therefrom are not important provided the anaplastic nature of these cells is recognized by the pathologist and he reports this information in a manner understood by the clinicians concerned. This pragmatic approach to the problem is recognized in the Kernohan classification (Kernohan and colleagues, 1949), which allocates the glial tumours of astrocytic, ependymal and oligodendroglial origin to four grades of increasing anaplasia. The first two grades include the differentiated tumours which can be said to have a reasonably sound attribution to an origin from a particular type of glial cell. The third and fourth grades include tumours of increased anaplasia. No system of classification overcomes the sometimes insoluble problem of separating tumours showing Grade IV anaplasia into those of astrocytic, ependymal and oligodendroglial derivation and this is the major practical difficulty encountered by pathologists in pursuing the classification scheme of Kernohan and his colleagues at the Mayo Clinic.

It is proposed to discuss neuroectodermal tumours under the three main headings of Table 1. It is not intended to be a fully comprehensive list. Rare and debatable entities are for the most part excluded.

TABLE 1

Classification of Neuroectodermal Tumours

Differentiated glial tumours	Astrocytoma	20·5%
	Oligodendroglioma	5%
	Ependymoma	6%
	Choroid plexus papilloma	2%
Undifferentiated glial tumours	Glioblastoma multiforme	55%
Neuronal tumours		
—differentiated	Ganglioglioma	< 1%
—undifferentiated	Medulloblastoma	6%

Further general problems in classifying the glial tumours should be appreciated. First, the degree of differentiation is not uniform and impressions gained on the study of small biopsies prove often to be ill-founded, wider sampling of the same lesion revealing both anaplastic and differentiated areas. Because of this some authorities hold that grading is an exercise that should be carried out only on autopsy material. The second feature of glial neoplasms that causes difficulty is the tendency for mixed populations of differentiated glial cells to occur. For instance, it is not uncommon to observe areas of oligo-dendroglial cell predominance in neoplasms which are in greatest part astrocytic. It must be remembered that astrocytomas, grade I, examined in small biopsy samples, present the greatest difficulty to the pathologist in distinguishing neoplastic from reactive glial changes.

GENERAL CONSIDERATIONS

It is unfortunately true that, even when fully differentiated, glial tumours do not form well-marked boundaries with the remainder of the brain tissue. Margins seen naked eye are deceptive in the assess-ment of the extent of the tumour. Characteristically the histological boundary is even less sharp than that found between brain and most rapidly growing secondary carcinomas. Autopsy studies have shown the high frequency of occurrence of anaplastic areas in otherwise fully-differentiated tumours. This is particularly true of the cerebral astrocytomas. Nevertheless, the relatively long survival of some such examples and the results of serial biopsy in a few cases indicate that the development of anaplasia is sometimes a late event.

TUMOURS OF GLIAL DERIVATION

Differentiated Glial Tumours (Gliomas Grades i and ii)

Astrocytoma

These are the most common of the differentiated glial tumours and may be seen at all ages. They occur in the cerebral hemispheres, the brain stem and the cerebellar hemispheres, with a predilection for the mid- and hind-brain and cerebellum in children and adolescents and for the cerebral hemisphere in the adult. Astrocytomas can be slowly growing. Some are solid and form diffusely white, ill-defined swellings in the white matter. The neurosurgeon often recognizes them by their firmer resistance to the introduction of the brain needle than normal white matter. Some tumours undergo a central degenera-tion and, particularly in cerebellum and brain stem, appear honey-combed by very small spaces in histological sections. Particularly in the cerebellum large cysts can develop which contain yellow-coloured fluid and surviving tumour may be found only over a localized button-like area of the cavity wall.

Various histological patterns are recognized but all are notable for a general uniformity of the cell picture, in which they differ from the anaplastic group. The details of the histological picture have no

19

place in this account, but some explanation may be desirable of some of the terms applied to special examples of astrocytic tumours. These terms, protoplasmic, fibrillar, gemistocytic and pilocytic, refer to the particular morphology of the constituent astrocytes. Often this is a reflection of the site of the tumour, either because certain forms of

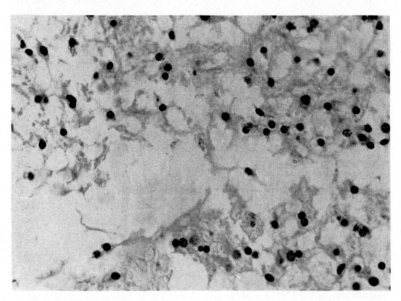

Figure 1. Differentiated astrocytoma of cerebellum. It shows the uniformity of appearance and the low cellularity of a differentiated tumour. Degeneration is resulting in the development of small cystic spaces (magnification × 300)

astrocyte predominate there or the site imposes a modifying effect upon the growing astrocytes. What is important in this context is to appreciate that there is no obvious connection between these variations of histological structure and the biological behaviour.

Oligodendrogliomas

These are a relatively uncommon form of primary neoplasm of the brain. They are generally tumours of early adult life, although occasionally seen at an earlier age. They are rarely found except in the cerebral hemispheres, particularly the frontal lobes. There are few distinctive gross features, except that cystic change is uncommon, the colour usually more pink than white, and the tumour masses are apparently well-defined. Calcification related to the blood vessels, especially those of the periphery, is a common and significant feature aiding in the radiological diagnosis of these tumours.

The cell picture is highly uniform and the constituent oligodendroglial cells are recognized on account of their swollen cell cytoplasm. The cells appear as rounded nuclei lying within a clear space three or four times the diameter of the nucleus. It seems that the oligodendroglia are particularly sensitive to alterations in their nutritional

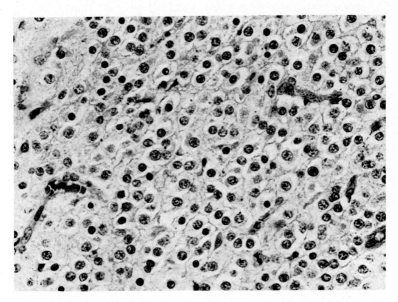

Figure 2. Area from an oligodendroglioma showing uniformity of pattern and the 'boxed' character of the tumour cells (magnification × 300)

conditions and it is therefore often artificially created factors which determine the customary histological picture. The oligodendrogliomata are generally slowly growing and, while there is considerable variation in the duration of these tumours, some span a long interval in a person's life. Prognostication of behaviour is difficult.

Ependymoma

Ependyma is the lining epithelium of the ventricular system and spinal canal. The tumours arise in or close to these sites, but it must be realized that not all gliomas so sited are of ependymal origin. Ependymomas comprise over half of the primary tumours of the spinal cord, whilst as intracranial growths they are a relatively small group. In the latter situation they are most common in the region of the fourth ventrical. Ependymomas are predominantly tumours of children or adolescence.

As might be expected from their sites of origin they frequently form projecting intraventricular tumours; sometimes they develop tongue-like extensions which protrude through the foramina.

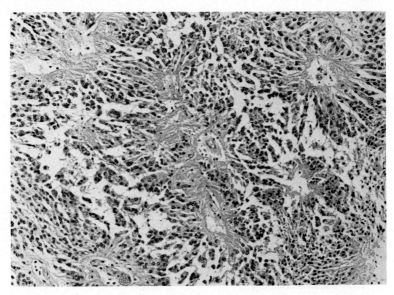

Figure 3. A well differentiated ependymoma. The radial orientation of the cells and their cytoplasmic processes is well demonstrated and in places canals form the centres of these arrangements (magnification × 120)

Growth into the brain tissues varies in amount but, in some instances, this is a more pronounced factor than the intraventricular protrusion. Many tumours have a contribution of astrocytic glial cells and in occasional examples this element predominates, giving rise to a histological sub-group, referred to as the sub-ependymomas. Differentiated ependymomas are a relatively benign neoplasm and, because of their situation, they are prone to declare their presence early.

Papillomas of the Choroid Plexus

These uncommon tumours of young adults, occasionally young children, are seen most frequently in the fourth ventricle, and slightly less often in the third ventricle. They are classified by some persons with the tumours of ependyma (Kernohan and Fletcher-Kernohan, 1937). While the lining epithelium has an obvious affinity with ependyma, the abundant vascular connective tissue stroma—which takes the place of the astrocytic component of the classical ependymoma—is a point of difference.

The intraventricular papilloma is amenable to surgical removal since it protrudes in cauliflower pattern into the ventricular cavity, held by a narrow stalk. For technical reasons, however, the removal may be difficult and no doubt accounts for the recurrence rate.

ANAPLASTIC GLIAL TUMOURS (GLIOBLASTOMA MULTIFORME AND TUMOURS OF KERNOHAN GRADES 3 AND 4)

The only difference between the use of the bracketed titles lies in the one being a non-committed and the other a committed opinion regarding the basic glial cell family from which origin has occurred. Some tumours are wholly anaplastic and can only be accommodated by such non-committal title as 'glioblastoma multiforme' (Ringertz, 1950). Others may have areas which are better differentiated, from which it may be reasonable to predict the cell type concerned in the anaplastic part.

Glial tumours with anaplastic features comprise the largest group of tumours of the adult. They occur in the cerebral hemispheres a decade or so later than the cerebral astrocytomas. It is possible that the relative proportion of glial tumours that fall into this category rises with increasing age (Moersch, Craig and Kernohan, 1941). They show a deceptive appearance of circumscription forming expansive masses which deform the adjacent structures. They are notably variegated in appearance as a result of haemorrhage and necrosis. Extensive vascularity due to the development of a pathological circulation is an interesting feature of the group of anaplastic gliomas, diagnostically of help to the pathologist and the radiologist. Concomitant with the glial proliferation occurs a proliferation of vascular endothelium. This results in an excess of newly-formed blood channels, many of which have a grossly abnormal structure because the growth of endothelial cells exceeds that needed to form a simple lining. Solid cords of vascular endothelium are quite commonly formed.

Accurate histological appraisal of anaplasia in glial, as in other tumours, comes from an analysis of the cellular characteristics. Pleomorphism, the formation of tumour giant cells, hyperchromatism of nuclei, a high frequency of mitoses and the occurrence of abnormal mitoses are the qualities used in this assessment. A caution must be voiced against the paired features of pleomorphism and tumour giant-cells being accepted alone as evidence of anaplasia, using the term as synonymous with tumours of a high growth rate. Both these qualities occur in the rare benign gliomas of tuberose sclerosis and, more importantly, may arise in response to irradiation of gliomas in general.

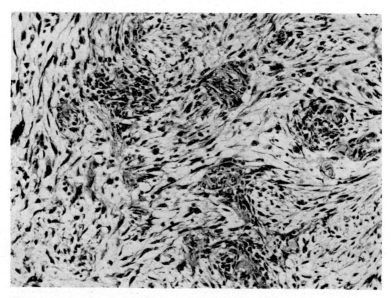

Figure 4. The pleomorphic character of the tumour cells, their hyperchromic nuclei and the presence of many mitoses mark this out as a glioblastic tumour (grade IV). Many of the cells forming the clumps in this picture are centres of proliferated endothelium (magnification × 120)

Neural Tumours

Medulloblastoma of the cerebellum is the only frequently occurring tumour of the brain with the potential to differentiate along a nerve cell line. It is essentially a primitive tumour and adult type ganglia are only rarely formed. Differentiated neural tumours are rarities.

Gangliogliomas and Gangliocytomas

These tumours which include in their structure mature nerve cells, are spread over a spectrum in which this feature is combined with an inactive or a proliferating glia. The latter, the gangliogliomas, have an importance which their rare occurrence does not entirely justify. They form relatively circumscribed tumours usually deep within the forebrain. Their progress is notably slow. It is desirable to separate them accurately from some astrocytic tumours with which, in view of the shared feature of astrocytic proliferation, they can be confused. First, tumour ganglion cells must be distinguished from ganglion cells incorporated in a purely astrocytic neoplasm. Secondly, one of the morphological forms of the astrocyte to which I have already referred—the gemistocyte—has a slightly similar appearance to the neoplastic ganglion cell and can therefore be falsely interpreted.

Medulloblastoma

Seen most commonly in the first few years of life and only occasionally in adults, the medulloblastoma is a tumour confined to the structures lying in the roof of the fourth ventricle. It grows rapidly

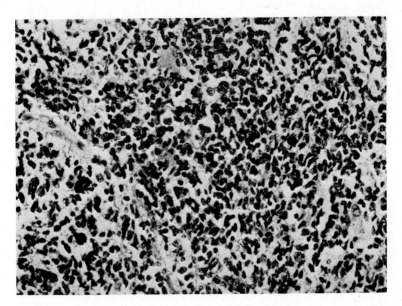

Figure 5. A tumour of closely-packed, densely hyperchromatic, tumour cells which in this field show no special arrangement. The tumour occurred in the vermis of the cerebellum of a three-year-old child. It is the typical histological picture presented by the medulloblastoma of this region (magnification × 300)

and this, combined with its position, determines a short course. The few adult examples occupy a more lateral position than the common central tumour site of childhood. The medulloblastoma forms a soft, expanding tumour mass of pink to grey colour, growing out of the lateral recess of the ventricle and seeding early by the cerebrospinal fluid.

Histologically, the majority of tumours are totally undifferentiated and composed of small, oval, hyperchromatic cells which differ in the density of their nuclear chromatin from tumour cells of the glia. Medulloblastomas are notably radio-sensitive tumours. The degree to which their neural derivation is apparent varies but a few of those which show a classical rosette arrangement of cells will have demonstrable axon fibres if specially stained for this purpose. Even less common have been reported examples in which adult-type ganglion cells have been identifiable.

THE GROWTH AND SPREAD OF NEUROECTODERMAL TUMOURS

Most glial tumours, even of the best differentiated types, seed by the cerebrospinal fluid once the brain-pial barrier or the ependymal surface is breached. Intraventricular tumours, such as the ependymoma and the medulloblastoma, are prone to show this development at an early stage giving rise particularly to seedling spread at the bottom of the spinal theca.

Under natural circumstances neuroectodermal tumours do not spread outside the central nervous system. However, operative exposure carries a slight risk of extracranial growth. Systemic spread, usually to the bone, has been reported following cerebrospinal fluid by-pass procedures carried out for blockages in the region of the hind-brain caused by medulloblastoma.

REFERENCES

Bailey, P. and Cushing, H. (1926). *A Classification of Tumours of the Glioma Group*. Philadelphia; Lippincott.

Kernohan, J. W. and Fletcher-Kernohan, E. M. (1937). *Proc. Ass. Res. nerv. ment. Dis.*, **16**, 182.

— Mabon, R. F., Svien, H. J. and Adson, A. W. (1949). *Proc. Mayo Clin.*, **24**, 71.

Moersch, G. H., Craig, W. McK. and Kernohan, J. W. (1941). *Archs Neurol. Psychiat.*, **45**, 235.

Ringertz, N. (1950). *Acta path. microbiol. scand.*, **27**, 51.

Russel, D. S. and Rubinstein, L. J. (1971). *Pathology of Tumours of the Nervous System*, 3rd ed., p. 13. London; Edward Arnold.

3—Diagnosis

I—Radiological Diagnosis

G. du Boulay

INTRODUCTION

For the radiotherapist an interest in the radiodiagnosis of tumours of the central nervous system is not merely intellectual curiosity: he needs to weigh practical considerations about the reliability of diagnosis of tumour type and extent. The presence or absence of associated coning is important to him.

It is not the purpose of this short chapter to describe technique or choice of investigation in detail but a list of those in use at the present time will illustrate that the neuroradiologist will often have helpful advice to offer on the order and method of diagnostic management.

Tumours in the supratentorial compartment of the skull are commonly diagnosed by a selection of the following tests: plain x-rays, including tomography and stereoscopy: soon computerized axial tomography will have a large role; carotid angiography; vertebral angiography; scintigraphy (scanning or gamma camera studies); pneumoencephalography; gas ventriculography; and positive contrast ventriculography.

The sequence of the list is intended to emphasize the author's belief that, in spite of all that has been said to the contrary, scintigraphy is not yet either a definitive examination for most tumours or an acceptable early screening test. It has immense value as a back-up to angiography and is discussed in another chapter. Vertebral angiography may be necessary to show the posterior cerebral artery. Gas ventriculography is reserved for patients in whom pneumoencephalography would be considered too dangerous because of severely raised intracranial pressure. Positive contrast ventriculography is sometimes employed in tumours extending upwards from the brain stem.

Tumours in the region of the sella are usually delineated by plain x-rays and pneumoencephalography, but carotid angiography and vertebral angiography provide helpful signs in some cases. Scintigraphy, though commonly carried out, has very little bearing on the management of the case. Gas ventriculography is sometimes an obligatory step when a suprasellar mass has caused obstructive hydrocephalus or in differential diagnosis between these two conditions. Venography may be used to show the lateral extent of a pituitary adenoma.

Infratentorial tumours are commonly investigated by plain x-rays, vertebral angiography, carotid angiography, pneumoencephalography, gas ventriculography, positive contrast ventriculography, scintigraphy, and myelo-encephalography.

There seems no doubt that the effectiveness of scintigraphy will increase with the general adoption of computer assisted analysis. For the moment, however, it is unreliable in the posterior fossa.

Carotid and vertebral angiography are often performed together, the former showing the degree of ventricular dilatation and the presence of trans-tentorial coning upwards or, rarely, downwards.

Tumours of the foramen magnum often require a combination of spinal and cranial investigation: plain x-rays, vertebral angiography, pneumoencephalography, jugular venography, gas myelography, positive contrast myelography, and myelo-encephalography.

Spinal tumours are usually shown by: positive contrast myelography (non-miscible), gas myelography, spinal angiography, and water-soluble contrast myelography (water-soluble myelography is restricted to the cauda equina, and is not widely practised in Great Britain).

THE CARDINAL SIGNS OF LOCATION

In addition to a great mass of detail there are certain localizing signs which are both frequently seen and especially reliable.

Plain X-rays

Pressure

Between 10 and 20 per cent of patients with cerebral tumours exhibit changes in the sella turcica; but they are very easy to misinterpret. Their primary diagnostic use is in screening patients with obscure symptoms who have slow-growing or benign neoplasms (*Figure 1*).

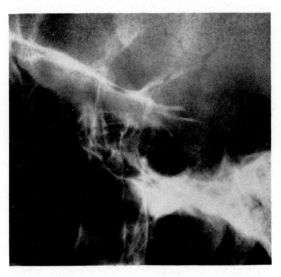

Figure 1. Severe changes in the sella turcica due to raised intracranial pressure of many months' duration. Not only has the cortical bone lining the pituitary fossa disappeared in places, but the planum sphenoidale has suffered the same effect

Erosion

Actual erosions are usually due to secondary deposits within the bone or to involvement by meningioma. Expansion of the various foramina of the skull and spine may be produced by new growths which pass through them, notably, of course, neurinomas and, much less commonly, ganglioneuroma. *Figure 2* shows a chemodectoma.

Tumours of the brain and spinal cord themselves only transgress the meninges and invade the bone on very rare occasions. Therefore, obvious bone destruction of the skull generally means an extracerebral lesion (meningioma or malignant growth) and, if a pedicle or vertebral body is destroyed, it generally implies the presence of a carcinoma metastasis.

29

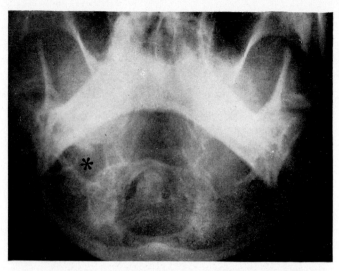

Figure 2. Erosion of the jugular foramen by a glomus jugulare tumour. The normal jugular foramen is marked with an asterisk. The arrow points to the abnormal side where most of the margin of the jugular foramen has been destroyed

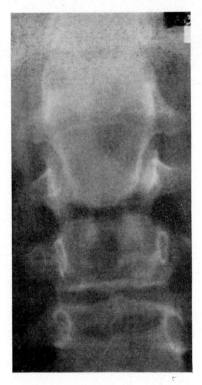

Figure 3. Spinal neuroenteric cyst. Plain x-ray antero-posterior view; dorsi-lumbar spine. The spinal canal is greatly widened over several segments by this long-standing mass

Expansion

Very slow-growing tumours, although remaining within their meningeal covering, are able to cause remodelling of the overlying bone so that a local expansion of the skull or spinal canal takes place (*Figure 3*), the only condition for the occurrence being the essential slowness of the process, so that 'benign' gliomas and non-neoplastic cysts are two of the more common causes of a moderately rare appearance.

Hyperostosis

New bone may be laid down as a result of stimulation by the presence of meningioma cells; thus an increase in bone density or a bony spur or thickening in the vicinity and particularly at the point of attachment of a meningioma is a helpful radiological sign (*Figure 4*).

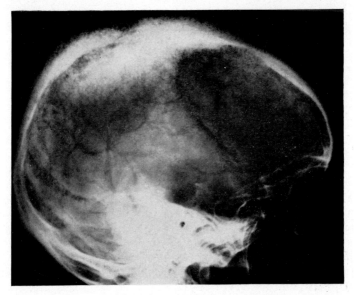

Figure 4. Very large hyperostosis due to a meningioma

It may be seen in roughly half of all meningiomas. Confusion between meningiomas and secondary carcinoma invading both skull and brain is very rare but possible (*Figure 5*). Much more common causes of confusion are the normal irregularities of ossification of the inner table and irrelevant plaques of calcification in a normal dura.

31

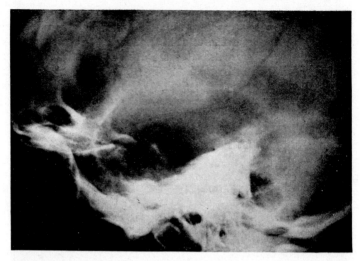

Figure 5. Increased density of the sphenoid bone, due in this case to a nasopharyngeal carcinoma

Calcification

The pineal.—The pineal or habenula commissure, or both, are sufficiently heavily calcified to be visible in lateral and axial views in about 40 per cent of the adult population and are not infrequently, also, calcified in children.

The pineal moves with adjacent structures, and pineal displacement is therefore a good sign of displacement by tumours, either the rather rarer tumours in its immediate neighbourhood or those which, by their bulk, cause sub-falcine herniation. Lateral displacement of the pineal greater than 3 mm from the midline generally indicates a supratentorial mass.

Some tumours, which are not large or are distant—in the temporal lobe for instance—do not, however, cause such midline shifts.

Upward and downward displacements of the pineal also occur (*Figures 6* and *7*), together with backward and forward dislocation, as a result of trans-tentorial herniation upwards or downwards due to infra- or supratentorial masses; a point of some importance in radiotherapy since added brain or tumour swelling may cause critical brain stem damage.

Choroid plexus calcification.—The glomus of the choroid plexus of the lateral ventricles is a common situation for calcification; severe displacements are recognizable.

32

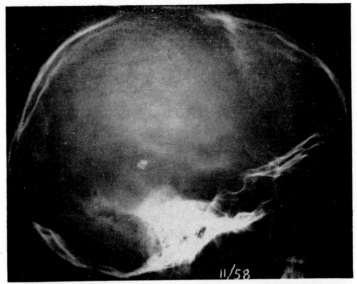

Figure 6. Downward displacement of the pineal as a result of hydrocephalus due to a quadrigeminal plate tumour

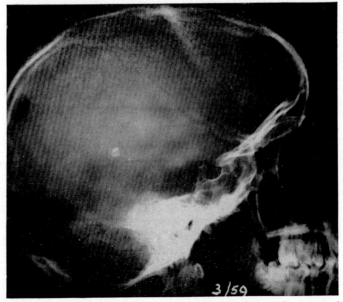

Figure 7. After ventriculo-cisternostomy the lateral ventricles are much smaller and the pineal has risen

33

Tumour calcification.—The most common pathological calcification visible in plain x-rays of the head is in atheroma of the carotid arteries. The second most common is the calcification which takes place in glial tumours (9–14 per cent) (*Figure 8*). It is found both in adults and in children above and below the tentorium; but is certainly more commonly seen in supratentorial tumours of slower

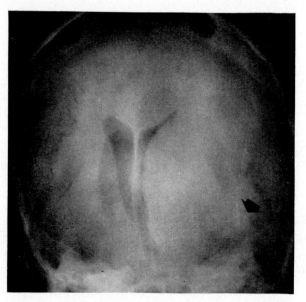

Figure 8. Calcification in an oligodendroglioma. Note, also, the displacement of the ventricular system shown at ventriculography. There is a deep indentation in the lateral ventricle, suggesting that the tumour is lying close to it

growth. For instance, calcification of a particular wavy, banded form is found in 20 per cent of oligodendrogliomas; and in 16 per cent of slow-growing astrocytomas. Speckled or amorphous calcification is found in many more of the glial tumours. Of course, as is well known, part of a 'benign' glioma may change and start to grow very rapidly so the presence of calcification is of little help in prognosis, nor does it give the slightest indication of extent.

Plaques or masses of calcium are seen in 4 per cent of meningiomas, 16 per cent of angiomas have small, calcified dots and shells. Ten per cent of chromophobe adenomas exhibit a partly calcified capsule. Craniopharyngioma, so commonly thought of as a calcified tumour, is so in childhood, but in only about 20 per cent of those cranio-pharyngiomas which present in adult life can calcification be demonstrated. In my experience only a small proportion of all tumours diagnosed from their situation as 'pinealoma' are calcified.

In the spinal canal, meningiomas may almost invariably be shown to contain calcium by x-raying the specimen removed at operation: but it is very rare to recognize *in situ*. Overlying bony shadows also interfere with the demonstration of calcification, if it occurs, in other spinal masses.

Angiography

Arteries, capillaries and veins each play their parts in localization, and locality may sometimes give clues to pathology. The cardinal signs of particular pathologies, however, are the character of tumour circulation and its sources.

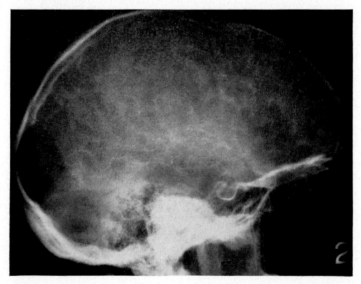

Figure 9. Parietal intracerebral tumour. Carotid angiogram, lateral view 'capillary' phase. The region of the tumour is relatively avascular and the capillary shadows of surrounding convolutions are displaced by the mass

The capillary phase of the carotid (and, less easily, the vertebral) angiogram often provides the best localization of avascular tumours since it shows the empty area of the tumour, the crowding of surrounding gyri and the displacement of the ventricular system (*Figure 9*).

Arterial and venous phases are interpreted together. Some of the most useful combinations of signs are listed here; but interpretation is very much a matter of common sense.

Frontal Tumours

The anterior cerebral artery is displaced in a curve away from the midline or sometimes directly backwards. The main trunk of the middle cerebral and the anterior part of the Sylvian triangle are often pushed down (*Figures 10* and *11*). The internal cerebral vein is usually displaced laterally less than the anterior cerebral artery, and its anterior end may be pushed backwards.

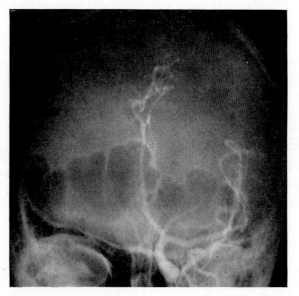

Figure 10. Frontal meningioma. The lateral displacement of the anterior cerebral is minimal because the tumour is bilateral

Parietal Tumours

Lateral displacement of the anterior cerebral artery is matched by that of the internal cerebral vein. The posterior part of the Sylvian triangle is depressed.

Occipital Tumours

The posterior parts of the middle cerebral branches are stretched

36

and splayed (as branches usually are in the immediate vicinity of a tumour). The Sylvian triangle is squashed forwards. Lateral displacement of the internal cerebral vein is usually greater than that of the anterior cerebral artery.

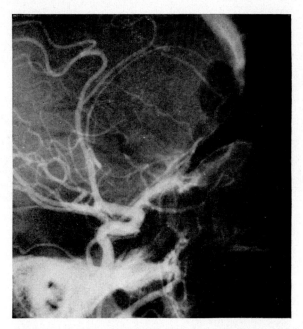

Figure 11. The same patient showing extreme backward displacement of the anterior cerebral artery

Temporal Tumours

Midline displacement may be small. Most of the middle cerebral branches are elevated, although the posterior temporal artery may be stretched over an intracerebral mass and thus not elevated throughout its course.

Parasagittal Tumours

Lateral displacement of midline structures may be small but the pericallosal artery is nearly always depressed (*Figure 12*). The pericallosal and calloso-marginal arteries may be seen to be separated in an antero-posterior view.

37

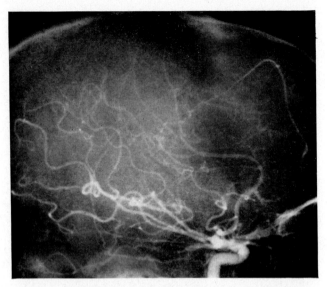

*Figure 12. A frontal parasagittal mass depressing the pericallosal
artery and stretching the calloso-marginal*

Central Tumours (*Corpus Callosum*)

When the tumour mass, perhaps in both parietal lobes, is equal on
two sides there will be little or no lateral displacement of midline
structures. The symmetry of the dislocation of vessels in the two
hemispheres may disguise the condition. Superimposition of the
arterial and venous phases of the lateral angiogram should show an
unnaturally wide gap between the line of the pericallosal artery above
the corpus callosum and the uppermost ends of the subependymal
veins on the roofs of the lateral ventricles (*Figures 13* and *14*).

Thalamic Tumours

The lateral ventricles may well be dilated, giving the angiographic
signs associated with hydrocephalus (*see below*). The important signs
of swelling in the thalamus are lateral and upward displacement of
the internal cerebral vein, the lateral displacement usually being out
of proportion to any lateral displacement of the anterior cerebral
artery. At the same time, the basilar vein is usually depressed, the
lateral posterior choroidal artery takes a widened sweep around the
inferior, then the posterior borders of the thalamus itself.

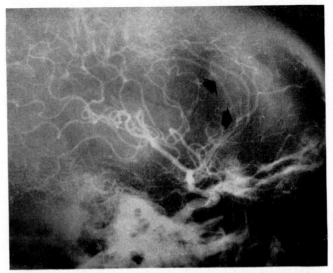

Figure 13. Anterior corpus callosum tumour invading the frontal horns.
The pericallosal artery is wide-swept

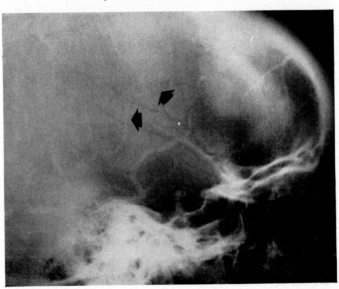

Figure 14. The same patient shows displacement of ventricular veins away
from the sweep of the pericallosal artery. This tumour is predominantly in
the genu. When the mass lies in the body of the corpus callosum the
ventricular veins will by displaced downwards

Cerebellar Hemisphere Vermis Tumours

It is usual to find hydrocephalus and reversed tentorial herniation. Tonsillar herniation at the foramen magnum is equally likely. Cerebellar hemisphere tumours displace the vermian and supra or medial tonsillar segments of the posterior inferior cerebellar artery across the midline. The choroidal point is likely to be pushed forwards and so are the arteries and veins on the anterior surface of the pons (the basilar artery, the anterior ponto-mesencephalic veins and their immediate tributaries). The upper anterior margin of the cerebellum outlined by the pre-central cerebellar vein and artery will also probably be displaced anteriorly.

Vermis tumours result in the same forward displacements without a lateral shift.

Brain stem Tumours

Hydrocephalus is quite uncommon. The maximum vascular displacements depend upon the position of the tumour in the medulla, pons or midbrain. Swelling of these structures will be shown directly by the vessels which surround them; the medullary loops of the posterior inferior cerebellar artery, the pontine arteries, the posterior and lateral mesencephalic veins, the superior cerebellar and posterior cerebral arteries (*Figure 15*). Vessels posterior to the brain stem but not in direct contact, such as the choroidal branch of the posterior inferior cerebellar artery, the veins of the lateral recesses of the fourth ventricle and the lower part of the pre-central vein, will be pushed backwards. Vessels anterior to the brain stem go forwards.

Fourth Ventricle Tumours

These commonly cause hydrocephalus. Vessels behind the fourth ventricle, like the choroidal branch of the posterior inferior cerebellar artery, go backwards. Brain stem vessels go forwards and the tonsils, carrying with them the arteries and veins on their medial surfaces, are pushed laterally. The veins of the lateral recesses are also squashed laterally.

Cerebello-pontine Angle Tumours

Large tumours cause hydrocephalus and also lateral and posterior displacement of both brain stem and fourth ventricle, carrying with them the vessels already described. There may also be upward displacement of the superior cerebellar artery and, indeed, of all the other vessels near it in the tentorial hiatus, such as the posterior

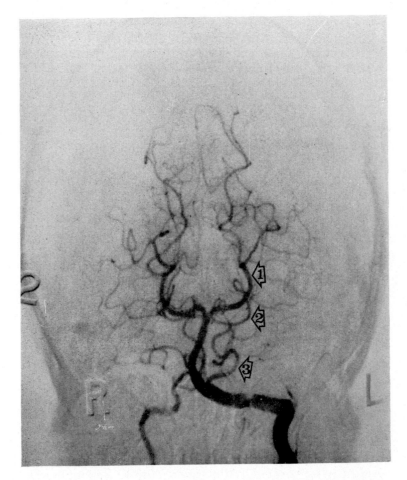

Figure 15. Vertebral angiogram. Angled antero-posterior views: (1) posterior cerebral artery; (2) superior cerebellar artery; (3) posterior inferior cerebellar artery

cerebral artery, the basilar vein and the posterior mesencephalic vein. The vessels more intimately in contact with the angle are displaced also by much smaller tumours. Thus, the petrosal vein is elevated from the petrous bone, the anterior inferior cerebellar artery is also pushed away and may appear in antero-posterior and Towne's views to be displaced upwards or downwards.

41

Clivus Tumours and Extracerebral, Middle Fossa Masses

Clivus tumours push the brain stem vessels backwards. They often extend onto the floor of the middle fossa where they cause displacement upwards of the anterior choroidal artery, the anterior parts of the basilar vein and the temporal branches of the middle cerebral artery.

Suprasellar Tumours

Angiography is not usually the best investigation for these; but in a proportion the pre-communicating parts of the anterior cerebral arteries are elevated, the peduncular veins pushed backwards, the top of the basilar artery pushed downwards or backwards and the anterior choroidal arteries displaced laterally.

Hydrocephalus is caused by sufficiently large masses.

Hydrocephalus

Wide-sweeping of the anterior cerebral artery is a good sign of hydrocephalus if a callosal tumour (q.v.) can be excluded. More reliable is an estimate of the width of the lateral ventricles from the position of the thalamostrite vein. Most reliable of all is the direct visualization of the floor of the lateral ventricle by capillary filling in the adjacent caudate nucleus as seen in the antero-posterior views. In the lateral view a good 'cast' of the frontal horn, body and trigone can be constructed by joining all the most peripheral points of the ventricular veins.

Severe hydrocephalus also elevates the middle cerebral group of branches because the temporal horns are dilated.

Tentorial Herniation

Upward and downward herniation through the tentorial hiatus is revealed by the positions of the vessels which lie close to the midbrain, third ventricle and uncus. Interpretation is a most useful skill but requires practice.

The vessels are: the posterior cerebral artery, the basilar vein, the internal cerebral vein and the anterior choroidal artery (*Figures 16* and *17*).

Tonsillar Herniation

The lower margin of the cerebellar tonsil is commonly crossed by an artery, either the main trunk of the tonsillo-hemisphere branch of the posterior inferior cerebellar artery or a small tonsillar branch

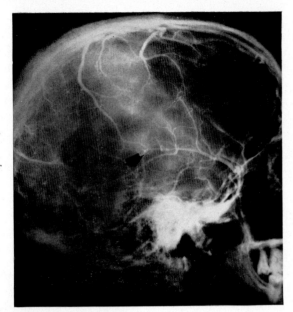

Figure 16. Aqueduct stenosis. The internal cerebral vein is flattened and depressed to a point where it must lie below the level of the tentorial opening

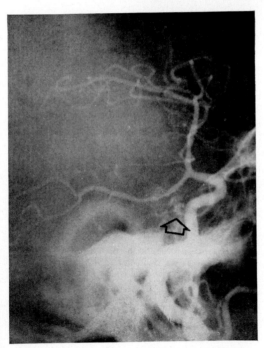

Figure 17. A pterion meningioma. The arrow points to tumour circulation. Note, also, the downward displacement of the posterior cerebral artery by tentorial herniation of the uncus

derived from it or derived from the retro-tonsillar segment of the posterior inferior cerebellar artery. The lower margin of the tonsil should not transgress a line joining the anterior and posterior margins of the foramen magnum. Tonsillar herniation may be diagnosed in error if one of the medullary loops of the posterior inferior cerebellar artery is mistaken for the tonsillar loop or branch.

Tumour Circulation

The recognition of tumour circulation is dealt with at the end of this chapter.

Air and Positive Contrast Studies of the Head

It is not possible in so short a space to discuss the choice of investigation. Pneumoencephalography, gas ventriculography, positive contrast ventriculography and myelo-encephalography all outline the cerebrospinal fluid spaces with different aptitude.

Frontal, Parietal, Occipital and Temporal Tumours

In each case the lateral ventricle betrays the situation of the tumour; that part of the ventricle which is nearest to the mass being most displaced. Air in the basal cisterns and the cortical spaces is not very helpful in localization, although it does give evidence of the presence of a cone (if one undertakes a pneumoencephalogram in such a patient).

The distinction between superficial and deeply extending tumours may not be easy; but displacement apart of the temporal horn and body of the ventricle is a reliable sign of deep extension. Very clear and prominent abnormal indentations into the ventricular shadows are also reliable signs (*see Figure 8*).

The 'elevation' of a mass (on a coronal section) may be determined partly by whether it sharpens or blunts the angle between the roof and floor of the lateral ventricle and partly by the tilt given to the septum pellucidum. Subfalcine herniation of brain also causes its own impression on the roof of the lateral ventricle, which should not be confused with tumour identation.

Cerebellar Tumours

Hydrocephalus is generally severe but the third ventricle is not depressed. The aqueduct and fourth ventricle are pushed forwards by vermis tumours or forwards and laterally by hemisphere masses.

Intraventricular (Fourth Ventricular) Tumours

Hydrocephalus may be extreme; but may sometimes be accompanied by downward herniation of the third ventricle. Small parts of a dilated fourth may be visualized around the mass it contains (*Figure 18*). The aqueduct will be shortened and widened.

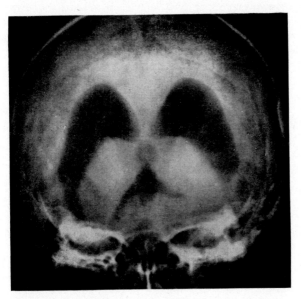

Figure 18. Ventriculogram. Medulloblastoma in the floor of the fourth ventricle

Brain-stem Tumours

The aqueduct may be patent and hydrocephalus mild or absent. the floor of the fourth ventricle will be unduly separated from the front of the pons. In axial views, during pneumoencephalography, the lateral margins of the brain-stem will also show its expansion.

Cerebello-pontine Angle Tumours

Large tumours cause hydrocephalus and displace the aqueduct and fourth ventricle backwards and away from the side of the lesion, twisting the ventricle on its long axis. The third ventricle may be elevated. Both large and small tumours obliterate the cerebello-pontine angle cistern and its extension into the internal auditory meatus. If the brain stem is displaced, cisterna ambiens on the side of the tumour is widened.

Suprasellar Tumours

The shadow of the tumour is seen surrounded by air in the distorted chiasmatic cistern and third ventricle. Most tumours above and in front of the sella are meningiomas. Chromophobe adenoma, optic chiasm glioma and metastasis also occur in this situation, pushing the anterior end of the third ventricle backwards and downwards.

Tumours above and behind the sella are usually chromophobe adenomas or craniopharyngiomas. Other pathologies in this situation, elevating the anterior end of the third ventricle, are very rare but include extension of clivus meningiomas and chordomas.

Tumours of the Floor of the Middle Fossa

These elevate the whole of the lower parts of the ventricular system at the appropriate site and largely obliterate the cisterns into which they extend. At their edges there may be collections of air.

Spinal Tumours

Myelography.—Whatever contrast medium is used, two views at right angles are needed to determine the position of a mass. It may be intramedullary, intrathecal but extramedullary, like meningiomas and many neurofibromas, or extradural when it will often be found to be a metastasis. Intramedullary masses widen the cord in all directions. Intrathecal, extramedullary masses widen the subarachnoid space above and below themselves by pushing the cord to one side. The compressed cord may look narrow in one plane but widened in the other. Extramedullary masses compress the whole theca as well as the cord.

In special situations there are special problems of diagnosis. For instance, the capacious posterior subarachnoid space at C1 not only conceals tumours at positive contrast myelography unless very special care is taken in the supine position, but also allows intramedullary masses to extrude lumpy prolongations which look very like intrathecal but extramedullary masses. They may also resemble the lower poles of herniated cerebellar tonsils, drawing, therefore, Chiari malformation with and without a syrinx and cerebellar tumour into the differential diagnoses.

At L2 and below, an intrathecal mass may be one of the benign tumours of meninges or nerve roots; but may also be an ependymoma growing downwards from the conus or arising from the filum terminale.

A very long expansion of the cord may be a solid tumour or a cyst and the latter may be a developmental syrinx or a syrinx which has formed in association with a comparatively small intramedullary neoplasm.

Spinal angiography.—Because of the possibility of surgery spinal angiography has been developed for the diagnosis of spinal angiomas; it is now beginning, also, to have an impact on spinal tumour diagnosis.

SOME CHARACTERISTICS OF PARTICULAR TUMOURS

Intracranial Glioma

At the benign end of the spectrum astrocytomas are so like normal brain that they defy radiological detection for years. Eventually they may declare themselves because of a malignant alteration or because of extraordinarily widespread, minor distortion and compression of the ventricular system, extending perhaps from one temporal horn across the midline in the frontal lobes to the other temporal horn.

Astrocytomas, grades 3 and 4, have within them blood vessels and spaces which can be seen and recognized for what they are on carotid angiography in as many as 40 per cent of cases (*Figure 19*). The vessels are irregular in calibre and distribution; many are wide. The tumour edge is rarely distinct. Circulation time through the tumour is reduced to a point where veins may be seen in the first two seconds of an angiogram. Such an appearance accords well with the histology of most glioblastomas, but there is also a proportion of these tumours which, for one reason or another, show vascular displacement but not vascularity at angiography.

No radiological method provides a reliable guide to the position of the tumour's outermost edges. With experience allowances may be made for likely lines of spread (to the corpus callosum, from temporal to frontal lobes or between the frontal lobes for instance); but the margin cannot actually be seen.

In the posterior fossa tumour circulation may also be demonstrated, though less readily, and less is known about tumour type distinction by vertebral angiography.

The author has not been able to provide reliable recognition signs from plain x-rays and air studies by which astrocytomas, medulloblastomas or ependymomas may be labelled before operation.

Tumour recurrence and spread after excision or treatment are usually best recognized at angiography.

Almost exactly the same criteria apply to spinal gliomata but, since spinal angiography is such a lengthy and complex examination, reliance has usually to be placed on myelography.

Because a cord glioma alters the smooth cord surfaces in some

47

cases, and also sometimes results in dilatation of superficial cord vessels, Myodil may show that the pia is not normal, but has trapped many droplets. Small excrescences may be individually recognizable.

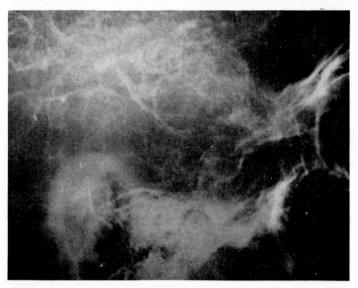

Figure 19. The circulation of a glioblastoma multiforme at angiography

Meningioma

Characteristic tumour circulation is found in about 50 per cent of cases. It consists of a rather homogenous capillary 'blush' having a clear margin and longer persistence than the capillary filling of the brain (*Figure 20*). There are no early filling veins. Wide vessels sometimes ramify over the tumour surface. External carotid branches provide part of the blood supply in 60 per cent of cases. One of the pitfalls of ventriculography in cases of meningioma is the frequent coincidence of cerebral oedema which makes the tumour appear larger than it actually is.

Although meningioma is benign in most senses and rarely penetrates the pia, it is an infiltrating tumour as far as bone is concerned and in bone its radiological appearances are more like those of malignancy; nor can its extent in bone be easily gauged by the radiologist.

In the spinal cord, however, because of the different relationship of dura and bone, meningiomas are nearly always vèry sharply demarcated from all other structures.

48

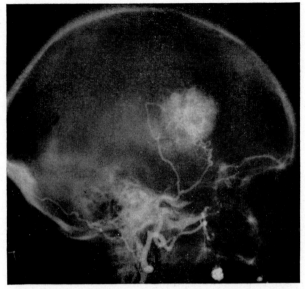

Figure 20. A meningioma. External carotid angiogram: observe that this meningioma gets almost all its blood supply from branches of the external carotid

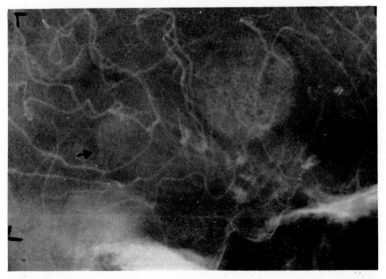

Figure 21. Typical circulation of a cerebral metastasis from carcinoma of the bronchus

Metastases

The most helpful diagnostic sign is, of course, the multiplicity of the lesions; but a solitary metastasis may have a mixture of the angiographic characteristics of glioma and meningioma (*Figure 21*). Even when multiple tumours are present they do not necessarily all show the same tumour circulation.

The very fact of multiplicity may catch the unwary because it tends to prevent displacement of normal landmarks.

Brain and skull metastases rarely seem to be present in the same patient, at least at the time when he comes for radiological tests.

Intrathecal spinal metastases are rare, but they do occur.

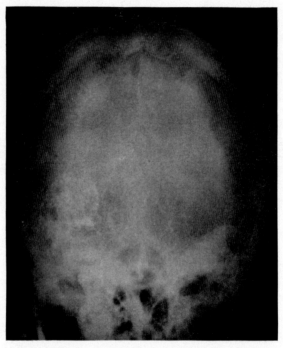

Figure 22. The circulation of an haemangioblastoma shown at vertebral angiography

Other Tumours

Other tumours also have characteristic findings and 'radiological natural histories'. There is no space to discuss them here; but attention should be drawn to the characteristic nature of haemangioblastoma vessels (*Figure 22*) and the possible multiplicity of these tumours in the posterior fossa and spinal canal.

A comment about chemodectomas in the jugular canal may also be helpful. Air studies for them and the other tumours which grow in the same general region, neurinomas of the ninth, tenth and eleventh nerves, are usually only fractionally abnormal, but internal and external carotid angiography, vertebral angiography and jugular venography give a lot of assistance.

II—Radionuclides

A. S. Bligh

INTRODUCTION

The investigation and localization of cerebral tumours by isotope studies has many advantages as far as the patient is concerned. It is painless, quick and can be carried out as an out-patient with the minimum of preparation. However, no method of investigation of a patient suspected of having an intracranial tumour replaces the need for proper history taking and a full neurological examination. Nor do isotope studies replace the need for plain films of the skull and chest. It is often true that a decision on treatment can be made on the basis of a cerebral scan alone but in many cases, angiography or air-studies are required to provide a more definite diagnosis (Di Chiro, 1962).

When the order in which to perform these investigations is considered, cerebral isotope studies (scans) are second only to the plain radiological studies. Many lesions of the skull and scalp can give rise to changes in cerebral scans which could be misinterpreted (Kieffer and Loken, 1969). Conversely it is interesting to note that Holmes and Walker (1971) have reported seven cases of primary and metastatic tumours which gave rise to positive scans but had negative cerebral arteriograms.

In the early days of isotope studies the complexity, cost and time consumed by the methods then available were responsible for the failure of the technique to develop (Moore, 1948; Brownell and Sweet, 1953). Two factors were responsible for the development of cerebral scanning as a useful diagnostic technique. The first of these was the development of a rectilinear scanner with a large detector and the ability to record the results as a photoscan on conventional x-ray film.

The second was the availability of isotopes with a short half-life which enabled the activity given to the patient to be increased and resulted in a corresponding increase in resolution and a shorter scanning time. The short-life isotopes necessitated some method of generation and consequently isotopes were stored and became available on site and could be dispensed in response to clinical demand. The simplicity of the techniques involved, the lack of discomfort and pain to the patient and the reported accuracy of these techniques (Davies and colleagues, 1966; McAfee and Taxdall, 1961) have led to a wide increase in demand.

SCANNING INSTRUMENTS

Essentially these are of two types: the moving rectilinear scanner and the stationary gamma-camera.

The rectilinear scanner has a crystal of sodium iodide varying in diameter from 7 to 20 cm which traces a grid pattern over the organ to be investigated. The resulting information may be recorded as a photoscan or on Teledeltos paper. Alternatively, a colour output may be obtained either on colour film or as a print-out with each colour representing a specific count rate.

The gamma-camera has a much larger crystal between 28 and 33 cm in diameter. This views the whole organ at once and is in turn viewed by a bank of photo-multipliers which position the signal on the display.

It is not the purpose of this chapter to discuss the construction of these instruments but a comparison of the two was thought to be useful (Table 1).

TABLE 1

Function	Gamma camera	Rectilinear scanner
Cost	Comparable. Basic camera is cheaper than dual head scanner	Comparable. Simplest is cheaper than basic camera
Views obtainable	Crystal can be placed at almost any angle in relation to target	Most instruments scan in one plane only
Dynamic studies	Dynamic studies available with basic camera. 16 per sec available with tape and data processor	Static studies only possible
Field size	Limited, but diverging collimators available. Pinhole collimator for magnification	Whole body scanning possible

TABLE 1–*continued*

Function	Gamma camera	Rectilinear scanner
Visual record	Usually by Polaroid ($8\frac{1}{2} \times 10\frac{1}{2}$ cm). Full size attachment available	Full size, dot, colour print out or photo
Field uniformity	Within $\pm$ 10 per cent	Within $\pm$ 2 per cent
Smallest detectable lesion	Approximately 2 cm	Approximately 2 cm
Tomography	Attachment available	Collimator has limited effect, dependent upon crystal size and depth of focus
Data processing	Easily coupled to MCA or computer, preferably on line	Probably best done off line using paper or magnetic tape
Speed	Limited by permissible activity. Can compensate for low count rates by increasing time	Limited by mechanical speed but this can be 500 cm/min. Time per view is usually longer than with camera
Ease of operation	Energy window easily set and operation extremely simple. Movable but not mobile	Energy window setting is more complex and there are many controls to be adjusted. Modern development is toward automation. Simple scanners are mobile
Reliability	Mechanically and electronically reliable. Uniformity is checked monthly	Electronically reliable. Mechanical problems do occur and regular servicing is required
Energy range	Approx. 80–500 keV. Efficiency falls above 200 keV	Approx. 25–500 keV. Efficient at higher energies
Positioning of target organ	Easy with use of persistancescope	Time consuming and can be very difficult with low counts

Speed

The rectilinear scanner takes approximately 20 minutes per projection if 7–10 mCi of technetium-99m is given intravenously. At least three views are taken and on many occasions four are required. Thus a total time of $1–1\frac{1}{2}$ hours may be required for this study.

Dual-headed scanners are able to take both lateral views, and then anterior and posterior views, at once, decreasing the total examination time. The gamma-camera takes 3–4 minutes for each projection and is set to record either a certain number of counts per projection or for a predetermined time. This investigation may therefore only take half an hour.

Resolution

In a comparison of 40 cerebral scans carried out by both instruments no lesion was believed to have been seen by one method that was not seen by the other (Bligh, 1970). Neither method will detect a lesion much smaller than 2 cm in size. The normal cerebral scan, by either method, shows areas of high and low activity (*Figure 1a* and *b*) and the possibility of 'hiding' a lesion under the normal areas of increased activity is common to both. The gamma-camera has the advantage that when only very low counts are available, the time factor can be increased. The speed of travel of a rectilinear scanner can be decreased but then each projection can take up to 45 minutes to produce and few patients are able to lie still for this time.

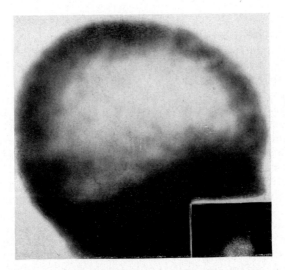

Figure 1. (a) Lateral projection. A rectilinear and gamma-camera scan with the same degree of geometrical reduction

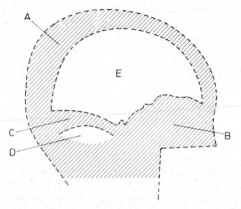

A: Superior sagittal sinus, scalp and skull. Note this activity is thinner over frontal area

B: Temporalis muscle

C: Transverse sinus and torcula

D: Cerebellar hemisphere

E: Cerebral hemisphere

Figure 1. (b) A tracing of Figure 1a with the main 'anatomical' features labelled

Operation

The rectilinear scanner is a more complex instrument to operate than the gamma-camera although there has been some improvement in more recent models. It is easier to adjust the crystal of a gamma-camera to obtain the exact projection required than to adjust a rectilinear scanner.

The gamma-camera has two main disadvantages. First the bank of photo-multipliers detecting the gamma rays must be balanced so that a uniform response is obtained over the whole of the crystal. Even after final adjustment some drifting may occur so that false 'hot' or 'cold' areas are produced on the resultant scan. This fault can be diagnosed by noting that the abnormal area bears a constant relation to the crystal and not to the organ investigated.

The second disadvantage of the gamma-camera is that it is less efficient with the higher energy isotopes. The optimum energy level for a gamma-camera appears to be about 140 keV which coincides with the gamma energy of technetium-99m.

Some clinicians feel that the final scan record produced by a gamma-camera is too small. Especially is this true if the model available provides three records at different photographic stops on the one polaroid print measuring 8·5 × 10·5 cm. The rectilinear scanner produces a life-size scan. This criticism is not valid, for it can be shown that no information is lost and that with increased experience the smaller gamma-scan is found to be totally adequate.

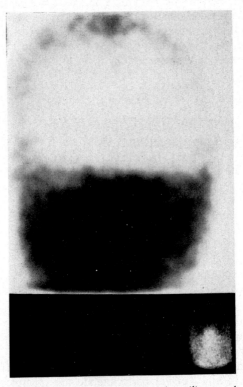

Figure 1. (c) Anterior projection. A rectilinear and gamma-scan with the same degree of geometrical reduction

A life-size rectilinear scan and a gamma-camera scan are shown (*Figure 1a* and *c*). These are both reduced by the same geometric scale for publication.

Finally the cost of the two pieces of apparatus is much closer than is generally realized. A basic gamma-camera is more versatile than a more complex model of a rectilinear scanner, certainly in the study of the central nervous system.

These comparative functions are tabulated (Table 1) but it is believed that the speed and ease of use of the gamma-camera makes it the instrument of choice not just for the study of the central nervous system but in any busy isotope scanning department.

For the sake of completeness a third type of apparatus should be mentioned. This is a much smaller detector with a heavily collimated crystal. A number, usually between 8 and 16, are applied to the skull and each measures regional activity limited to its own area. By this method regional cerebral blood flow may be investigated. At the present time, this is largely a research investigation and appears to be more of value in vascular lesions than in tumour investigation.

ISOTOPES

An ideal scanning agent should:

(1) Be free from beta activity.
(2) Have a single gamma energy.
(3) Have a short half-life (measured in hours).
(4) Have a good range of stable radio pharmaceuticals.
(5) Have a high critical organ affinity.
(6) Provide a high tumour/background ratio.
(7) Have a suitable photon energy (100–120 keV).
(8) Be carrier free, i.e. all atoms should be radioactive.
(9) Be available from a generator on site.
(10) Be competitive in cost.

As yet no such isotope exists although it is probably true to say that there are two main contenders for this title, technetium-99m and indium-113m.

For cerebral work, many scanning agents have been used, chlormerodrin, radio-iodinated serum albumin, arsenical compounds, technetium and indium compounds amongst them. Of these, Hg-197 chlormerodrin and Tc-99m pertechnetate are in greatest universal use. Some recent work with indium DTPA compound has been disappointing (Brookerman and Williams, 1970). Hg-203 chlormerodrin has been largely dropped because of the dose to the kidneys, which could be as high as 17–19 rads, even with a pre-screening blocking dose of non-active chlormerodrin (Blaue and Bender, 1962). Mercury-197 gives a high percentage uptake per gram of tumour, provides a good tumour/brain ratio and is stated to be of especial value in metastatic lesions (Sodee, 1968). For many departments specializing only in studies of the central nervous system, this is perhaps the isotope of choice. However, for departments with wider interests Tc-99m is more versatile.

Technetium-99m is a break-down product of molybdenum-99 (from which it is generated) and as an isomer it has no beta emission. It has virtually a single gamma energy of 140 keV. This is well suited for work with either a rectilinear scanner or a gamma-camera. Its half-life of six hours is ideal. As a simple saline eluate it can be given into the ventricles or intra-thecally. Albumin macroaggregates can be used for pulmonary scans and as a sulphur colloid it can be used for liver and splenic scans. As a compound with iron and vitamin C functioning renal tissue can be demonstrated and in its simple per-technetate form it is absorbed by the thyroid but not metabolized. Its universality of use provides a large economic factor as the isotope of choice in a busy general department. In particular, in cerebral work, a high degree of accuracy can be obtained with both neoplastic and non-neoplastic lesions.

PATIENT PREPARATION

Apart from a simple description of the investigation and a statement that a small venepuncture is required, little mental preparation is necessary.

If the technetium is to be given orally it should be given to a patient who has not eaten for the previous 12 hours. This improves absorption of the isotope from the gut. If given intravenously starvation is not necessary. Two hours before the isotope is given the patient is given 200 mg of potassium perchlorate by mouth. Witcofski and colleagues (1967) and Mandel and colleagues (1968) have both re-corded evidence of activity in the choroid plexus after scans with technetium. The demonstration of such 'hot' areas can confuse the interpretation of a cerebral scan. Silberstein and Levy (1970) have measured the concentration of pertechnetate in the choroid plexus, brain and cerebrospinal fluid in two groups of rabbits. One group was given potassium perchlorate (15 mg/kg i.v.) 15 minutes before the technetium-99m was administered. The other group was not given perchlorate. These workers were able to show a plexus/brain ratio of 8:1 in group 1 and 70:1 in group 2, thus demonstrating that perchlorate can block the intake of technetium by the choroid plexus in the rabbit. Similarly, perchlorate can be shown to block absorption of the pertechnetate ion by the thyroid and in this way protect the thyroid from unnecessary radiation. With very young children or those whose mental constitution make it impossible for them to co-operate, sedation or anaesthesia may be required. It is obviously important that the patient's head is kept still during each projection.

59

Some authorities state that the optimum time for scanning is about three hours after the intravenous administration of pertechnetate (Ramsey and Quinn, 1971) but suitable data can be obtained within 30 minutes. If the technetium is given orally, then a period of at least one hour is required to obtain a good count rate. This delay before scanning is a factor governing the turn-over in a busy department. The preferred policy is to scan at 30 minutes and if this is negative in a case with high clinical suspicion of a lesion, to re-scan three hours after the injection.

THE NORMAL CEREBRAL SCAN

To carry out an adequate investigation of the brain at least four views need to be taken. These are: both lateral views, an anterior and a posterior view. To obtain a posterior view it is necessary, with most rectilinear scanners, for the patient to lie prone. Therefore this view may be reserved for those patients where there is a clinical suspicion of a posterior fossa lesion. With a gamma-camera the posterior view should be a routine projection and an attempt made to show the posterior fossa with this view rather than just the occipital lobes. To do this the neck must be flexed and the crystal adjusted to the plane of the posterior fossa. Similarly with the anterior view, a Towne's projection with the chin tucked well down is more useful as a routine. Other views such as a true anterior view, with Reid's base line at right angles to the crystal, may be required for orbital and retro-orbital lesions or a superior view to determine the relationship of a lesion to the falx. It is obvious that what is needed is to demonstrate any given lesion and quite unorthodox views may be of value.

As has been said, the gamma-camera is an easy instrument to use. If pre-set count levels determine when sufficient data have been collected then 500,000 counts per projection is a satisfactory level. With refractory patients or young children, a lower level of counts may have to be accepted but a loss of data density is always to be avoided wherever possible. Care must be taken in positioning the head in the lateral projection so that large numbers of counts are not recorded from areas of little interest (mouth and pharynx). This is one reason why some centres carry out cerebral scans on a pre-set time basis.

The normal cerebral scan does not show a uniform uptake (*Figure 1*). Increased activity is visible in areas of relatively high vascularity. The skull and scalp with the superior sagittal sinus provide such an area and give a halo-like shadow in all projections. In the lateral projection this halo should be thinner over the frontal pole than elsewhere and if this is not so a possible clue to underlying pathology may exist. However, rotation of the head or an unbalanced photo-multiplier in the gamma-camera are alternative explanations.

The transverse venous sinus and the torcular can be seen on all posterior scans and provide very useful landmarks. However, it must be remembered that in normal cases the right transverse sinus is more prominent in a greater percentage than the left and that they are symmetrical in only about 15 per cent of patients (Holmes and Golle, 1971). Choroid plexus uptake may occasionally be visible in the trigonal area of the lateral ventricle even after premedication with potassium perchlorate. The oro- and nasopharynx, the tongue, temporalis and occipital muscles all provide areas of increased uptake. With a gamma-camera the Sylvian group of vessels can just be seen end-on in both lateral projections.

In this manner a composite picture of areas of differing activity is seen and soon recognized as normal. The essential feature must be that a technically satisfactory normal scan should show the cerebral and cerebellar hemispheres as virtually devoid of activity. The ability to recognize the normal anatomy as demonstrated by the areas of increased activity is the most convincing method of demonstrating the veracity of a scan. It is undoubtedly true that small lesions can be masked by normal increased activity but the routine four views nearly always give some suggestion of their existence and it is not suggested that a negative isotope scan should over-ride abnormal clinical findings. With the present-day apparatus lesions of 2–2·5 cm in diameter represent the smallest size that can be detected.

THE ABNORMAL SCAN

Isotope scans are of great value in the diagnosis of non-tumorous conditions but this aspect is outside the scope of this chapter which considers only the value of cerebral scanning in tumours.

When positive a cerebral tumour is shown on the scan by an area of increased activity. This increase in activity is probably due to two factors. First, the tumour process causes an interference in the blood/brain barrier allowing the isotope to be taken up by the tumour cells. Secondly, the tumour circulation gives rise to an increase in vascularity in an area which is normally relatively avascular.

From these facts it can be seen that a small increase in activity could be hidden by an area of normally high activity such as the sagittal sinus, torcula or temporalis muscle. This latter structure obscures most pituitary tumours and is one of the reasons why isotope scans are of little value in the investigation of pituitary tumours. If there is an absent or poor uptake of the isotope by the tumour cells then there may be an insufficient increase in activity above background to allow of localization. The latter factor is particularly true of the more slowly growing astrocytomas and accounts for the false-negative scans that are often obtained with this tumour (Moreno and Deland, 1971).

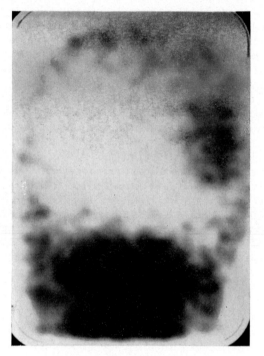

Figure 2a

These then are the main reasons for failure of the method to demonstrate space-occupying lesions. Various investigators have reported between 10 and 15 per cent of false-negative scans. It should not be forgotten than an isotope scan is only one part of the total investigations in a patient with clinical symptoms. A negative scan in the face of positive clinical findings should be ignored and not allowed to influence the further investigation of a patient. Occasionally a second scan at a later date will reveal a positive finding.

The diagnosis of cell type from a scan is fraught with danger. The meningioma is always quoted as the example that such an exercise is possible. It is undoubtedly more true of some meningiomas than of any other cell type. As Bull and Marryat (1965) pointed out, the combination of a well defined area of high uptake in an anatomical site where such tumours are known to occur enables a type diagnosis to be made with a fair degree of certainty (*Figure 2*). In spite of this many neurosurgeons request an angiogram to demonstrate supplying and draining vessels.

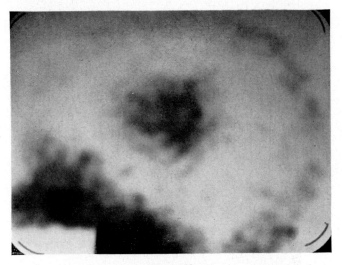

Figure 2b

*Figure 2. Anterior and lateral projection. The high, well defined activity
in the tumour which is shown to lie in a peripheral position suggests a
meningioma (proven)*

The gliomas take up the pertechnetate less avidly but with a range of activity approaching the meningioma at one end (*Figure 3*) and often showing a failure of uptake at the other, represented by the astrocytoma grade I. Again the diagnosis of cell type may sometimes be suggested. The anatomical situation may be of help as, for example, in those cases of corpus-callosum tumours where an extension of the abnormal frontal activity is shown to either side of the mid-line. The shape of glioma uptakes is not a diagnostic feature as they can adopt almost any pattern. However, a rounded lesion on a lateral projection which, in the anterior or posterior view, is shown to extend deeply with a wedge shape is very suspicious of a malignant glioma. In a patient with a short and rapidly progressive clinical

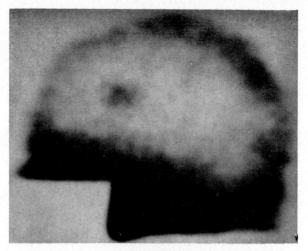

Figure 3a

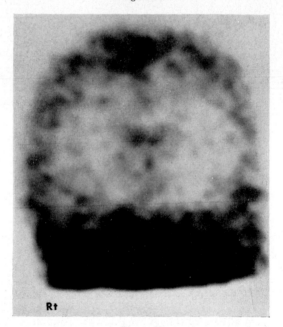

Figure 3b

*Figure 3. Anterior and lateral projection. Compare the
activity level with Figure 2b. This lesion is not peripheral
and suggests a glioma (proven)*

64

history with abnormal neurological signs suggesting a lesion in a dominant site, some neurosurgeons are prepared to act upon evidence of the scan alone and confine their operation to a burr hole with biopsy. This can save the patient an uncomfortable and unpleasant angiogram, a major craniotomy and possibly two anaesthetics. This factor, by permitting an earlier diagnosis and the earlier institution of radiotherapy, will also allow an increased turn-over from the neurosurgical wards.

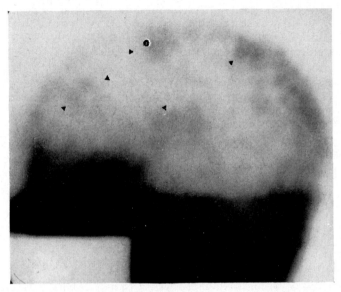

Figure 4. Lateral projection. Multiple areas of increased activity (arrowed); suggests multiple metastases (proven) but can be due to multiple emboli

The finding of multiple lesions or an intracerebral lesion in a patient who has a known neoplasm in some other site is very suggestive of metastatic disease and this knowledge can result in a radical alteration in treatment plan (*Figure 4*). Multiple intracranial lesions can be of vascular origin and in such very difficult cases even the clinical history may be confusing. However, the clinical progress of the patient and a follow-up scan may help. An area of increased activity but with variations in uptake in different parts may be explained by a large cystic tumour enclosing a small active nubbin which provides the 'hotter' or more active part of the scan.

Posterior fossa tumours are more difficult to localize than supratentorial lesions especially if a rectilinear scanner is used (Takahashi, 1965). This is because the cerebellar hemispheres are surrounded by structures which in the normal scan give rise to areas of increased activity. The occipital muscles, the torcular and the transverse sinuses cause much overlap in this region. Only small areas of low uptake remain, within which any area of pathological activity could be seen. However, with a gamma-camera the crystal can be more easily adjusted to be parallel to the coronal and sagittal planes and a better data density can be obtained. It is doubtful if a posterior view is worthwhile as a routine projection with a rectilinear scanner. It can be reserved for patients with clinical suspicion of a posterior fossa lesion, for with a size limitation of 2 cm few patients with a posterior fossa tumour of this size are likely to be missed by clinical and other investigative methods.

The value of follow-up scans to show the effect of therapy is difficult to assess. Especially is this true if a major cranial operation has been performed. Surgical interference to the skull and scalp produces increased activity on a cerebral scan which may persist for many months. The absence of a positive uptake in a previously abnormal scan can be demonstrated but this only reveals the macroscopic removal of tumour and obviously does not exclude microscopic remnants which can give rise to a recurrence. Deep x-ray therapy up to a dose of 6,000 rads in six weeks does not seem to affect the scan (McCready, 1967).

RADIO-ISOTOPE ARTERIOGRAPHY

For those departments equipped with a gamma-camera a dynamic technique is possible (Maynard and colleagues, 1969; Penning, Front and Beckhuis, 1971).

The patient is positioned under the crystal, either as for an anterior view or for the relevant lateral view.

The isotope is injected intravenously and a serial study is made. There are eight films in a polaroid pack and with an assistant pulling each film from the pack the camera can be re-set approximately every two seconds. Obviously longer time intervals are possible. With an anterior projection flow to the two hemispheres can be compared. If the lateral projection is used flow within a hemisphere can be studied. The anterior view is of greatest value in suspected vascular lesions and here the early arterial pattern is of greatest importance. Blocked vessels can be suspected from a diminished activity in their anatomical territory. An angiomatous process will show early increased activity and a hypertrophy of the supplying vessels. Tumour circulation can best be seen in the lateral projection and the progression of activity from an arterial pattern to the cerebral tissue uptake may be demonstrated if the technique is prolonged for 30 minutes with films every 3–5 minutes. Recent work has shown that by correlating the findings by this form of dynamic scan with the findings of a static scan more information concerning the blood supply and the activity of the tumour can be obtained.

SUMMARY

In summary it can be said that cerebral isotope studies are a potent diagnostic aid in the localization, and are of some value in the identification, of malignant cerebral tumours. The technique is relatively simple and has a high degree of accuracy. Some authorities carry out more and more complex techniques, attempting to make the method self-sufficient. It is felt that, whereas research to expand the scope of isotope studies is obviously required, increasing complexity can only add to the time required and increase the patient discomfort (Gottschalk, 1971). Then two of the most valuable aspects of cerebral scanning are lost for a slight increase in the percentage accuracy of the method.

REFERENCES

Blaue, M. and Bender, M. A. (1962). 'Radio-mercury (Hg 203) labelled neohydrin. A new agent for brain tumour localisation.' *J. nucl. Med.*, 3, 83.
Bligh, A. S. (1970). 'Radioactive isotope scanning. Part 2.' *X-ray Focus (Ilford)*, 10, 8.
Brookerman, V. A. and Williams, C. M. (1970). 'Brain scintigrams with Tc 99m iron D.T.P.A. complex in experimental metastatic disease.' *J. nucl. Med.*, 11, 733.
Brownell, G. L. and Sweet, W. A. (1953). 'Localisation of brain tumours with positron emitters.' *Nucleonics*, 11, 40.
Bull, J. W. D. and Marryat, J. (1965). 'Isotope encephalography. Experience with 100 cases.' *Br. med. J.*, 1, 474.
Davies, H. C., Alexander, E., Witcofski, R. L. and Maynard, C. D. (1966). 'Brain scanning with technetium.' *J. Neurosurg.*, 24, 987.
Di Chiro, G. (1962). 'How reliable is neuro-radiology?' *Neurology*, 12, 93.
Gottschalk, A. (1971). 'Brain scanning—is it becoming unnecessarily complicated?' (Editorial). *Am. J. Roentgenol.*, 111, 851.

Holmes, R. A. and Golle, R. (1971). 'Appearance of the transverse sinuses in brain scanning.' *Am. J. Roentgenol.*, **111**, 340.
— and Walker, A. G. (1971). 'When is the brain scan the primary diagnostic test?' *J. nucl. Med.*, **12**, 439.
Kieffer, S. A. and Loken, M. K. (1969). 'Positive brain scans in fibrous dysplasia and other lesions of the skull.' *Am. J. Roentgenol.*, **106**, 731.
McCready, V. R. (1967). 'Review article—clinical isotope scanning.' *Br. J. Radiol.*, **40**, 401.
Mandel, P. R., Saxe, B. I. and Fayenburg, D. (1968). 'Demonstration of the choroid plexus with technetium 99m brain scan.' *Am. J. Roentgenol.*, **102**, 97.
Maynard, C. D., Witcofski, M. M., Janeway, M. D. and Bowden, M. D. (1969). 'Radio-isotope cisternography as an adjunct to the brain scan.' *Radiology*, **92**, 908.
Moore, G. E. (1948). 'The use of radio-active diiodofluorescein in the diagnosis and localisation of brain tumours.' *Science*, **107**, 569.
Moreno, J. B. and Deland, F. H. (1971). 'Brain scanning in the diagnosis of astrocytomas of the brain.' *J. nucl. Med.*, **12**, 107.
Penning, L., Front. D. and Beckhuis, J. (1971). 'Differentiation of brain lesions by sequential gamma-camera studies.' *J. neurol. Sci.*, **14**, 1.
Ramsey, R. and Quinn, J. L. (1971). 'Comparison of the accuracy of initial and delayed 99m Tc Pertechnetate brain scans.' *J. nucl. Med.*, **12**, 389.
Silberstein, A. N. and Levy, L. M. (1970). '99m technetium localisation in the choroid plexus.' *Radiology*, **95**, 529.
Sodee, D. B. (1968). 'Comparison of Tc 99m pertechnetate and chlormerodrin 107 for brain scanning.' *J. nucl. Med.*, **9**, 645.
Takahashi, M. (1965). 'Comparison of scintillation scanning with other neuro-radiologic procedures in the diagnosis of posterior fossa tumours.' *J. Can. Ass. Radiol.*, **16**, 248.
Witcofski, R. L., Janeway, R. and Maynard, C. D. (1967). 'Visualisation of the choroid plexus on the technetium 99m brain scan.' *Archs Neurol.*, **16**, 286.

III—The Use of Ultrasound

Douglas Gordon

INTRODUCTION

It is a little known fact that the earliest attempts to use ultrasound for diagnostic purposes in Britain were those made in the Radiotherapy Department of what was then the Royal Cancer (now the Royal Marsden) Hospital, London, beginning in 1951 (Durden-Smith, 1972).

Dr Joan Durden-Smith and Dr Richard Walton, both radiotherapists, and Dr Turner, a physicist, embarked on a research project to see whether isotopes or ultrasound held out more promise in observing the effect of radiotherapy on cerebral tumours.

They used a modified industrial flaw detector produced by Henry Hughes & Son Ltd for this purpose (*Figure 1*). At that date quartz was the only suitable material available for transducers of tnis type and amplifiers were virtually those used in war-time radar apparatus. Looking back now after 20 years of experience and the development on the technical side that has been made in this period, it is remarkable that any echoes at all were obtained from within the cranial cavity.

It is not surprising that the outcome of the project went very much in favour of isotopes but, although both Dr Durden-Smith and Dr Walton left the Royal Cancer Hospital in 1953, Dr Turner in 1954 demonstrated the apparatus at the Physical Society's Annual Exhibition held that year at Imperial College, London.

It was this exhibit that first drew the writer's attention to the possibility of using ultrasound in neuroradiology and it was an industrial flaw detector of this type which he first used.

ECHO-ENCEPHALOGRAPHY

Durden-Smith, Walton and Turner, like many others since, assumed that the large mid-line echo was derived from the falx cerebri which was expected to be displaced with the brain by a tumour. So far as the great majority of patients are concerned this was a mistaken idea. Although it is unwise to draw too close a parallel between optical reflection and acoustic reflection it is still true that a reflecting surface should be very nearly perpendicular to a beam of ultrasound if a detectable echo is to be produced. It is only in the dolichocephalic that it is possible to obtain adequate contact with the scalp high enough up for the falx cerebri to contribute to the echo-pattern.

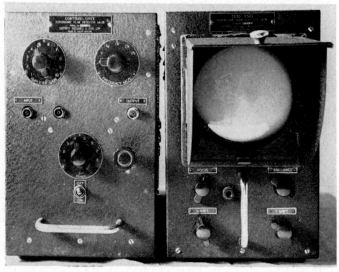

Figure 1. The first ultrasonic flaw detector used for medical diagnosis

In the normal anatomy there are below the falx cerebri, the lowest part of the longitudinal fissure, the pineal body, the septum pellucidum and the third ventricle which contribute to the so-called 'M-echo' that indicates the position of the median plane of the brain. Naturally the two lateral walls of the third ventricle can produce separate echoes when they are far enough apart for the acoustic system to resolve them. In practice the higher the probe position the more likely the 'M-echo' is to appear as a single large echo attributable to the septum and the lower the position the more likely is the appearance of two equal echoes from the walls of the third ventricle.

Leksell of Lund (1956) attributed the 'M-echo' solely to the pineal at first but it is only thought to be a contributory factor now by most workers.

While the detection of the displacement of the brain by a haematoma in cases of head injury has undoubtedly become widely accepted as a useful diagnostic procedure, the value of echo-encephalography in cerebral tumours is much less accepted.

After more than 19 years of experience the writer still has a very considerable proportion of unsatisfactory diagnostic results in tumour cases, in striking contrast to the very low proportion of false-negative results in trauma cases.

As long as a tumour, such as a meningioma of the convexity, behaves very much as does a sub-dural haematoma it can be lateralized satisfactorily. When, however, it is intracerebral and particularly if it is invasive and slow growing, the anatomy becomes so altered that it is quite impossible to attribute any particular echo signal to any particular intracranial structure with any certainty.

The falx will resist all but extreme violence, but with the slow growth of a tumour it softens and becomes tilted so that it is much easier to detect from the side of the tumour than from the other side. It is impossible, however, to say that any particular signal is derived from the tilted falx and not from a tilted septum or from the lateral wall of the lateral ventricle.

It is therefore easy to understand why Durden-Smith, Walton and Turner rapidly came to the conclusion that it was not possible to obtain accurate anatomical information of the type needed for the control of radiotherapy.

Even with the very great improvement in both probes and amplifiers in a period exceeding 20 years, it is only in small children that the effect of the skull bone is small enough to permit something like the correct anatomy to be demonstrated. A very large number of research projects have been undertaken, all with the hope of demonstrating the brain anatomy by ultrasound to the same standard as can be obtained by pneumoencephalography. Nobody has achieved anything that would justify the large sums expended. The most elaborate of these known to the writer is that developed by the Frys at the University of Illinois (Kossoff, Fry and Eggleton, 1971) in which a large computer, a highly focused transducer and a waterbath failed to produce results that were more than 'interesting' in the presence of the skull bones.

Makow in Ottawa, de Vlieger in Rotterdam, Houdart in Paris, Brinker in St Louis, Mo., and Taylor in London have each produced their variations in the basic technique but none can claim to produce results comparable with those obtained by x-ray techniques. It has been a depressing result to so much effort and such high hopes.

THE LIMITED USE OF ECHO-ENCEPHALOGRAPHY

Although the high hopes have been dashed, echo-encephalography does have some limited contribution to make. The place in initial diagnosis hardly falls within the scope of this book but once the diagnosis has been made and radiotherapy has begun, it can provide useful aid. It is hardly permissible to perform repeated air-studies or angiograms to control the progress of a case but there is absolutely no objection to repeated ultrasonic investigation.

Where the tumour causes obstruction in the cerebrospinal fluid system, it is undoubtedly possible to demonstrate progressive changes in the ventricular size but with diminishing accuracy as age advances. The thin uniform skulls of small children present none of the problems of the adult skull. Echoes derived from tumours and cysts above the tentorium are frequently detectable but Japanese claims to identify posterior fossa tumours have never been confirmed.

As age advances fewer and fewer cases will benefit from echo-encephalography but where there are lacunae left by the surgeon a window is provided for the ultrasonic probe, and in such cases it would be worth while to perform serial examinations with a view to detecting a recurrence after operative removal without having to submit the patient to the significant risk of x-ray methods of diagnosis.

As radiotherapy is rarely housed in the same building or even the same complex as the neurosurgical unit, a practical point arises that there is not likely to be a sufficient volume of cases for any member of the radiotherapy staff to become experienced in conventional echo-encephalography. The logistic problem of transferring suitable cases between widely separated units makes it unlikely to prove popular.

In recent years the invention of the computerized echo-encephalo-graph, the Midliner (*Figure 2*) by Williams of Lexington, Mass., has at last made it possible for a technician, after a very brief instruction period, to obtain the same results as the experienced operator (Gordon, 1973). This instrument has a very sophisticated system of discrimination between individual echo-signals and measures the position of the largest mid-line signal to the nearest 2 mm.

ULTRASONIC DIAGNOSIS APART FROM THE SKULL

If the skull presents difficulties for ultrasonic diagnosis, the vertebral column presents even more, because of the extreme complexity of the bone shapes. It is impossible to believe that tumours of the spinal canal can usefully be examined by ultrasound.

There is undoubtedly a very large place for ultrasound in improving the accuracy of radiotherapy beam alignment in the rest of the body (Brascho, 1971) but this will be of importance for other systems much more than for the central nervous system and will be better left to another volume of this series. In the near future it will be possible with ultrasound to make a major contribution to radiotherapy by making it possible to outline the skin surface accurately and quickly in any plane chosen and to indicate within that plane the sites of organs and often the site of the actual tumour.

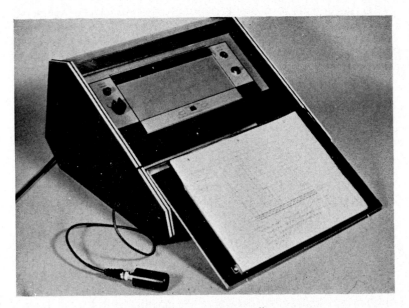

Figure 2. The Midliner automatic midline computer

ULTRASONIC SURGERY

In the diagnostic uses of ultrasound the harmlessness of the method has been stressed. It may seem paradoxical therefore to discuss now the use of ultrasound as a destructive agent in its own right. However, the intensities used in diagnosis are measured in milliwatts per square centimetre while in the surgical use the intensity is of the order of hundreds or even thousands of watts per square centimetre. In passing it should perhaps be mentioned that the intensity used in physical medicine is at most three watts per square centimetre.

These intensities can only be achieved by using a high degree of focusing and this produces the small deep trackless lesion that is so useful to the physiologist. The method of producing these lesions is the subject of considerable dispute. The pioneer work in the field carried out at Urbana, Illinois, by Fry, Fry, Kelly and Dunn over a period of years and at Iowa City, Iowa by the same team in association with Meyers, was deliberately planned to use very high intensities and short exposure times so that the removal of heat by the unpredictable circulation of blood would have minimal effects (Meyers and colleagues, 1960).

At these intensities the mechanical hysteresis of the tissues is sufficient to raise the temperature of the focal zone to a lethal figure. The later work of Ballantine, Lele and Basauri at Massachusetts General Hospital, Boston, used intensities of the same order (Basauri and Lele, 1962). When they kept the intensity down to rather lower levels or restricted the time of irradiation, it was shown that there was a mixture of effects some attributable to heat and some purely 'ultrasonic'.

In the meantine in Padua, Italy, Arslan, an otologist, had developed his technique for the ultrasonic surgery of Menière's disease (Arslan, 1955). This was at the other end of the intensity spectrum from the Urbana group. Arslan sought a method of destroying the vestibular apparatus in the semicircular canals without damage to the cochlea. If this could be achieved it would be possible to relieve the tinnitus and vertigo long before total deafness justified a complete surgical destruction of the labyrinth. The fact that both cochlea and canals have a common endolymph and perilymph system made this an inherently very difficult problem.

An earlier attempt in Vienna to use ultrasound by filling the external meatus with water and applying a transducer in the axis of the meatus had failed. The air in the middle ear restricted transmission to the inner ear to the tiny amount transmitted by the ossicles but this may well have given Arslan the basic idea.

Arslan realized that the transducer must be applied directly to the semicircular canal system and for this surgical exploration of the middle ear was essential. He ground away sufficient bone over the lateral semicircular canal so that a flat instead of a convex surface was available. With a transducer coupled to a metal cone and rod with a 5 mm tip, he was able to apply the ultrasound with only 0·5 mm of bone between the active metal surface and the cavity of the lateral canal. Providentially the ultrasound, once in the lymph space, appears to be trapped as in a wave-guide and the energy is nearly all absorbed within that space. The angulation between the cochlear system and the canal system is such that there is very little transfer of energy from one to the other.

Arslan's original equipment suffered from a major disadvantage in that the use of metal to transmit the ultrasound was very inefficient and the metal rose in temperature to such an extent that facial paralysis was produced in a significant proportion of cases. The significant fact was, however, that the patients derived so much relief of their Menière's disease that they accepted the transient facial paralysis as a price well worth paying.

The writer introduced water transmission in place of metal and this, with a reduction in the active area to about 2 mm in diameter, has made the operation a major contribution to the management of a rare but crippling disease (Gordon, 1964).

The significant aspect so far as dosage is concerned is the very low level employed. Cases have been recorded where a total acoustic power of less than a quarter of a watt for about 20 minutes achieved total destruction of the vestibular apparatus. With modern apparatus the total power is of the order of a watt but as the area is only a twentieth of a square centimetre the intensity produced is 20 watts per square centimetre.

Arslan later extended his method to attack the pituitary by the sphenoidal route (Arslan, 1968). The removal of a small amount of bone from the anterior wall of the sphenoidal sinus exposed the bone forming the anterior wall of the pituitary fossa. The latter can be removed leaving the dura mater intact. Irradiation of the pituitary by a long hollow applicator can be performed through the nose and the writer developed an applicator 8 mm in diameter which enables the whole pituitary to be irradiated in two fields (Gordon, 1964). This method was not developed until the enthusiasm for pituitary ablation in the palliation of carcinoma had much abated.

Unfortunately ultrasonic methods are much less useful for pituitary tumour than for palliative surgery. Once the tumour extends above the anatomical fossa and particularly when the posterior bony wall of the fossa has been eroded, there is no way of restricting the irradiation to the pituitary tissue and the vital brain centres would be at risk.

The team at Iowa City had earlier used the focused transducer through a very large craniotomy to attack the pituitary in palliative surgery. Unfortunately approaching from above, the ultrasound had reached a high intensity by the time the cranial nerves were reached and though the pituitary was destroyed there was such a high incidence of cranial nerve palsies that the method was abandoned.

There appears to be no reason to believe that tumour cells are more susceptible to ultrasound than normal grey or white matter. A direct ultrasonic attack on cerebral tumours through a craniotomy is therefore unlikely to become a serious alternative to the ionizing radiations. The writer, however, did embark on animal experiments with focused ultrasound with the intention that ultimately it would be possible to destroy tumours in the pons or medulla oblongata.

Another possible application of focused ultrasound is to perform an ultrasonic cordotomy after laminectomy but without opening of the dura. A very high degree of accuracy of placement of such focal lesions is possible and the absence of any track makes this a very attractive method.

It would be rash to forecast the place in the palliative treatment of malignant disease that ultrasonic techniques will achieve but they certainly merit more consideration than they have so far received.

REFERENCES

Arslan, M. (1955). 'Applikation des ultraschalles auf das labyrinth: ein beitrag zur therapie der labyrinthose.' *Arch. Ohren-, Nasen- u. Kehlkopfheilk.*, **167**, 559.

— (1968). 'Ultrasonic selective hypophysectomy.' *Proc. R. Soc. Med.*, **61**, 7.

Basauri, L. and Lele, P. (1962). 'A simple method for production of trackless focal lesion with focussed ultrasound. Statistical evaluation of the effects of irradiation of the central nervous system of the cat.' *J. Physiol. Lond.*, **160**, 513.

Brascho, D. (1971). 'A proposal for the utilisation of B-scan sonography in computerised radiation treatment planning of malignant disease.' Program of Sixteenth Annual Meeting. American Institute of Ultrasound in Medicine. Denver, Colorado, U.S.A.

Durden-Smith, J. (1972). Personal communication.

Gordon, D. (1954). 'The use of ultrasonic rays in diagnostic radiology.' Paper given at Fourth Symposium in Neuroradiologicum, London. Text published as Appendix 2 of *Ultrasound as a Diagnostic and Surgical Tool* (1964), pp. 350–353, Ed. by D. Gordon. Edinburgh; Livingstone.

— (Ed.) (1964). *Ultrasound as a Diagnostic and Surgical Tool*, pp. 233–251, 309–323. Edinburgh; Livingstone.

— (1973). 'Objective echo-encephalography using a computer technique.' Paper read at Symposium Neuroradiologicum, Gothenburg, 1970. *Acta radiol.* (In press).

Kossoff, G., Fry, F.J. and Eggleton, R.C. (1971). 'Application of digital computers to control of ultrasonic visualization equipment.' *Ultrasonographia Medica*. Proceedings of 1st World Congress on Ultrasonic

Diagnostics in Medicine, Vienna 1969. Vienna; Wiener Medizinischen Akademie.

Leksell, L. (1956). 'Echo-encephalography: detection of intracranial complications following head injury.' *Acta chir. scand.*, **115**, 301.

Myers, R., Fry, F. J., Eggleton, R.C. and Schultz, D. F. (1960). 'Determination of topological human brain representations and modifications of signs and symptoms of some neurologic disorders by the use of high level ultrasound.' *Neurology*, **10**, 271.

IV—Localization by Electro-encephalography

I. M. S. Wilkinson

The electro-encephalogram certainly has a place in the detection and localization of intracranial tumours, but its value in very accurate localization has proved disappointing. Localization is less precise than might be imagined from theoretical considerations, and is certainly less accurate than that which can be achieved by other atraumatic methods, such as radioactive brain scanning, and by neuroradiological investigations such as angiography and air-encephalography.

EEG abnormalities found in association with·intracranial tumours are of two main types: those due to the presence of raised intracranial pressure, which are of a generalized nature; and those due to the presence of a focal lesion interfering with the normal local cerebral electrical activity.

The generalized EEG abnormalities occurring in association with raised intracranial pressure take the form of continuous or intermittent, bilateral and symmetrical, slow waves. These are usually in the delta range (less than 4 cycles/sec) but are sometimes in the theta range (4–7 cycles/sec). The appearance of such abnormalities in the record correlates reasonably well with the degree of intracranial hypertension, and they are almost constantly present when the pressure is of such a degree as to cause impairment in the conscious level of the patient.

Posterior fossa or infratentorial tumours, and deep midline supratentorial tumours (e.g. of the pineal gland, hypothalamus, third ventricle or thalamus) tend to produce the EEG abnormalities of raised intracranial pressure early, since they produce obstruction to the cerebrospinal fluid pathways (*see Figure 2*). They do not produce focal features in the EEG record and thus precise localization of the tumour cannot be achieved by this investigation.

Supratentorial tumours situated in the cerebral hemispheres produce localized abnormalities in the EEG. These abnormalities will be described in detail further, but it must be mentioned at the outset that once the supratentorial tumour has commenced to produce significant elevation in intracranial pressure, then diffuse bilateral abnormalities will appear in the EEG and the localized abnormalities caused by the cerebral tumour will become less evident. It follows, therefore, that the EEG is likely to be of better localizing value in the investigation of a cerebral hemisphere tumour early in its clinical presentation, in an alert patient who does not have the clinical hallmarks of raised intracranial pressure—headaches, vomiting, depression of conscious level and papilloedema.

We have now narrowed the application of the EEG in the localization of cerebral tumours to patients with tumours within the cerebral hemisphere which are unassociated with severe intracranial hypertension. It is in this group of patients that the EEG is useful, but it is important to be clear whether the EEG is being used for tumour detection or for very accurate tumour localization. In such patients the EEG is very commonly abnormal, showing localized, or at least lateralized, abnormalities, and is therefore reasonably reliable in the detection of such lesions. It would indeed be unusual for the EEG to be normal in such circumstances. Frequently, however, the EEG abnormalities are not very well localized, and tend to be diffuse throughout the affected hemisphere, sometimes associated with minor abnormalities over the other hemisphere. Moreover, there may be none of the characteristic wave forms (phase-reversal, *see* page 84) in the affected hemisphere which permit very precise determination of the site of the lesion. It is for these reasons that the EEG is more satisfactory as an investigation in cerebral tumour detection than in tumour localization of the degree of accuracy which is required for the planning of surgical or deep x-ray treatment.

From a more theoretical point of view it might be imagined that a destructive and compressive cerebral lesion such as a tumour should produce relatively localized interference of cerebral electrical activity, destroying normal rhythms and replacing them with abnormally slow and high voltage wave forms in the theta or delta ranges. Perhaps the discovery of rather more widespread electrical abnormalities throughout the affected cerebral hemisphere, and sometimes in the contralateral hemisphere, is a reflection of the spreading of abnormal impulses through the very considerable numbers of association fibres linking one part of the cerebral cortex with immediately adjacent parts by subcortical white matter loops, with more remote groups of neurons in the same hemisphere by well recognized specific fibre pathways in the cerebral white matter, and with cortical areas in the contralateral hemisphere by means of fibre

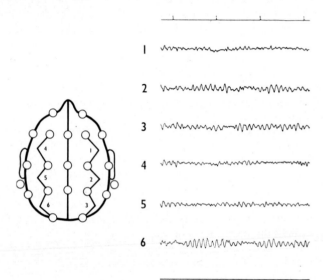

Figure 1. A normal EEG record. Note the low amplitude, fast activity over the anterior parts of the brain, and alpha activity over the post-central regions (the time marker at the top of all illustrations represents 1 sec intervals)

pathways in the corpus callosum. It seems likely that the abundant interconnection of neuronal function within the cerebral hemispheres by myelinated nerve fibre pathways is responsible for the difficulty in obtaining confined focal electrical abnormalities in the EEG record, even of those patients with sharply defined, focal cerebral lesions.

The characteristic EEG changes over the site of a cerebral hemisphere tumour consist of suppression of normal cerebral rhythms, i.e. the fast (beta range) activity over the anterior regions and the 8–13 cycles/sec alpha activity found over the postcentral regions (*Figure 1*), and the appearance of slow waves, generally in the delta range. Though often rather poorly localized there is a tendency for the slow wave activity to be most continuous and of highest voltage over the actual tumour region (*Figures 3–5*). During an EEG recording the bipolar scalp electrodes can be linked together in various combinations, to produce a series of traces which enable the greatest degree of localization of the slow wave disturbance produced by a

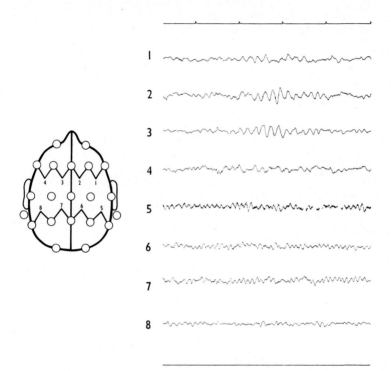

Figure 2. Abnormalities in the EEG associated with raised intracranial pressure, due to a posterior fossa tumour (pontine astrocytoma). The outstanding feature is the short run of bilateral slow wave activity (theta range) seen over the frontal regions. This recurred at intervals throughout the record

supratentorial cerebral tumour. Although these technical manoeuvres are often helpful in indicating the site of maximal electrical disturbance, it is uncommon for very precise localization of the lesion to be achieved. Often one can only conclude that the disturbance is maximal in one fronto-temporal region, or some region of the hemisphere of similar magnitude. It is very unusual for categorical localization to more specific regions to be possible, e.g. anterior third of temporal lobe, or inferior aspect of frontal pole.

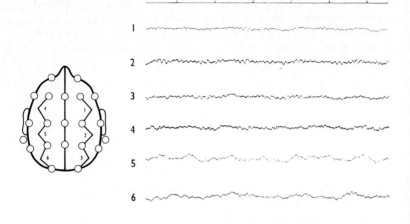

Figure 3. The EEG in a case of a left parieto-occipital metastasis from a bronchial carcinoma. The cerebral rhythms over the right hemisphere are relatively normal. On the left side there is a suppression of the normal alpha rhythm accompanied by continuous moderate voltage delta wave activity, maximal in channel 5

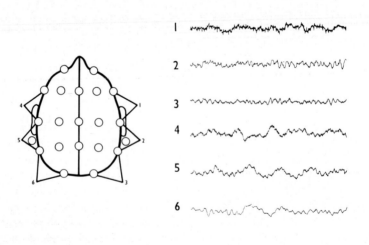

Figure 4. The EEG record of a patient with a left posterior frontal metastasis from a bronchial carcinoma. The principal abnormal features are the suppression of normal rhythms and the presence of moderately high voltage delta waves over the left cerebral hemisphere. Localization is poor, but the delta activity is most evident in channels 4 and 5

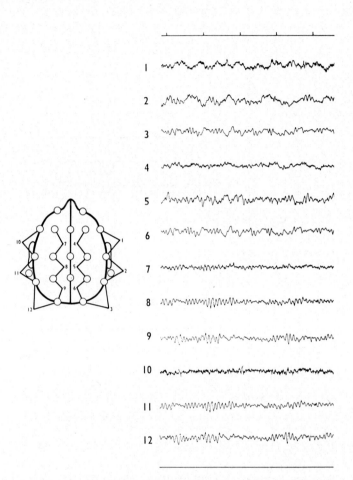

*Figure 5. The record from a patient with a right sphenoidal wing menin-
gioma. All the right-sided leads show abnormal slow wave activity in
the theta and delta range. Although not entirely normal the left hemisphere leads are much more satisfactory. Localization is very poor in
this case*

In addition to this identification of the region in which the slow wave activity is most continuous and of highest voltage, localization may be assisted by the appearance of 'phase-reversal' in the abnormal wave forms in the EEG record. This phenomenon results from monitoring a relatively localized electrical discharge by several

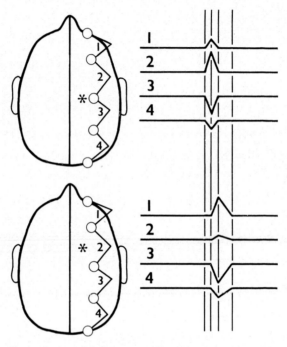

Figure 6. A model diagram to illustrate phase reversal. In the two instances illustrated the discharging focus is indicated by a star

bipolar scalp electrodes simultaneously (*Figure 6*). The wave forms from electrodes situated on one side of the focal disturbance will have a deflection of opposite direction to those from electrodes situated on the other side of the lesion. Phase-reversal in two planes at right angles gives the best possible localization of an abnormally discharging focus. Unfortunately phase-reversal giving this degree of localization is not common in the case of cerebral tumours (*Figure 7*), although phase-reversal about a less well defined area is sometimes observed.

The site of maximum electrical disturbance is sometimes best shown by the technique of unipolar recording. In this, each scalp electrode is not connected to an adjacent one (as in bipolar recording) but to a common reference point such as the nose or contralateral ear. Although subject to rather more artefact the electrical traces

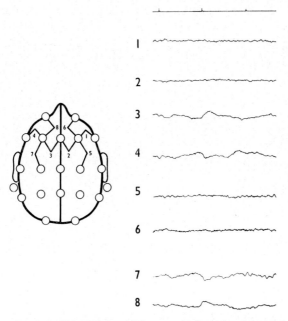

Figure 7. The EEG record from a patient with a left-sided anterior temporal glioma (grade 2). All four recordings from the left anterior quadrant are abnormal but phase reversal is seen between leads 3 and 4, and between leads 7 and 8. This suggests a discharging electrical focus at the point common to leads 3, 4, 7 and 8, which is not far from the site of the lesion in the anterior temporal region

obtained in this way sometimes highlight the region of highest voltage slow wave activity. The principal limitation of this technique, like that encountered with bipolar recording, is the tendency for the abnormal discharges from a focal lesion to be diffuse and not confined to the region of the lesion itself. Thus several unipolar leads tend to record the abnormal slow wave activity, which may reach similar voltage in more than one trace (*Figure 8*).

Provocation techniques, such as recording the EEG during hyperventilation, photic stimulation or sleep, do not have a very large part to play in the localization of cerebral tumours by the EEG. Some-times hyperventilation may accentuate the slow wave activity in the record, but it is exceedingly rare for significant focal slow wave abnormalities to appear in the region of a tumour for the first time during hyperventilation after recording a normal resting record.

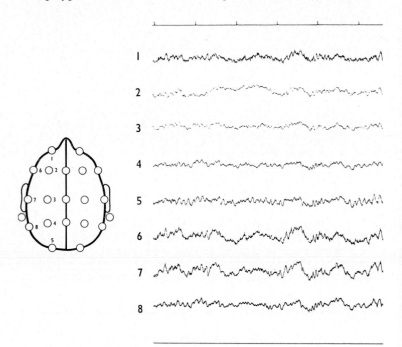

Figure 8. Unipolar recording in a patient with a left temporal glioma (grade 3). Slow wave (delta range) abnormalities can be seen throughout the left hemisphere, but are most pronounced in leads 6 and 7

It is not possible to obtain any reliable indication of the patho-logical nature of a tumour from the abnormalities obtained in an EEG. In general the more malignant the tumour, the more marked are the EEG abnormalities, so that high grade malignancy gliomas and rapidly growing metastases tend to be much more evident in EEG records than meningiomas, low grade gliomas and oligodendro-gliomas. This, however, is only a general rule with numerous exceptions. It is exceptional to see evidence of more than one focal disturbance, such as phase-reversals, occurring about two separate cerebral foci, indicative of more than one cerebral lesion and suggesting the presence of cerebral secondaries rather than a primary cerebral tumour.

In conclusion it may be stated that although the EEG is usually abnormal in the presence of a supratentorial tumour, it is rare for the EEG abnormalities to be sufficiently localized to define the position of the lesion adequately for the planning of treatment. Precise localization is better achieved by careful attention to the clinical phenomena, and by other investigations, including brain scanning and neuroradiological procedures. Posterior fossa and deep midline intracranial tumours, and any tumour complicated by marked increase in intracranial pressure, are not localized by the EEG at all.

ACKNOWLEDGEMENT

I am indebted to the Department of Medical Illustration, Manchester Royal Infirmary, for their great help in the preparation of the illustrations.

4—Surgery of the more Common Intracranial and Spinal Tumours

J. M. Rice Edwards

INTRODUCTION

The surgery of brain and spinal tumours is now less formidable than in the past. Within living memory is the era when there was no effective method of controlling haemorrhage or intracranial pressure and when localization was established by clinical evaluation alone. Patients with symptoms suggestive of brain tumour were often examined daily for the onset of localizing signs. Even then the surgeon, as well as experiencing poor conditions, might operate at the wrong site.

Nowadays operations are hopefully less dramatic. This is due to development in many fields. The surgeon virtually never operates until the tumour has been displayed by the elegant techniques used by the neuroradiologists. The exact location, size and usually the pathology of the tumour is known before operation, enabling precise siting of the craniotomy.

The problem of blood loss is nowadays less serious. For many years the neurosurgeon has used diathermy and small silver clips to occlude cerebral vessels. The clips were introduced by Harvey Cushing in the United States and brought back to this country for the use of surgeons by Sir Charles Symonds. These classical methods are still used. Haemorrhage has been much reduced by modern anaesthetic techniques which allow arterial hypotension and effective control of the intracranial pressure.

The methods of controlling the intracranial tension as outlined in Chapter 5 also ensure that the brain does not herniate through the wound and facilitate access to deep tumours without undue retraction on the brain. Sometimes it is necessary to excise either the tip of one frontal or temporal lobe for adequate exposure but this causes no demonstrable disability.

The improvements in operating conditions has encouraged the introduction of more refined techniques. The use of bipolar coagulation (which enables small vessels to be occluded without damage to the surrounding area) and of magnification undoubtedly helps in the dissection of benign tumours where they are adherent to important vessels or nerves.

THE SURGERY OF MENINGIOMAS

Meningiomas account for only 10–15 per cent of intracranial neoplasms but have a wide and favourable reputation because of their nature which is usually benign. This is broadly justified but results of surgery are sometimes marred by difficulty in surgical access, incomplete removal, recurrence or malignant change. They should usually be removed as soon as they are diagnosed but this attitude is not so rigid that the occasional elderly patient presenting with mild symptoms may be better left alone, especially if the lesion is dangerously placed.

The great principle of meningioma surgery is one that is not usually applied to the removal of tumours in the rest of the body: the tumour should be removed piece meal to avoid undue retraction on the brain. Theoretically a few cells may be spilled in doing so and lead to recurrence in the future but better this than a crippled patient, for the brain is delicate and does not withstand heavy retraction. Another principle is that, where possible, the dural origin with an adequate margin should be removed to prevent recurrence. This may not always be feasible but should be applied where possible.

From the surgical point of view the meningiomas are classified according to favoured sites of origin.

Convexity Meningiomas

Convexity meningiomas may present with epilepsy or focal neurological signs, depending upon the site. If the tumour overlies a 'silent' area such as a frontal lobe it may grow as large as an orange before presenting with mental slowness and evidence of raised intracranial pressure.

Initially the dura is opened close around the edge of the tumour in order to avoid herniation of the brain should the intracranial tension be high. The centre of the tumour is removed first so that the outer portion, rendered thin and pliant, can be dissected gently from the surrounding brain. The tumour is retracted away from the brain and not vice versa. At the completion of removal one of two policies may be adopted: the dural defect may be repaired with a dural substitute and the bone flap replaced, or the dura may be completely excised back to the bone edge and the bone flap temporarily left out. Logue introduced the latter technique and has achieved a mortality rate in the region of 3 per cent for convexity meningiomas (Logue, 1972). It has three advantages:

(1) It ensures wide removal of the tumour origin.

(2) It prevents herniation of brain through a small dural defect.

(3) It gives a large decompressive area through which the brain can bulge slightly in the post-operative phase of cerebral oedema.

The technique does involve replacement of the bone flap at a later date, involving a second operation and a slight risk of infection, but this is minimal nowadays if the bone flap is stored below freezing point in antibiotic solution.

Parasagittal Tumours

Parasagittal tumours are by definition attached to the sagittal sinus and cannot always be removed completely. It is safe to excise the anterior third of the sagittal sinus, and parasagittal tumours growing in this region can be totally eradicated without much difficulty. However, the price of sudden occlusion of the posterior two-thirds of the sagittal sinus is venous infarction of large and important areas of the cerebral hemispheres and this must be avoided at all cost. Removal of tumours in this region may therefore be incomplete but there are certain circumstances where total excision may be attempted: (a) sometimes the tumour is merely adherent to the sinus, in which case all macroscopic tissue can be removed even though some cells may be left behind in the dura; (b) if the sinus has been invaded over a limited area and this does not coincide with the entry of a major cerebral vein it may be possible to excise the tumour origin and repair the sinus with pericranium or some other dural substitute; (c) on the other hand, should the sinus be completely occluded by tumour it may be removed, for the occlusion will have occurred gradually and alternative channels such as the inferior sagittal sinus enlarged. However, where the sinus is heavily invaded, but not occluded, or where the tumour is adjacent to important cerebral veins, complete excision should not be attempted. The patency of the sinus can usually be assessed from the pre-operative angiogram but, if this is not adequate, a sinogram may be performed at surgery.

90

Sphenoidal Ridge Tumours

The difficulty of tumours arising from the sphenoidal ridge usually increases as they become more medially placed. It is difficult to generalize about them as they pose any one of a number of problems. Those growing from the outer portion are usually easily dealt with but sometimes they may be extraordinarily vascular, in which case preliminary ligation of the external carotid artery may help. Some tumours spread along the meninges, presenting the problem of a meningioma-en-plaque. A meningioma at any site may affect the underlying bone in different ways. It may cause thinning, reactive hyperostosis or the tumour may invade bone. Sphenoidal wing tumours frequently cause thickening of the roof of the orbit and proptosis. Gradual depression and protrusion of one eye may in fact be the presenting clinical feature. Hyperostosis may or may not imply penetration of the bone by tumour but, should extensive invasion occur, removal may be impossible. If the tumour arises from the inner part of the sphenoidal ridge it may become adherent to, or actually surround, the optic nerve, ocular motor nerve or carotid artery. Alternatively the tumour may dissect open the sylvian fissure and become attached to the middle cerebral artery. If there is involvement of any of these important structures safe total removal is unlikely.

Olfactory Groove Meningiomas

Olfactory groove meningiomas often attain a very large size before presenting with mental dullness, incontinence and raised intracranial pressure. It is usually necessary to excise the overlying lip of frontal lobe to remove them. The origin from the basal dura is excised or heavily coagulated.

Suprasellar Meningiomas

On the other hand suprasellar meningiomas usually present when they are small for they compress the optic chiasm at an early stage. Access here is difficult and the ease of removal largely depends on consistency. If the tumour has a soft centre, it can be sucked out, thereby rendring the capsule thin and malleable and a total excision is fairly easily achieved, but in cases where the tumour is hard and calcified it may be a very major procedure.

Middle Fossa Tumours

In the treatment of those tumours arising from the base of the middle fossa it may be necessary to excise a small portion of the overlying temporal lobe. Here again the centre of the tumour is 'gutted' first before the outer portion is dissected from the brain. The dural origin is usually treated by heavy coagulation but where the tumour arises from the tentorium this may be incised around the perimeter of the tumour unless it has involved the peritorcula region. Encroachment on the free edge of the tentorium is serious as the tumour is likely to be adherent to the posterior cerebral artery, mid-brain and other important structures.

Posterior Fossa Tumours

Meningiomas may occur in any part of the posterior fossa. They may involve the third to twelfth cranial nerves, otherwise they usually present with increasing ataxia and mental dulling due to hydrocephalus. Where the tumour arises from the posterior or lateral wall of the posterior fossa the dural origin can be removed as it can be in those attached to the under-surface of the tentorium. More commonly the tumours occur in the cerebello-pontine angle and here their entanglement with cranial nerves and important branches of the basilar artery (in particular the anterior inferior cerebellar artery) present a major problem. The operating microscope is undoubtedly a help in dissecting the tumour away from these small and delicate structures.

Clivus Meningiomas

In the past, clivus meningiomas were considered inoperable. Very many of them still are, for their position anterior to the brain stem and their adherence to the basilar artery result in a very cramped surgical exposure and a hazardous dissection. With the aid of arterial hypotension and the use of the operating microscope some of them may be removed by a lateral posterior fossa approach. Otherwise the only hope lies in the treatment of any associated hydrocephalus by a shunting operation.

Mortality and recurrence

Published figures of mortality and morbidity are difficult to compare for the results depend upon the era. However, the trend of the years has been forward and Logue, in a series of over 350 cases, has achieved a mortality rate of 3 per cent for convexity, parasagittal and falx tumours and 7 per cent for basal tumours (total 5 per cent). Of the survivors 87 per cent were able to carry out their previous employment.

In this series 60 per cent had pre-operative epilepsy and over half were relieved of it by surgery. Only 4 per cent of those without epilepsy gained it as a result of surgery. Altogether 27 per cent continued to suffer from post-operative epilepsy. All patients undergoing surgery for a supratentorial meningioma are treated with anti-convulsants and these are continued at least for some years, often indefinitely. It is wise to discontinue anti-convulsants only when the patient has been free of fits for some years and the EEG shows no 'spike' activity.

From what has been said it will be apparent that, although tumour removal is the ideal, it cannot always be achieved. The dural origin cannot always be removed. Knobs of tumour may have to be left in a venous sinus or attached to important arteries or nerves. Bone infiltrated with tumour may have to be left behind and, in the case of clivus meningioma, it may be impossible to remove the tumour at all. It is questionable whether radiotherapy influences the rate of recurrence following these incomplete removals. Radiotherapy has sometimes been given as a preliminary to surgery where the tumours are exceptionally vascular but, here again, the effect is questionable and with the help of arterial hypotension highly vascular tumours can be successfully removed.

Simpson (1957) assessed the risk of recurrence in a period of 17–27 years after surgery and found that the recurrence rate depended upon the type of removal: where there had been apparent total removal, 9 per cent recurred; where there had been diathermy of dural origin, 16 per cent recurred; without treatment of dura or sinus attachment, 22 per cent recurred; with incomplete removal, 39 per cent recurred.

In Logue's series the recurrence rate was: convexity, 7·5 per cent; falx, 15 per cent; parasagittal, 20 per cent; basal, 5·6 per cent; total, 9 per cent.

THE SURGERY OF GLIOMAS

General Principles

The gliomas have an evil reputation which for the most part is fully justified. The word tends to conjure up memories of the devastating progress of the most malignant type—the glioblastoma multiforme: deeply penetrating, incurable and often untreatable.

The range of tumour morphology and behaviour is considerable, however, and some gliomas, unfortunately the minority, may behave well. No astrocytoma is truly benign for they all infiltrate, but the growth of the optic nerve glioma of childhood may be so indolent that it eventually seems to stop spontaneously. This is also true of some cerebellar astrocytomas in children and, as this tumour is more circumscribed than most, it can often be removed completely. The ependymoma of the spinal cord is another tumour which occasionally may be totally excised. For the most part, however, the part of surgery of gliomas is diagnostic and palliative because most of them infiltrate deeply into vital areas of the brain. If a cure for these is to be achieved in the future it will not be by the development of more radical operations.

Cerebral Hemisphere Gliomas

Can an astrocytoma ever be cured when it involves the cerebral hemisphere? In practice it is not possible to diagnose these lesions until they have infiltrated widely. Longevity following surgery seems to depend on the intrinsic behaviour of the tumour rather than the surgical operation. Growth may be so slow that the patient lives for 20, even 30 years after the diagnosis or so fast that gross neurological disablement occurs within five or six weeks. In the exceptional case long survival may occur after radical excision of a glioblastoma multiforme but these cases are of extreme rarity. For practical purposes operation is palliative.

The surgical policy will depend on the site of the tumour and the degree of malignancy which can usually be assessed from the rapidity of clinical progression and the appearance of the angiogram. The best policy may sometimes be to postpone surgery. Should a patient present with fits or with very minor symptoms, and be shown by radiology to have an intracerebral mass which is deep or involves especially 'eloquent' regions of the brain such as the speech area, it is likely that operative intervention will only inflict damage earlier than it would naturally occur. The ominous progression of symptoms and signs will soon justify an operation, the purpose of which may be purely diagnostic.

The purpose of surgery is not to preserve life at any price. Where the patient is severely disabled by hemiplegia or dysphasia by a widely infiltrating malignant tumour no operation is likely to achieve a worthwhile result. In fact where the angiogram leaves no doubt, by demonstration of malignant circulation deep within the brain, that the tumour is a glioblastoma multiforme, even biopsy may be withheld. In all other cases, however, the surgeon must confirm that the tumour is what he fears it to be. The pathological circulation in a meningioma may be mistaken for a glioblastoma. I have on three occasions encountered unsuspected cerebral abscesses, in one instance in the basal ganglia. It is important, therefore, to obtain histological verification in nearly all cases even where no definitive treatment is envisaged. This may be done by passing a brain cannula via a burr hole into the tumour and sucking a little out. Haemorrhage

94

within the tumour cannot be controlled by this method and occasionally the technique causes some deterioration but this is surprisingly infrequent.

The best results of palliative surgery are obtained where the greater portion of tumour can be removed without inflicting additional neurological damage. This allows an internal decompression, thereby taking pressure off the surrounding brain. If the tumour is situated in the frontal or temporal lobe this can be achieved by performing the relevant lobectomy. Gliomas less commonly involve the occipital lobe but here a lobectomy can also be performed at the cost of persisting hemianopia. In other areas as much of the tumour as possible is removed without encroaching upon important areas of the brain.

Slow growing gliomas are likely to have a white and waxy appearance which blends imperceptibly into the surrounding brain. There may be a cyst which usually contains clear yellow fluid and aspiration of this helps in achieving an internal decompression. As much of the tumour as possible is removed but if important gyri are involved (such as those near the Sylvian fissure of the dominant hemisphere or the Rolandic fissure) they must be left strictly alone, for tumour may infiltrate brain that is still functioning.

The more malignant tumours have an ugly appearance and, if cystic, the fluid tends to be turbid rather than clear yellow. They may be tough or soft and often contain areas of haemorrhage, necrosis and thrombosed vessels. Occasionally they are adherent to dura and may superficially appear to be circumscribed, in which case they may look very similar to a meningioma. There is no doubt that the best results are obtained where the removal of these active tumours is as radical as possible. In the more circumscribed tumours removal may look complete but it never is, and recurrent symptoms usually return within months. However, radical removal may result in good quality survival for two years in about 13 per cent (Jelsma and Bucy, 1967).

Optic Nerve Glioma

Highly malignant gliomas of the optic nerve are very rare. They occur in adults and are resistant to any form of treatment.

The commoner tumour is a very slow growing astrocytoma almost invariably occurring in childhood which causes a gradual onset of visual failure or proptosis. Sometimes these ophthalmic abnormalities come to light during a routine medical examination or investigation into some other illness. There is a strong association with neurofibromatosis. The tumour may be limited to one optic nerve but usually there is evidence that it has spread to the optic chiasm.

Occasionally the hypothalamus is involved causing diabetes insipidus, somnolance and mental deterioration. If these signs are severe the prospect for survival is not good but in the majority of cases, where the lesion is restricted to the visual apparatus, the outlook is much more encouraging.

The combination of unilateral disc pallor, neurofibromatosis and an enlarged optic foramen without cortical destruction on x-ray makes a safe diagnosis of optic nerve glioma. Where necessary further confirmation can be obtained by air encephalography to show the enlarged intracranial portion of the optic nerve or optic chiasm. Only in doubtful cases need diagnosis rest on biopsy.

Treatment of these slow growing tumours of childhood is controversial but a good case has been made for conservative management (Glaser, Hoyt and Corbett, 1971; Hoyt and Baghadassarian, 1969). In most cases vision remains static for many years without treatment, the visual fields 'monotonously stable'. About 25 per cent show some deterioration but it is usually mild. A few may experience spontaneous improvement in vision and even proptosis may naturally improve. These factors make evaluation of treatment difficult. Radiotherapy does not appear to influence the natural history (Hoyt and Baghadassarian, 1969).

Where the tumour is localized to one optic nerve it is possible to resect it leaving the eye-ball intact (Housepian, 1969) but it must be rare for a tumour to be eradicated in this way for the cut end of the optic nerve usually shows a significantly increased population of astrocytes. The operation is done at the expense of the remaining vision in the affected eye. It is highly likely that the majority of tumours are self-limiting and surgery should probably be restricted to cases where there is marked proptosis and gross impairment of visual acuity in one eye.

Cerebellar Astrocytomas

In general the cerebellar gliomas are exceptionally favourable. Malignant tumours may occasionally occur in adults and the outcome is predictably bad, but the common tumour is a slow growing astrocytoma of childhood or young adults. The indolent growth is mirrored in the history which is usually one of progressive headache, vomiting and ataxia extending over several months. Symptoms may be neglected because of this slow evolution and result in visual failure due to secondary optic atrophy, but this is happily rare nowadays due to a greater awareness of the problem.

It has been asked why the prognosis is so much better than for astrocytomas of the cerebral hemisphere. This may be partly a factor of age. Astrocytomas of the cerebral hemisphere are exceptionally rare in children but when these tumours do occur they are also relatively benign (Gol, 1962). Another factor is that the cerebellar tumours tend to be more circumscribed. About half are cystic in which case the solid portion of tumour presents into the cystic cavity as a mural nodule. Less frequently the whole of the cystic cavity is surrounded with tumour. Usually the mass can be removed completely and, in patients where complete removal has been obtained, a life-long cure can be expected. Even in cases where the removal has been partial exceptionally long survival without recurrence of symptoms is frequent (Geissinger and Bucy, 1971). The tumour should always be removed completely if possible but if there is attachment to the side of the brain stem or to the floor of the fourth ventricle it is wiser to leave these portions alone rather than risk the hazard of total removal. These patients may still live for many years or even a normal life span.

Brain Stem Gliomas

Clearly these intrinsic tumours of the brain stem cannot be removed surgically and, whether fast or slow growing, they are uniformly depressing. There is usually a progressive and tragic disablement due to cranial nerve involvement, gaze palsies, dysphagia, dysarthria, ataxia, spastic weakness and sensory impairment. Characteristically, raised intracranial pressure due to hydrocephalus occurs late. Many of these tumours are treated with radiotherapy without preliminary biopsy. There must be clear radiological evidence, however, that the tumour is intrinsic, for benign extra-axial lesions may cause similar signs and symptoms.

Recently there has been a tendency to explore brain stem tumours in the hope of finding a cystic glioma which may improve after aspiration (Poole, 1968; Lassiter and colleagues, 1972). In younger patients it may be reasonable to propose exploration before radiotherapy. It must be admitted, however, that the chance of aspirating a cyst is not great, that operation carries some risk and that effective palliation is rare.

Oligodendrogliomas

These tumours occur in the cerebral hemispheres, more usually in the frontal region. The neurological history is quite long, averaging about a year, and the diagnosis may be suspected because of characteristic calcification seen on skull x-rays in 50 to 70 per cent of cases.

The operative appearance is of a purplish or grey tumour which may fungate through the pia and has a highly malignant look. It is therefore pleasant to receive histological confirmation that the tumour is an oligodendroglioma. Average survival is about five years after operation but it appears to be better in those patients where a radical removal of the tumour has been possible and some exceptionally long survivals have been recorded (Weir and Elvidge, 1968; Roberts and German, 1966).

Recurrent tumours may be excised a second time if good palliation has been achieved by the first operation. The histological appearance of the tumour may be identical on the second occasion but sometimes the appearance becomes that of glioblastoma multiforme.

Ependymomas

It might be thought that these tumours have a good prognosis for most are histologically benign and, to the surgeon, they may appear well circumscribed. However, almost 70 per cent occur in the posterior fossa and these are attached to the floor of the fourth ventricle making total removal impossible or hazardous. Thus they are 'benign tumours in a malignant situation'. Supratentorial ependymomas are less common. They also characteristically involve the ventricular system and form masses deep in the brain which are difficult to remove. They tend to be more anaplastic than the infratorial tumours. Added to these difficulties is the fact that ependymomas tend to seed in the subarachnoid pathway.

Thus surgery usually involves subtotal removal and is seldom curative although some exceptionally long survivals occur. It is probable that the results are best in those who have a course of postoperative radiotherapy (Fokes and Earle, 1969).

Post-operative survival depends more on the position and extent of the tumour than the histological appearance. Supratentorial ependymomas in general cause severe neurological disablement because of their deep situation and the results of surgery are generally poor. Infratentorial ependymomas usually cause less brain damage and present because of hydrocephalus which can be relieved. Post-operative survival appears to depend on the extent of the tumour. The average post-operative survival for infratentorial ependymomas is far better (10 years) in those where the tumour is limited to the fourth ventricle than in those where it extends beyond the cisterna magna (five years) or whether it invades the cerebellum (two years) (Kricheff and colleagues, 1964).

Pinealoma

Some of the tumours occurring in the pineal gland are undoubtedly teratomas but there is controversy concerning the pathological nature of the 'pinealoma'. Gliomas, meningiomas and metastatic deposits also occur in this region at the back of the third ventricle. Most of the tumours are invasive but simple benign cysts also occur. They all give rise to a similar clinical picture: raised intracranial pressure, due to hydrocephalus, and Parinaud's syndrome (that is, failure of upward eye movement, failure of convergence and convergent nystagmus) due to the effects of pressure or invasion on the tectal plate region of the mid-brain.

These tumours, poised within the tentorial opening, may be approached either from above or below the tentorium and some surgeons have advocated removal (Jamieson, 1971; Suzuki and Iwabucki, 1965). In the experience of most, however, radical operation is associated with heavy mortality and morbidity. The majority of surgeons recommend treatment of hydrocephalus by a shunting procedure, usually either ventriculo-artrial or ventriculo-cisternal, followed by radiotherapy (Poppen and Marino, 1968). This is one of the few occasions where radiotherapy without histological verification is justified. It is possible to perform stereotactic biopsy of tumours in the pineal region as a preliminary to radiotherapy but fear that this may encourage seeding of the tumour, though not proved, would seem justified on commonsense grounds.

Most of the patients are considerably improved after a shunt operation combined with radiotherapy and these results justify the few undoubted cases where radiotherapy is given for a benign cyst. Without histological verification it is difficult to evaluate the results of surgery statistically. Most of the tumours are slowly invasive and subsequent deterioration within months or years may be expected in the majority.

Radical surgery may be considered where the primary treatment fails but this is likely to involve the more malignant forms of tumour and heavy morbidity must be expected.

Medulloblastoma

The surgeon has never been able to treat this tumour adequately and his role nowadays is mainly to diagnose the tumour as a preliminary to radiotherapy. This is humiliating because, apart from the exceedingly rare ganglioneuroma, it appears to be the only brain tumour that actually arises from neural rather than supporting cells. Medulloblastomas probably arise from primitive granular layer cells in the cerebellum.

The vast majority of posterior fossa tumours in childhood are astrocytomas or medulloblastomas; the former largely benign, the latter highly malignant. Medulloblastomas tend to occur in the midline and therefore cause truncal, rather than limb, ataxia and raised intracranial pressure. The history is characteristically shorter than in the case of cerebellar astrocytoma but this is not reliable and definitive diagnosis depends on biopsy. They are purplish or grey tumours which tend to spread in every direction within the posterior fossa. Their tendency to seed within the subarachnoid space is well known and they are irremovable. Enough tumour should be removed, however, to 'unblock' the fourth ventricle and allow normal cerebrospinal fluid circulation. In the past the eventual outcome of surgical treatment has been 100 per cent mortality. This gloomy prospect has been enlivened in recent years by astonishing results achieved with new techniques of radiotherapy. It remains to be seen how many cures can be achieved.

Medulloblastomas occasionally occur in young adults and here the natural history is more favourable, the patients usually living for many years.

INTRACRANIAL METASTASES

One should be pessimistic about the surgical treatment of intracranial metastases for most of these tumours originate in the lung and few patients live long. The surgery of cerebral metastases from lung carcinoma is a gloomy chapter and radiotherapy appears to provide the best palliation (Deeley and Rice Edwards, 1968).

The surgeon usually encounters patients with intracranial metastases as problems in diagnosis. Where angiography shows multiple deposits characteristic of cerebral metastases, the diagnosis may sometimes be accepted without pathological verification but these cases constitute a minority. In most cases histological proof is mandatory and biopsy of the cerebral lesion is usually the quickest route to diagnosis. The choice of surgical procedure (between burr hole biopsy and palliative excision of the deposit) is made on the same criteria as those used in the surgery of gliomas. Where there is marked neurological disablement due to involvement of important areas of the brain, palliative surgery is unlikely to be successful and biopsy via a burr hole the sad but necessary choice. Where the tumour is favourably placed and appears to be single, excision may be justified. This also applies in the case of secondary deposits from a known primary neoplasm. A palliative excision in selected cases may give worthwhile improvement, particularly relief of headache, until the patient dies of some other manifestation of his disease. Excision of a single secondary deposit from a slow growing tumour such as a hypernephroma may give a favourable result for some years. Overall about 13 per cent of operated cases live over a year, the lung tumours faring worst (3 per cent) and tumours of the genito-urinary tract the best (37·5 per cent) (Veith and Odom, 1965).

SURGERY OF PITUITARY AND PARA-PITUITARY TUMOURS

The common effects of tumours growing in the pituitary region are that they are likely to present with endocrinological disturbances or visual failure due to chiasmal compression. The differential diagnosis includes pituitary adenoma, craniopharyngioma, suprasellar meningioma, chordoma, metastasis and giant carotid aneurysm. The latter is particularly important because it should usually be excluded by performing bilateral carotid angiography before surgery is undertaken. This avoids embarrassment for the surgeon or, at worst, a surgical catastrophe.

Pituitary Adenomas

These tumours may be excised by an intracranial subfrontal approach or by a trans-sphenoidal operation employing the operating microscope. The latter method is particularly indicated where the lesion is small. Thus the approach is vastly superior to the intracranial one for removal of a normal pituitary in the treatment of carcinoma of the breast or diabetic retinopathy. It is the operation of choice in the treatment of acromegaly for the adenoma is usually small and rarely causes chiasmal compression. There is a good case to be made for treating acromegaly. The life expectation is halved by the disease (Wright and colleagues, 1970) and removal of the adenoma may be expected to improve this. It also often alleviates the depressing disfiguration. Cure of headache when it occurs is achieved in most. In some cases it is possible to remove the adenoma while preserving normal pituitary tissue (Hardy, 1968).

Chromophobe adenomas of the pituitary usually cause signs of hypopituitarism long before visual failure but they often come to notice because of the latter. Should the patient present purely with hypopituitarism without any abnormality of vision and where the diagnosis of chromophobe adenoma tends to be upheld by characteristic 'ballooning' of the sella tursica on x-ray, it is usual to treat him with replacement hormone therapy alone and await events because many of these tumours progress so slowly that they never cause visual disturbance. Such patients, however, should be followed up carefully with visual field charting.

If there is even mild impairment of the visual fields due to chiasmal compression surgery should not be delayed. The trans-sphenoidal approach may be used for the smaller tumours. The optic nerves are not seen but they are protected by the diaphragma sellae which is pushed up by the adenoma and lies between it and the nerves. As the tumour is removed the diaphragma can be seen to drop down towards the sella. The advantage of this approach is that the adenomas can be removed completely and there is probably no need to give post-operative radiotherapy.

Adenomas with large supra-sellar extensions, however, cannot be reliably removed by the trans-sphenoidal approach particularly if they extend upwards and anteriorly. The intracranial operation is then indicated and it has the advantage that the optic nerves can be seen. The operation involves a right frontal craniotomy and upward retraction of the right frontal lobe. The incidence of pre-fixation of the chiasm is low and the tumour can be seen between the optic nerves stretching them and the chiasm upward. A needle is first passed into the tumour to make sure that it is not an aneurysm and the 'capsule' incised between the optic nerves. The adenoma is then removed by suction and parts of the 'capsule' underneath the optic nerves removed to give a complete decompression. The excision of the 'capsule' is taken as far back as the pituitary stalk but this is not interfered with because of the high incidence of post-operative diabetes insipidus when it is damaged. As the sella itself is not inspected removal is usually incomplete and operation should be followed by a course of radiotherapy.

This is not the place to give details of hormonal management of pituitary surgery but this is undoubtedly the main item which has made both approaches increasingly safe. The mortality rate for the intracranial approach should be extremely low and improvement in vision occurs in about 75 per cent of cases (Ray and Patterson, 1971).

Craniopharyngioma

These congenital tumours arise in the region of the pituitary stalk but may spread into the sella tursica and the middle or posterior fossae, or they may extend up into the hypothalamus and third ventricle. Not only may they cause endocrine dysfunction and chiasmal compression but the upward extension may also block the foramen of Monro leading to hydrocephalus and raised intracranial pressure (a common presentation in childhood) or cause hypothalamic damage. In adult life the tumour may present with disturbance of memory and increasing dementia (Ross Russell and Pennybacker, 1961).

The surgical problem is different to that of the pituitary adenoma.

102

The latter arises within the sella and, as it increases in size, pushes the diaphragma sellae upward. This membrane separates it from the under-surface of the chiasm and hypothalamus; not so the craniopharyngioma, which may become densely adherent to the hypothalamus. Therefore total excision carries the risk of severe hypothalamic damage and operations in the past have been associated with heavy mortality. There has thus been a tendency to avoid radical surgery. The majority of the tumours are cystic and tapping a cyst can often lead to temporary improvement.

In children, however, the tumour appears to be less adherent to the hypothalamus and in some cases a complete removal can be obtained (Matson and Crizler, 1969). The recurrence after partial removal is usually rapid in children and total excision the only hope of permanent cure.

The policy to be adopted in adults is controversial and must depend upon the degree of attachment to the hypothalamus. In the majority of cases total removal is impossible, in which case the surgical treatment will consist either of tapping a cyst and attempting no more or performing as radical a removal as possible (Kramer, Southard and Mansfield, 1968; Hoff and Patterson, 1972).

Acoustic Neuroma

For some reason these benign tumours, which grow from the vestibular branch of the eighth nerve, arise constantly at the mouth of the internal auditory meatus. When they are quite small they cause deafness but the British public bears this disability with fortitude and patients seldom present before other symptoms develop. By this time the tumour usually indents the pons and this distortion of the brain stem may block the aqueduct and cause hydrocephalus. Important cranial nerves and branches of the basilar artery are stretched around the perimeter of the tumour. It is for these reasons that the acoustic neuroma presents the surgeon with a challenging task.

In the past controversy centred round the question of whether the acoustic neuroma should be totally or partially removed. Partial removal carries less immediate risk but a second operation for recurrent tumour presents such a formidable hazard that there is no doubt that it should be completely removed at the first operation. An exception to this is in the case of an elderly patient.

A more recent controversy centred round the timing of surgery, some holding the opinion that the risk of operation did not justify surgery in those with minor symptoms. Operation was deferred until the effects became life-threatening. With developments in technique the results have improved, however, and there is no doubt that the operative mortality rate is much lower when the tumour is small. Consequently, early operation should usually be advised.

A great contribution was made by House (1964, 1968) who popularized the trans-labyrinthine removal of acoustic neuromas. The approach is not suitable for large tumours but his results with the small ones have encouraged neurosurgeons. It is not necessary to use the trans-labyrinthine approach. Small tumours can also be effectively dealt with via the posterior fossa (Drake, 1968) and with the aid of magnification it may be possible to preserve the facial nerve.

Saving the facial nerve becomes of secondary importance in the removal of large tumours. Here the problem is to save the patient's life by dissecting the medial wall of the tumour away from the brain stem without jeopardizing the vital blood vessels particularly the anterior cerebellar artery. Magnification is very useful for this part of the operation and a mortality rate in the region of 10 per cent may be achieved; for small tumours it should be considerably lower.

Thus early and total removal is usually advocated and radiotherapy plays no part.

SPINAL TUMOURS

Extradural Metastases

In this country the most common cause of a rapidly progressive spinal compression is an extradural metastatic deposit, but a malignant cause must not be assumed. In some parts of the world the most common cause of progressive paraplegia is tuberculosis and spinal compression due to this is now being encountered in Great Britain. Multiple sclerosis and rare but important causes of spinal compression such as a pyogenic extradural abscess may also cause a rapidly progressive paraplegia and may be mistaken for spinal metastases. Therefore, surgical decompression is often a diagnostic as well as a therapeutic manoeuvre.

Another important aspect of spinal compression is speed. The patient who developed pins and needles in the feet a week ago, noticed weakness three days ago and is unsteady today will probably not walk at all tomorrow. The results of decompression are far better in those who are not already seriously disabled.

Extradural metastases may present when the primary tumour has already been diagnosed and choice of treatment will then primarily depend on the radio-sensitivity of the tumour. Recent evidence suggests that, in the case of compression by lymphoma, the best results are obtained by radiotherapy using a high initial daily dose without laminectomy (Verity, 1968; Rubin, Mayer and Poulter, 1969).

In the management of spinal compression due to secondary carcinoma the treatment has traditionally been a combination of surgical decompression followed by radiotherapy. The results of surgery of course depend upon the pre-operative disability and the type of tumour. In general about two-thirds can be expected to remain walking if they were doing so before surgery and one-third to walk following surgery if they were not before. Only one in ten recover significant use of their legs if they have been totally paralysed (White, Patterson and Bergland, 1971).

In the treatment of radio-resistant tumours such as prostate and renal carcinoma there is little doubt that a laminectomy should be done. There has been some controversy regarding the primary treatment in the case of partially radio-sensitive lesions such as breast or lung carcinomata (Rubin, Mayer and Poulter, 1969). The results of using high initial daily dose radiotherapy need to be compared with surgery in a prospective controlled trial.

There are some occasions when palliative surgery holds so little chance of improving the patient's existence that decompression is unjustified. Where the patient's general condition is poor or where there is evidence of complete cord transection by marked vertebral collapse palliative surgery is usually contra-indicated provided that there is histological proof of the primary disease.

Neurofibroma and Meningioma

Although these benign tumours may occasionally occur extra-durally they are usually intradural. The neurofibroma is the more common, arising in relation to a nerve root and often forming a dumb-bell shaped tumour extending through an intervertebral foramen to become partly intra- and partly extraspinal. Thus radiological bone changes are common. The tumours may sometimes be multiple and there may be evidence of generalized neurofibromatosis but usually the tumours are single.

Meningiomas virtually always occur in middle-aged women in the thoracic region. The results of surgery are usually spectacularly successful.

Intramedullary Tumours

These present a formidable problem and very often the surgeon is apprehensive about operating before the patient is significantly disabled on the grounds that the procedure may cause deterioration. In

the past this waiting period has sometimes been occupied by adminis-
tering a course of radiotherapy. However, this probably makes
surgery more hazardous and should be postponed until after surgery
when the histological diagnosis of the tumour has been confirmed.

The intramedullary tumours are usually astrocytomas or ependymomas. Lipomas and dermoids occasionally occur within the cord.
In most cases little can be done but ependymomas are sometimes
circumscribed and may be removed completely with the aid of
magnification (Greenwood, 1963). There is usually no clear line of
demarcation between tumour and spinal cord in the case of astrocytomas but they are sometimes cystic and temporary improvement
may be obtained by aspiration or by partial excision. Dermoids
growing within the cord cannot usually be removed completely and
any attempt to remove lipomas is usually attended by disaster.

REFERRAL FOR RADIOTHERAPY

Collaboration between the neurosurgeon and his radiotherapeutic
colleague should be a close one. The surgeon is often grateful for the
radiotherapist's opinion and referral is not necessarily a demand for
treatment. If treatment is to be undertaken, operative details should
always be forwarded to the radiotherapist and he should expect
discussion of the x-rays or simple diagrams illustrating the extent of
the mass.

The criteria for referral of patients varies. In the past patients with
incompletely removed meningiomas were referred but seldom nowadays as little evidence has accumulated that radiotherapy does any
good. In the case of gliomas, radiotherapy is usually regarded as a
prophylactic measure. On the whole only those patients who have
had a tolerable result of surgery are referred in the hope that radiotherapy will prolong the period of palliation. It is less seldom considered where the patient is already considerably disabled, for past
experience has not led us to expect dramatic results. In the case of
the relatively benign growth such as the cerebellar astrocytoma
radiotherapy is usually not given.

In the surgery of pituitary adenomas radiotherapy has a most
important role. Usually the tumour is incompletely removed and
there is good evidence that treatment of this radio-sensitive tumour
reduces the recurrence rate. Primary treatment of these tumours by
planted radioactive seeds is being assessed and a careful comparison
will have to be made between this and conventional surgery in the
future.

The most promising advances have been in the treatment of meduloblastomas and spinal compression due to lymphomas—tumours where the surgeon has had less success than the radiotherapist. The primary treatment of radio-sensitive carcinomas causing spinal compression will have to be assessed.

On the whole it has been a fruitful collaboration.

REFERENCES

Deeley, T. J. and Rice Edwards, J. M. (1968). 'Radiotherapy in the management of cerebral secondaries from bronchial carcinoma.' *Lancet*, 1, 1209.

Drake, C. G. (1968). 'Surgical treatment of acoustic neuroma with preservation or reconstitution of the facial nerve.' *J. Neurosurg.*, 26, 459.

Fokes, E.C. and Earle, K. M. (1969). 'Ependymomas: clinical and pathological aspects.' *J. Neurosurg.*, 30, 585.

Geissinger, J. D. and Bucy, P. C. (1971). 'Astrocytomas of the cerebellum in children.' *Archs Neurol.*, 24, 125.

Glaser, J. S., Hoyt, W. F. and Corbett, J. (1971). 'Visual morbidity with chiasmal glioma.' *Archs Ophthal.*, 85, 3.

Gol, A. (1962). 'Cerebral astrocytomas in childhood.' *J. Neurosurg.*, 19, 577.

Greenwood, J. (1963). 'Intramedullary tumours of the spinal cord.' *J. Neurosurg.*, 20, 665.

Hardy, J. (1968). 'Transphenoidal microsurgery in normal and pathological pituitary.' *Clin. Neurosurg.*, 16, 185.

Hoff, J. T. and Patterson, R. H. (1972). 'Craniopharyngiomas in children and adults.' *J. Neurosurg.*, 36, 299.

House, W. F. (1964). 'Transtemporal bone microsurgical removal of acoustic neuromas. Monograph I.' *Archs Otolar.*, 80, 599.

— (1968). 'Acoustic neuroma. Monograph II.' *Archs Otolar.*, 88, 576.

Housepian, E. M. (1969). 'Surgical treatment of optic nerve gliomas.' *J. Neurosurg.*, 31, 604.

Hoyt, W. F. and Baghadassarian, S. A. (1969). 'Optic glioma of childhood.' *Br. J. Ophthal.*, 53, 793.

Jamieson, K. G. (1971). 'Excision of pineal tumours.' *J. Neurosurg.*, 35, 550.

Jelsma, R. and Bucy, P. C. (1967). *J. Neurosurg.*, 27, 388.

Kramer, S., Southard, M. and Mansfield, C. M. (1968). 'Radiotherapy in the management of craniopharyngiomas.' *Am. J. Roentgenol.*, 103, 44.

Kricheff, I. I., Becker, M., Schneck, S. A. and Taveras, J. M. (1964). 'Intracranial ependymomas: factors influencing prognosis.' *J. Neurosurg.*, 21, 7.

Lassiter, K. R. L., Alexander, E., Davis, C. H. and Kelly D. L. (1972). 'Surgical treatment of brain stem gliomas.' *J. Neurosurg.*, 34, 719.

Logue, V. (1972). Personal communication.

Matson, D. D. and Crigler, J. F. (1969). 'Management of craniopharyngi-oma in childhood.' *J. Neurosurg.*, **30**, 377.

Pool, J. L. (1968). 'Gliomas in the region of the brain stem.' *J. Neurosurg.*, **29**, 164.

Poppen, J. L. and Marino, R. (1968). 'Pinealomas and tumours of the posterior portion of the third ventricle.' *J. Neurosurg.*, **28**, 357.

Ray, B. S. and Patterson, R. H. (1971). 'Surgical experience with chromo-phobe adenomas of the pituitary gland.' *J. Neurosurg.*, **34**, 726.

Roberts, M. and German, W. J. (1966). 'A long term study of patients with oligodendrogliomas: follow-up of 50 cases, including Dr. Harvey Cushing's series.' *J. Neurosurg.*, **24**, 697.

Russell, R. W. R. and Pennybacker, J. B. (1961). 'Craniopharyngioma in the elderly.' *J. Neurol. Neurosurg. Psychiat.*, **24**, 1.

Rubin, P. (1969). 'Extradural spinal cord compression by tumour. Part I. Experimental production and treatment trials.' *Radiology*, **93**, 1243.

— Mayer, E. and Poulter, C. (1969). 'Extradural spinal cord compression by tumour. Part II. High daily dose experience without laminectomy.' *Radiology*, **93**, 1248.

Simpson, D. (1957). 'The recurrence of intracranial meningiomas after surgical treatment.' *J. Neurol. Neurosurg. Psychiat.*, **20**, 22.

Suzuki, J. and Iwabuchi, T. (1965). 'Surgical removal of pineal tumours (pinealomas and teratomas). Experience in a series of 19 cases.' *J. Neurosurg.*, **23**, 565.

Veith, R. G. and Odom, G. L. (1965). 'Intracranial metastases and their neurosurgical treatment.' *J. Neurosurg.*, **23**, 375.

Verity, G. L. (1968). 'Neurological manifestations and complications of lymphoma.' *Radiol. Clins N. Am.*, **6**, 97.

Weir, B. and Elvidge, A. R. (1968). 'Oligodendrogliomas. An analysis of 63 cases.' *J. Neurosurg.*, **29**, 500.

White, W. A., Patterson, R. H. and Bergland, R. M. (1971). 'Role of surgery in the treatment of spinal cord compression by metastatic neo-plasm.' *Cancer*, **27**, 558.

Wright, A. D., Hill, D. M., Lowry, C. and Frazer, Russell T. (1970). 'Mortality in acromegaly.' *Q. Jl Med.*, **39**, 1.

5—Raised Intracranial Pressure

J. M. Rice Edwards and C. Pallis

INTRODUCTION

Before modern methods of controlling intracranial pressure (ICP) were introduced, the patient with a cerebral tumour and intracranial hypertension faced a serious ordeal. He would suffer from headache and vomiting, might become blind, and at any stage might lapse into coma. None of these symptoms would respond to medical treatment. If he came to surgery, the anaesthetic techniques caused a further increase in ICP and a serious risk of fatal brain stem compression. On incising the dura the surgeon would encounter swollen brain, which might herniate through the dural opening. If the tumour was not immediately located, the necessary retraction of the brain often caused further damage. Even following the successful removal of a benign tumour, severe cerebral oedema might persist into the post-operative period causing prolonged coma, at times aggravated by respiratory complications and CO_2 retention. The patient was lucky to survive.

Implied in the above description is the widely held assumption that symptoms such as headache, vomiting and various alterations of consciousness are directly related to raised ICP. This view has been challenged. Many years ago, during their investigations of various headache mechanisms, Schumacher and Wolff (1941) raised the ICP* to over 1,000 mm H_2O by injecting saline into the lumbar theca of humans. Their subjects suffered in no way from this manoeuvre, nor was there any change in pulse rate, respiration or blood pressure.

* The upper limit of normal CSF pressure, measured in lateral decubitus, is usually said to be 180 mm H_2O. According to Davson (1960) the mean pressure is of the order of 150 mm saline—i.e. 11 mm Hg.

Other facts are also relevant to this controversy. In the condition known as 'benign intracranial hypertension' patients may walk about, looking and feeling entirely well, even though their ICP may be over 500 mm H_2O. The raised pressure, in this strange and obscure condition, appears to be due to generalized swelling of the brain. There is no ventricular dilatation and no shift of brain tissue from one intracranial compartment to another. The raised ICP may persist for weeks or months and then usually subsides spontaneously. Headache is seldom severe and there is no vomiting. During this period, the only risk is to vision: the long standing papilloedema may be followed by gliosis of the optic papilla and consequent loss of sight.

It is useful to compare this clinical entity with another, namely 'normal pressure hydrocephalus' (Hakim and Adams, 1965; Adams and colleagues, 1965). This is a condition due to an abnormality of cerebrospinal fluid (CSF) dynamics, in which the patient does, in contrast, suffer severe symptoms and yet has a normal ICP. A communicating hydrocephalus* slowly develops and leads to progressive dementia, ataxia and incontinence. The development of hydrocephalus appears to be due to mild and intermittent increases of pressure, spread over a long period, and excellent results sometimes follow the permanent lowering of ventricular pressure by means of various 'shunting' procedures. From the point of view of symptoms, the significant difference between this condition and 'benign intracranial hypertension' is not the level of the ICP but the fact that in 'low pressure hydrocephalus' there is a distortion of brain tissue by the enlarged ventricles. We will return to this controversy after discussing the 'classical' features of raised ICP.

CLINICAL FEATURES

It is classically taught that headache, vomiting and papilloedema, occurring together, imply raised ICP. In fact many patients with raised ICP may have little or no headache, whereas headache may be a prominent feature of some cerebral tumours not associated with raised ICP. It is important to realize that patients with even large intracranial masses may fail to exhibit one or more features of the classical triad. Whether a mass causes *intracranial hypertension*, or not, is more often related to its site than to its size, strategically situated lesions being those that cause early obstruction to the circulation of the spinal fluid. Whether such a mass causes *headache* or

* By this we mean an obstructive hydrocephalus, in which the site of 'obstruction' is distal to the communication between the ventricular system and the spinal subarachnoid space.

not is probably related to its proximity to basal or meningeal blood vessels, well endowed with sensory nerve endings, or to well-innervated areas of dura. Traction on pain-sensitive structures—rather than raised ICP *per se*—seems to be the basis of most tumour headaches (Kunkle and Wolff, 1951; Wolff, 1963).

Headache

The headache of cerebral tumour is most often experienced in the mornings. It may be unilateral or bilateral, frontal, temporal or occipital, and may be characteristically aggravated by coughing, straining or stooping. Occasionally bursting in character, it is more often a deep, dull, aching pain only moderately troublesome, and certainly less severe than that associated with meningitis or ruptured aneurysm. It is often eased by analgesics. The most diagnostically helpful feature is its development and persistence out of a clear sky.

In young children, separation of the cranial sutures may delay the development of headache, even in the presence of considerably raised ICP. This 'diastasis of the sutures' is probably the basis of the 'cracked pot' sound heard on percussion of the head. In the elderly, brain atrophy may allow the cranial cavity to accommodate fairly large masses without the development of intracranial hypertension.

Vomiting

This is seen more often in children with intracranial hypertension than in adults. This may partly be due to the general tendency of children to respond by vomiting to any noxious stimulus but is probably also related to the greater frequency of infratentorial tumours in childhood. Posterior fossa lesions may, at an early stage, involve critical areas, such as the floor of the fourth ventricle, resulting in vomiting. Posterior fossa lesions will also cause early obstruction to the flow of cerebrospinal fluid. The vomiting may occur without antecedent nausea. Its very suddenness has given it a largely unwarranted reputation of being 'projectile'.

Papilloedema

This seldom causes symptoms until there is a serious threat of irreversible visual failure. There may then be repeated attacks of transient blindness, often related to changes in posture: the so-called amblyopic attacks. These only occur in cases of severe papilloedema. They will not, therefore, usually be confused with the amblyopic attacks due to platelet emboli, seen in patients with atheromatous disease of the internal carotid.

The ophthalmoscopic appearances of papilloedema are well

known and will not be recapitulated. They are indistinguishable from those of papillitis. The effects of the two conditions on the visual fields are, however, entirely different. Papilloedema is associated, at most, with some enlargement of the blind spot, whereas papillitis will produce a dense central scotoma and a gross reduction of visual acuity. Chronic papilloedema may be followed by secondary optic atrophy. The gliosis of papilla, in this condition, usually starts along the superior temporal border of the disc, causing an inferior nasal defect of the visual field. In many parts of the world where neuro-surgical facilities are scanty, secondary optic atrophy from unrelieved intracranial hypertension is still a common cause of blindness.

Papilloedema is rare in infants because, in the presence of raised ICP, the cranial sutures tend to 'spread'. A tense fontanelle is probably a more useful sign of intracranial hypertension in this particular age group.

Blurred discs may at times be encountered in the absence of any localizing or lateralizing neurological signs. This abnormal retinoscopic appearance may occasionally be due to a congenital malformation of the discs (pseudo-papilloedema). But it might also be due to genuine papilloedema and conditions such as arterial hypertension, chronic lung disease, mediastinal obstruction or hypocalcaemia would then have to be excluded.

In the absence of these conditions, isolated papilloedema could be due to 'benign intracranial hypertension', to bilateral subdural haematomas, to a large supratentorial mass affecting a clinically silent area (such as the non-dominant frontal lobe) or to a *mid-line block*. Lesions causing mid-line block may be intraventricular (colloid cysts of the third ventricle, aqueduct stenosis, lesions obstructing the exit foramina of the fourth ventricle). Or they may be external to the ventricular system, obstructing the circulation of CSF at the level of the tentorium (sequelae of meningitis or of subarachnoid haemorrhage, leukaemic infiltration) or at the level of the superior longitudinal sinus, which may even be occluded.

Papilloedema probably arises from an interference with the venous return from the eye. The tunica vaginalis of the optic nerve is a continuation, through the optic canal, of the cerebral subarachnoid space. Raised ICP may be transmitted along this channel, to the space around the optic nerve. This space is crossed, just behind the eyeball by the retinal vein, draining blood (via the superior orbital fissure) into the cavernous sinus. A tight optic canal may prevent the transmission of intracranial hypertension to the sheath of the optic nerve and may account for the undoubted cases, familiar to all neurologists and neurosurgeons, in which proved intracranial hyper-

112

tension is associated with normal fundi. Other mechanisms may also be operative in the production of papilloedema (Behrman, 1966).

BRAIN 'SHIFTS' AND 'FALSE LOCALIZING' SIGNS

The intracranial contents are separated by firm, unyielding structures such as the falx and tentorium. When a mass develops in the supratentorial compartment, brain tissue may be forced under the sharp edge of the falx (cingulate herniation) or through the tentorial opening (uncal herniation). When pressure rises in the infratentorial compartment the cerebellar tonsils may 'herniate' through the foramen magnum (tonsillar herniation). Upward shifts through the tentorium may also occur, with posterior fossa lesions. Each of these shifts causes distortion of brain substance and local compression of blood vessels which may lead to ischaemia and focal haemorrhage (*Figures 1–3*).

Tentorial Herniation

This usually results from supratentorial mass lesions. Two syndromes have been described by McNealy and Plumb (1962).

In the *'central'* syndrome the diencephalon is shifted in a caudal direction. The brain stem bears the brunt of the dislocation, showing a progressive impairment of function which fails in an orderly rostral–caudal sequence. Varying degrees of ptosis, often associated with abnormalities of conjugate upward gaze and a fluctuating level of consciousness are characteristic early signs.

In the *'uncal'* syndrome there is herniation of the uncus of the temporal lobe through the tentorial notch. This is more commonly seen with laterally placed lesions and may cause ipsilateral third nerve paresis, due to direct pressure on the third nerve. This may be followed by evidence of mid-brain compression and further deterioration of brain stem function, as in the 'central' syndrome. The phenomena are well described in the monograph of Plumb and Posner (1966).

Tonsillar Herniation

This may occur early with *infratentorial* lesions, or be a late result of a supratentorial lesion, in which case it is usually associated with a tentorial pressure cone.

The impaction of cerebellar tonsils into the foramen magnum will of course aggravate any pre-existing hydrocephalus. Characteristic signs of foraminal impaction include neck stiffness, abnormal postures of the head and abnormalities of respiratory rate of rhythm, sometimes of very sudden onset.

113

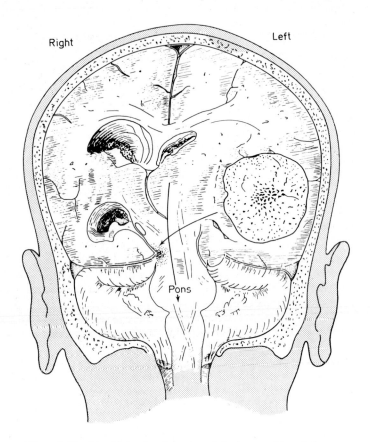

Right   Left

Pons

Figure 1. Combined lateral and downward displacement (semi-diagrammatic). Coronal slice of brain viewed from in front. A tumour is present in the left forebrain compartment. The arrows indicate the direction of the resulting displacement. The whole brain-stem is pushed downwards towards the foramen magnum. The lateral and downward displacement forces the right crus against the adjacent edge of the incisura tentorii. It also forces part of the left hippocampal region down through the incisura and thus the whole brain-stem is compressed at this level. The cerebrospinal fluid pathway is blocked by this tentorial impaction so that there is distension of the lateral and third ventricles. This distension is not uniform because the left-sided tumour has caused distortion of the ventricular system. (Reproduced by courtesy of Mr. Miles and Professor Dott)

114

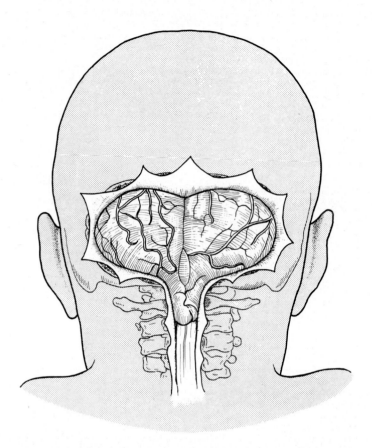

Figure 2. Foraminal impaction or cerebellar coning. The cerebellum and brain stem have shifted downwards and produced obstruction to the egress of cerebrospinal fluid from the fourth ventricle. This starts a vicious circle of obstructive hydrocephalus, particularly in tumours of the posterior fossa. In tumours arising above the tentorium cerebelli the cerebellar coning probably does not cause as much obstruction to the flow of cerebrospinal fluid as was originally thought. (Reproduced by courtesy of Mr. Miles and Professor Dott)

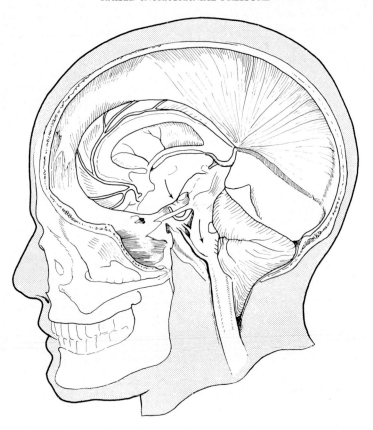

Figure 3. Paresis of the third and sixth cranial nerves by cerebral displacement. A space-occupying lesion, not shown, is present in the right forebrain compartment. The uncus on the right side has been forced down through the incisura tentorii. The right third nerve is pressed upon by this protrusion. The brain stem is dislocated downwards and the sixth nerve is subjected to angulation and to stretching. (Reproduced by courtesy of Mr. Miles and Professor Dott)

False Localizing Signs

A variety of other 'false localizing' neurological signs may also be encountered in patients with raised ICP.

Lateral rectus palsies, due to involvement of one or other abducens nerve, are common. Diplopia from this mechanism may in fact be the presenting sympton in 'benign intracranial hypertension'. An *ipsilateral hemiplegia* may develop, due to indentation of the

116

opposite crus cerebri by the free edge of the tentorium. *Anosmia* and *absent corneal* reflexes have less localizing significance, in the presence of raised ICP than they would otherwise have. A *bitemporal hemianopia*, in the presence of papilloedema, is sometimes a false localizing neurological sign. It is due to pressure on the optic chiasm by a dilated third ventricle, the obstructing lesion at times being in the aqueduct or even further back. (It is important to remember, in this context, that pituitary tumours tend to cause primary optic atrophy rather than papilloedema.) A *homonymous hemianopia*, in a patient with papilloedema, may also be a false localizing sign. The tentorial pressure cones associated with large supratentorial lesions may result in ischaemia of the visual cortex, from interference with its blood supply through the posterior cerebral artery (this vessel also has to 'negotiate' the tight tentorial bottleneck).

It may therefore be claimed that it is brain distortions, rather than generalized increases of ICP, that are responsible for most of the signs and symptoms encountered. It must be added, however, that differential pressures must have acted in the first place, to cause these distortions. Differential pressures between one part of the intracranial cavity and another may develop. This has recently been confirmed by simultaneously measuring tissue pressure over the temporal lobe of monkeys and pressure in the cisterna magna. Occlusion of the middle cerebral artery in monkeys sometimes causes a rise of local pressure before pressure is increased in the cisterna magna (Dorsch and Symon, 1972). Distortions of the brain appear to depend on the size of the abnormal mass, its site and the speed with which it developed. They appear to be independent of the supratentorial pressure (Weinstein and colleagues, 1968). The brain may indeed be distorted without the ICP rising although this is unlikely to be the case where brain stem compression is severe enough to be causing signs or symptoms.

It is not agreed by all, however, that a generalized increase in ICP is innocuous. Lundberg (1960) found that sudden, spontaneous rises of ICP were often associated with drowsiness, forced irregular respiration, headache, vomiting, restlessness, paraesthesiae in the limbs, flexor rigidity or clonus. Their findings were noted in three patients with meningeal carcinomatosis or sarcomatosis, in whom there was no evidence of hydrocephalus or intracranial mass. The intracranial hypertension, in these cases, was likely to be generalized and there was no shift. This suggests that, in raised ICP, symptoms may occur without brain distortion due to tentorial or foraminal herniation. However, others have noted no correlation between pressure changes

117

and symptoms in patients undergoing lower-term intracranial pressure monitoring.

The question of the association ·of symptoms with generalized intracranial hypertension has therefore not been completely resolved. The *cause* of the raised ICP may be relevant: cerebral oedema may have a different effect from directly raising the pressure in the sub-arachnoid space. Distortions caused by differential pressures are probably the more important factor, whether or not the overall pressure is increased. However, these shifts may be *lessened* if the ICP falls, for instance if the lateral ventricles are 'tapped' or *enhanced* if the ICP increases (for instance if there is respiratory obstruction). The effects of an overall increase in intracranial tension should clearly not be minimized. Raised ICP always means mischief and should be treated energetically, if only to save vision.

PHYSIOLOGY AND PATHOLOGY

Most considerations of the problem of raised ICP usually start with a reiteration of the Monro–Kelly doctrine, in its modified form. This proposes the simple concept that, as the skull and its dural lining constitute a 'closed' box and the three contents (brain, CSF and blood) are incompressible, the volume of one constituent can only be changed at the expense of that of one (or both) of the others. This is broadly true: the contents are for practical purposes incompressible. But there are two provisos. Although the skull is a closed box and cannot be expanded, this does not apply to the spinal intradural space, which is slightly distensible at the expense of extradural veins. CSF can therefore be displaced from the head into the spinal theca. The other proviso is that although the brain appears to be virtually incompressible by acute increases in pressure, prolonged compression may affect its substance (or at least the tissue water) leading to a reduction in cerebral volume. This whole area has yet to be explored.

Under normal circumstances, the volume of nervous tissue remains constant while intracerebral blood volume may vary from moment to moment. The intracranial venous volume can be increased by obstructing the venous return, as by pressure on the jugular veins. This volume change is large enough to cause a rise of intracranial pressure, as when doing the Queckenstedt manoeuvre. The rise of intracranial pressure is damped to a certain extent by 'venting' of CSF from the head into the distensible spinal theca.

When a subject coughs, the venous pressure increases both in the head and in the spinal extradural veins. In this instance, the rise in cerebral venous blood volume cannot be compensated by venting of CSF into the spinal theca. During coughing, CSF may in fact actually be shunted into the head causing, presumably, a transient reduction in intracranial blood volume (du Boulay and colleagues, 1973).

Since blood flow depends largely on arteriolar calibre, an increase in cerebral blood flow is normally accompanied by an increase in cerebral blood volume. This is also compensated for by 'venting' of CSF from the skull into the slightly distensible spinal theca. In fact CSF appears to be 'vented' in this way with each intracranial arterial pulsation (du Boulay and colleagues, 1973).

In the presence of an intracranial tumour certain compensatory changes will occur in the volumes of CSF and blood in the cranial cavity.

Effects on CSF Volume

If an intracranial mass develops acutely, a reduction of intra-cranial CSF volume may result from venting of the CSF into the spinal theca, as previously described. Furthermore the total CSF volume may be reduced, in the presence of raised ICP, by increased CSF reabsorption into the blood stream. CSF production normally averages 0·3 ml/min and, over short periods of time, appears to be independent of the ICP (Cutler and colleagues, 1968). Reabsorption, on the other hand, is closely related to pressure, rates of three or four times higher than the production rate having been recorded in the presence of intracranial hypertension (Katzman and Hussey, 1970). Thus the total volume of CSF may be reduced in patients with raised ICP.

Effects on Cerebral Blood Flow and Blood Volume

The effect of intracranial hypertension on cerebral blood flow (CBF) and volume are complicated. There is evidence in animals that cerebral blood flow remains constant in the face of increasing ICP owing to an autoregulatory mechanism. Many years ago it was noted (Wolff and Forbes, 1928) that increasing the ICP led to dilatation of cortical arterioles. This led to a reduction in cerebrovascular resist-ance and the maintenance of flow in the face of quite considerable intracranial hypertension. In the experimental animal, cerebral blood flow may remain constant when the CSF pressure is increased, even up to levels of over 1,000 mm H_2O (Zwetnow, 1970).

When raised ICP is due to a tumour, the findings are less predict-able, for here 'breakdowns' of autoregulation may occur. These may be purely focal phenomena, in the region of the tumour, or may involve the whole brain (Brock and colleagues, 1970). In the absence of autoregulation the cerebral blood flow will depend on the 'perfusion pressure', i.e. the difference between intracranial pressure and mean systemic arterial pressure. The Cushing response (the rise of arterial pressure in response to raised ICP) then assumes importance but it is not a constant phenomenon (Lundberg, 1960). There is some evidence that it only occurs when the brain stem blood supply

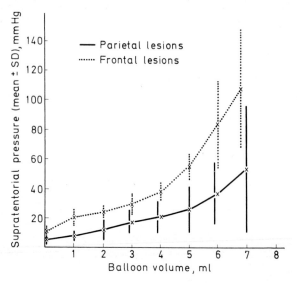

Figure 4. Variation of supratentorial pressure with volume for parietal and frontal lesions. (Reproduced by courtesy of Professor D. G. McDowell)

is critically involved (Zwetnow, 1970) but there is no general agreement on this point. Thus, in the absence of autoregulation the Cushing response, by maintaining the perfusion pressure, may keep CBF constant in the face of rising ICP: if the response does not occur CBF falls as ICP rises. However, if some other factor, such as a change in P_{CO_2} or the administration of volatile anaesthetics, directly affects the calibre of cerebral vessels, CBF and ICP will then rise or fall together.

Most experimenters have found a general reduction of cerebral blood flow in cases of brain tumour (Cronqvist and Lundberg, 1968; Brock and colleagues, 1970). Others have found evidence of maintained autoregulation up to pressures in the region of 400 mm H_2O, but reduction of blood flow when the pressures exceeded this level (Kety, Shenkin and Schmidt, 1948; Greenfield and Tindall, 1965).

The cerebral blood volume is generally decreased in the presence of raised ICP (Lowell and Bloor, 1971). Where the flow depends upon perfusion pressure this is easy to understand (as ICP rises, cerebral blood flow and volume fall) but even where autoregulation is still intact, the cerebral blood volume may be decreased, even though blood flow is maintained: the arterioles dilate but the much larger 'capacitance' vessels, i.e. the veins, are squeezed to produce an overall reduction of intracranial blood volume.

In summary, the effects of an expanding intracranial mass may be compensated by changes, both in intracranial CSF volume and in intracranial blood volume. The effect on brain tissue fluid itself has not been explored. The presence of a small intracranial mass can be compensated for, without any marked rise in ICP. With increasing size, however, each increment of volume leads to a much greater increase in pressure (*Figure 4*). On the 'vertical' limb of the volume/pressure curve, a very small increase in volume will lead to a large increase in pressure. At this stage the patient will be in a critical state: any disturbance such as an increase in cerebral oedema, or respiratory obstruction leading to CO_2 retention and an increase in cerebral blood flow, may precipitate disaster.

MEASUREMENT

It has already been pointed out that there is no constant or reliable correlation between symptoms and the level of the ICP. Direct measurement is therefore the only correct way of determining the ICP. In clinical practice this is usually done by lumbar puncture.

Lumbar Puncture

As far as pressure is concerned, the skull and spinal column act as an imperfectly closed tube, variations in intrathoracic and intra-abdominal pressure being imparted to the tube via the cerebral veins and spinal epidural venous network. The pressure, in various parts of this tube, is critically dependent on the patient's posture. In the recumbent posture (lateral decubitus) it is, as mentioned, of the order of 150 mm H_2O. In the sitting posture, cisternal pressure would be below atmospheric while the pressure in the lumbar subarachnoid space would be in the region of 400 mm H_2O.*

What is measured in the course of lumbar puncture is of course an approximate pressure. Some fluid escapes into the manometer thereby reducing the pressure in the subarachnoid space. This does

---

* For a fuller discussion of these interesting relationships see the papers by Carmichael, Doupe and Williams (1937) and Davson (1960).

not matter in clinical practice, where only a rough estimate is needed. The upper limit of normal CSF pressure (determined in the recumbent posture) is arbitrarily defined as 160, 180 and 200 mm H_2O, the middle figure being the one usually given.

The danger of performing a lumbar puncture in the presence of papilloedema, *or other evidence suggesting raised ICP*, is well known to most, but not apparently to all. The procedure is still carried out with depressing regularity. Where there is no shift of intracranial structures (as in 'benign intracranial hypertension' or in various conditions associated with communicating hydrocephalus) lumbar puncture may be performed quite safely. But this should only be done after careful assessment, preferably in a neurosurgical or neurological department. The real danger occurs when there is tentorial or tonsillar herniation. The pressure in the lumbar sac may then no longer reflect the true intracranial tension. There are many examples where enormously high supratentorial pressures have been recorded in the presence of a normal pressure in the lumbar sac. Any release of fluid below the block is likely to aggravate the impaction. The effects may not occur immediately. Fluid tends to seep out of the puncture hole in the dura for many hours. Dramatic clinical deterioration may first occur some ten hours or more after the lumbar puncture.

Measurement of Ventricular Pressure

When there is hydrocephalus, a neurosurgeon will often consider draining a lateral ventricle, either before, during or after the main intervention. Lundberg (1960) was the first to demonstrate that if a drain was placed into a lateral ventricle under scrupulously aseptic conditions, it could be left *in situ* for days or weeks, with only a small risk of infection. In his important monograph he described the long term measurement of ICP in such cases. He confirmed the fact that 'pressure symptoms' might occur, despite low ventricular pressure, and conversely that they might be missing, even when the ICP was extremely high.

The main contribution of Lundberg's work, however, was the recognition of the spontaneous 'plateau waves',* that may occur in patients with severe intracranial hypertension (*Figure 5*). These sudden increases in pressure, which may last for 10–20 minutes, may be associated with symptoms such as headache, nausea, vomiting and impairment of consciousness, though whether these symptoms

---

* 'Plateau waves', as well as being associated with the aforementioned symptoms, may possibly be the explanation of the sudden obscurations of vision that can transiently occur in patients with raised ICP.

are due to greater brain stem distortion or to the general effect of raised pressure is uncertain. The best way of abolishing 'plateau waves' is to drain CSF from the lateral ventricle. This remains the most effective way of lowering ICP in general.

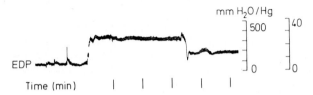

Figure 5. *A spontaneous 'plateau' (type A) wave occurring during apparently normal sleep. EDP = extradural pressure. (Reproduced by courtesy of Mr. Lindsay Symon)*

The 'plateau waves' are independent of arterial blood pressure. They may be provoked by a rise in PCO_2, but not necessarily so, and may also be triggered by injecting air into the ventricle. They usually occur without obvious precipitating cause. Investigations have shown that the waves are associated with a decrease in cerebral blood flow (Lundberg, Conqvist and Kjallqvist, 1968) and an increase in cerebral blood volume (Risberg, Lundberg and Ingrar, 1969). Angiograms suggest that arteries are more widely dilated during the occurrence of the 'plateau waves'. Whether or not these fluctuations in arterial calibre occur when the ICP is normal is unknown. They will clearly have a maximal effect when the pressure is already high—i.e. on the 'steep' part of the pressure–volume curve.

Extradural Pressure Transducers

An alternative approach to long-term measurement of ICP is to implant a device into the extradural space. This does not involve any injury to the brain or risk of ventricular sepsis. Insertion does involve a small operation, however. An additional disadvantage is that the patient is then restricted in his movements (by the wires passing between the transducer and the recording apparatus). The transducers tend to be unstable, and technical difficulties have been encountered in their use. These are being overcome (Dorsch, Stephens and Symon, 1971).

Extradural transducers have been used in experimental studies of ICP in animals. They have also provided useful information in the long term estimation of ICP in man, although, for technical reasons, they tend to record a higher pressure than that obtained by intraventricular measurement. In patients with so-called 'normal pressure hydrocephalus', long-term recordings demonstrate the occurrence of transient intracranial hypertension, particularly at night, illustrating that in this condition, the ICP is not 'normal' all the time (Symon and colleagues, 1972). The finding of an isolated lumbar CSF pressure below the arbitrary normal of 180 mm H_2O can therefore be misleading.

Continuous monitoring of intracranial pressure, either by intra-ventricular or extradural methods, provides much more reliable information than a single lumbar puncture. It has practical value in the diagnosis of raised ICP management of patients and assessing prognosis in head injuries (Jennett and Johnson, 1972). It will probably be used increasingly.

CONTROL OF RAISED INTRACRANIAL PRESSURE

In a patient with a cerebral tumour, the most effective way of re-ducing raised ICP is to remove the tumour. Pressure can also be lowered by measures aimed at reducing: (a) the P_{CO_2}; (b) any associ-ated cerebral oedema; and (c) any associated hydrocephalus.

Reduction of P_{CO_2} and Cerebral Blood Volume

The most important variable controlling both cerebral blood flow and cerebral blood volume is the arterial P_{CO_2}. An obstructed air-way is a most potent cause of a rise of intracranial pressure, this being due to an increase in both flow and volume. Management of the airway, in the unconscious patient is therefore of critical importance.

During anaesthesia, the P_{CO_2} may artificially be reduced by con-trolled hyperventilation. This is usually resorted to in neurosurgical operations. This controlled hyperventilation causes a considerable reduction of cerebral blood flow and of brain swelling. The reduction of cerebral blood flow does not seem to lead to significant hypoxia, until the P_{CO_2} is lowered below 20 mm Hg. These low levels are not reached in normal neurosurgical anaesthesia.

Treatment of Cerebral Oedema

Any brain insult (trauma, infarction, etc.) may be associated with cerebral oedema, which of course substantially contributes to raised ICP. Nowhere is this more apparent than in the case of cerebral metastases. Frequently a discreet metastasis may be surrounded by a wide area of oedema which contributes far more to the abnormal mass than the tumour itself. The cause is completely unknown.

If a *rapid* decrease in cerebral volume is needed, hyperosmolar solutions (such as urea or mannitol) are given, by rapid intravenous infusion. Mannitol is the substance in most common use nowadays: 40–80 g may be given over 10–20 minutes. This usually results in a rapid diuresis. The patient, usually stuporose, will have to have a catheter inserted. The hyperosmolar agents act by virtue of the fact that they only slowly pass through the blood–brain barrier (i.e. from the cerebral capillaries to the cerebral extracellular fluid). They therefore attract water by osmosis out of the brain. Short acting diuretics such as frusemide also have some effect on cerebral oedema, but the experience of most is that the clinical response is less predictable.

The introduction of dexamethasone has caused a revolution in neurosurgery. It may act by restoring to normal certain localized 'breakdowns' in the blood–brain barrier. The basis of the blood–brain barrier appears to be the fact that cerebral capillary endothelial cells are much more firmly welded together than capillary endothelial cells in other tissues. There are no 'pores' between these endothelial cells. In a wide variety of pathological circumstances changes may occur in these capillaries and the 'barrier' breaks down. This appears to be one of the causes of cerebral oedema (Klatzo, 1967). The effects of dexamethasone on cerebrovascular permeability have been discussed by Maxwell, Long and French (1971). Many facts still remain to be explained, the most puzzling of which is now mannitol may still act as a cerebral 'dehydrant' even in the presence of the postulated localized breakdowns of the blood–brain barrier.

There is no doubt, however, about the clinical observation that dexamethasone may produce quite striking improvement although this usually takes 12 hours or more. The introduction of this substance has vastly cut down the number of emergency operations for brain tumour—a result that should have a good effect on the long term survival of both patients and surgeons.

Management of Hydrocephalus

The effect of many brain tumours may be aggravated by the co-existence of hydrocephalus, due to obstruction of the ventricular system. This may be coped with by ventricular drainage which may either be temporary (i.e. into a bottle) or permanent (i.e. CSF may be shunted from the ventricle either into the cisterna magna—if the obstruction is in the ventricular system—or into the blood stream, if the obstruction is more distal). In fact permanent drainage may be the definitive treatment in the case of those deep tumours in the region of the third ventricle which are considered inoperable and which are producing most of their disturbance by causing hydrocephalus. The various 'short-circuit' procedures available—in the control of hydrocephalus—were reviewed by Logue (1968).

Hydrocephalus is sometimes treated as a prelude to removal of posterior fossa tumours but caution is needed. If the tumour is very large, ventricular drainage may lead to upward herniation of the mass through the tentorial opening.

Ventricular drainage during surgery is often very helpful. In the post-operative period it may be vital either to tide the patient over a period of temporary hydrocephalus, until the normal CSF pathways open up again, or as a preliminary to permanent ventricular drainage into the blood stream.

Overall Management of Patients with Raised ICP

To control ICP, a combination of the aforementioned techniques is often used, with 'interventions' before, during and after surgery. In practice, the combination of clinical symptoms and signs will give a good indication that there is an intracranial mass. Surgery may be undertaken. The reduction of mass and pressure will then, for practical purposes, be synonymous.

In the somnolent patient, maintenance of a good airway is mandatory. Where there is clinical evidence of brain stem compression, or the disease is progressing rapidly, it may be necessary to give intravenous mannitol as a preliminary to surgery. Hyperosmotic agents are not, however, usually used unless surgery is to be undertaken in the near future. Their effect seldom lasts for more than four to six hours, and with increasing use the effect of mannitol diminishes. Indeed when mannitol eventually does pass the blood–brain barrier, as it is likely to do in oedematous areas, a 'reversed effect' may develop. This tendency is probably more marked with urea, and is one of the reasons why mannitol is nowadays generally preferred. In less urgent circumstances, frusemide or dexamethasone will for a while control cerebral oedema.

The question of anaesthesia for neurosurgical investigations (such as pneumonencephalography or carotid angiography) is important. All the volatile anaesthetics, such as halothane or trilene, cause dilatation of intracranial vessels and a marked increase of ICP (Jennett and colleagues, 1969). In addition, halothane may cause a fall of blood pressure and thus reduce the perfusion pressure within the head. Whether or not this is important will depend upon whether autoregulation is still effective. If the intracranial pressure is very high, autoregulation may already have broken down. Under these circumstances, the perfusion pressure should not be reduced.

On the other hand, far better X-rays will be obtained under general anaesthesia. This is particularly noticeable in the case of carotid angiography, where induced hyperventilation will cause slowing of the circulation and much clearer definition of detail. For this reason anaesthesia is usually preferred. At the National Hospital, the usual technique is to induce anaesthesia with thiopentone (Pentothal) and to maintain it with nitrous oxide and oxygen, possibly supplemented by a small concentration of trilene (this agent does not cause much drop in blood pressure). A muscle relaxant is given and the patient is hyperventilated. This technique ensured that the intracranial pressure is not greatly increased and that the blood pressure does not fall alarmingly.

In the surgery of supratentorial tumours, hyperventilation is invaluable and is instituted as soon as the patient has been intubated and a drip set up. If the intracranial pressure is thought to be very high, mannitol is given before induction. This will lower the pressure during the short critical period before controlled hyperventilation can be established. The patient is placed on the table with the head slightly raised to encourage venous return.

After the intracranial tension has been reduced, a certain degree of arteriol hypotension can be allowed. Opening the dura will reduce raised ICP to atmospheric and ensure that the perfusion pressure will be reasonable, even in the presence of arterial hypotension. Tissue perfusion will be adequate, even in areas with defective autoregulation. Bleeding from the tumour will be reduced. At this stage halothane is a useful anaesthetic agent, in that it helps maintain this reduction of blood pressure.

Where access to deep tumours is needed, the brain can be 'shrunk' by the use of mannitol, even in the absence of raised intracranial pressure. Additional access can be obtained by spinal drainage or tapping a lateral ventricle. Before the skull is closed, the blood pressure is brought up to normal and spontaneous respiration allowed to return, so that effective haemostasis can be ensured under conditions similar to those that will pertain in the period following surgery.

In the surgery of posterior fossa tumours some surgeons feel that the advantage gained by induced hyperventilation is outweighed by the fact that the loss of spontaneous respiration means the loss of a valuable monitor. Surgery is often performed with the patient in the sitting position and intracranial pressure is controlled primarily by aspirating CSF from a lateral ventricle.

Unlike the situation described in the opening paragraph, the surgeon of today is therefore, hopefully, no longer faced with severe and intractable brain bulging. The control of raised ICP can, in the vast majority of cases, be effectively ensured. In the post-operative phase, the judicious use of mannitol, frusemide and dexamethasone will be supplemented, where necessary, by ventricular drainage which is probably the most effective way of lowering the ICP.

When radiotherapy is given to patients harbouring malignant brain tumours, dexamethasone has proved invaluable. Its use can be continued for long periods, although it has the usual drawbacks associated with steroid therapy. Some people are undoubtedly maintained on this drug for longer than is necessary.

REFERENCES

Adams, R. D., Fisher, C. M., Hakim, S., Ojemann, R. G. and Sweet W. H. (1965). 'Symptomatic occult hydrocephalus with "normal" cerebrospinal fluid.' *New Engl. J. Med.*, **273**, 117.

Behrman, S. (1966). 'Pathology of papilloedema.' *Brain*, **89**, 1.

du Boulay, G., O'Connell, J. E. A., Currie, J., Bostick, T. and Verity, P. (1973). 'Further studies of pulsatile movements in C.S.F. pathways.' In press.

Brock, M., Hadgidimos, A., Deriiaz, J. P. and Schurmann, K. (1970). 'Regional cerebral blood flow and vascular reactivity in cases of brain tumour.' In *Proceedings of Fourth International Symposium on Regulation of Cerebral Blood Flow*, pp. 281–284. London.

Carmichael, E. A., Doupe, J. and Williams, D. J. (1937). *J. Physiol.*, **91**, 186.

Cronqvist, S. and Lundberg, N. (1968). 'Regional cerebral blood flow in intracranial tumours with special regard to cases with intracranial hypertension.' *Scand. J. Lab. Clin. Invest.*, Suppl. 102.

Cutler, R. W. P., Page, L., Galicich, J. and Watters, G. V. (1968). 'Formation and absorption of cerebrospinal fluid in man.' *Brain*, **91**, 707.

Davson, H. (1960). In *Handbook of Physiology* (Section 1: Neurophysiology Vol. II). Washington; American Physiological Society.

Dorsch, N. W. C. and Symon, L. (1972). 'Intracranial pressure changes in acute ischaemic regions of the primate hemisphere.' In *Intracranial Pressure*, Ed. by M. Brock and H. Dietz. Berlin; Springer.

— Stephens, R. J. and Symon, L. (1971). 'An intracranial pressure transducer.' *Bio-med. Eng.*, **6**, 452.

Greenfield, J. D. Jnr. and Tindall, G. T. (1965). 'Effect of acute increase in intracranial pressure on blood flow in the internal carotid artery of man.' *J. clin. Invest.*, **44**, 1343.

Hakim, S. and Adams, R. D. (1965). 'The special clinical problem of symptomatic hydrocephalus with normal cerebrospinal fluid pressure.' *J. neurol. Sci.*, **2**, 307.

Jennett, B. and Johnson, I. H. (1972). 'The uses of intracranial pressure monitoring.' In *Intracranial Pressure*, Ed. by M. Brock and H. Dietz. Berlin; Springer.

REFERENCES

Jennett, B., Barker, J., Fitch, W. and McDowall, D. G. (1969). 'Effect of anaesthesia on intracranial pressure in patients with space-occupying lesions.' *Lancet*, **1**, 61.

Katzman, R. and Hussey, F. (1970). 'A simple constant-infusion manometric test for measurement of C.S.F. absorption.' *Neurology*, **20**, 534.

Kety, S. S., Shenkin, H. A. and Schmidt, C. F. (1948). 'The effects of increased intracranial pressure on cerebral circulatory functions in man.' *J. clin. Invest.*, **27**, 493.

Klatzo, I. (1967). 'Neuropathological aspects of brain oedema.' *J. Neuropath. expl. Neurol.*, **26**, 1.

Kunkle, E. C. and Wolff, H. G. (1951). 'Headaches.' In *Modern Trends in Neurology—1*, Ed. by A. Feiling. London; Butterworths.

Logue, V. (1968). 'Hydrocephalus.' In *Biochemical Aspects of Neurological Disorders*, Ed. by J. N. Cummings and M. Kremer. Oxford; Blackwell.

Lowell, H. M. and Bloor, B. M. (1971). 'The effect of increased intracranial pressure on cerebrovascular hemodynamics.' *J. Neurosurg.*, **34**, 760.

Lundberg, N. (1960). 'Continuous recording and control of ventricular fluid pressure in neurosurgical practice.' *Acta psychiat. neurol. scand.*, Suppl. **149**, 1.

— Conqvist, S. and Kjallqvist, A. (1968). 'Clinical investigations on interrelationships between intracranial pressure and intracranial dynamics.' *Progr. Brain Res. (Cerebral Circulation)*, **30**, 69.

McNealy, D. E. and Plumb, F. (1962). 'Brain stem dysfunction with supratentorial mass lesions.' *Archs neurol.*, **7**, 10.

Maxwell, R. E., Long, D. M. and French, L. A. (1971). 'The effects of glucosteroids on experimental cold-induced brain oedema. Gross morphological alterations and vascular permeability changes.' *J. Neurosurg.*, **34**, 477.

Plumb, F. and Posner, J. B. (1966). *Diagnosis of Stupor and Coma*. Philadelphia; Davis.

Risberg, J., Lundberg, N. and Ingvar, D. H. (1969). 'Regional cerebral blood volume during acute transient rises of intracranial pressure (plateau waves).' *J. Neurosurg.*, **31**, 303.

Schumacher, G. A. and Wolff, H. G. (1941). 'Experimental studies on headache.' *Archs Neurol. Psychiat.*, **45**, 199.

Symon, L., Dorsch, N. W. C. and Stephens, R. J. (1972). 'Long term measurement of extradural pressure in "low pressure" hydrocephalus.' In *Intracranial Pressure*, Ed. by M. Brock and H. Dietz. Berlin; Springer.

Weinstein, J. D., Langfitt, T. W., Bruno, L., Saren, H. A. and Jackson, J. L. F. (1968). 'Experimental study of patterns of brain distortion and ischaemic produced by an intracranial mass.' *J. Neurosurg.*, **28**, 513.

Wolff, H. G. (1963). *Headache and Other Head Pain*, p. 672. New York; Oxford University Press.

— and Forbes, H. S. (1928). 'The cerebral circulation. V. Observations of the pial circulation during changes in intracranial pressure.' *Archs Neurol. Psychiat.*, **20**, 1035.

Zwetnow, N. N. (1970). 'Effects of increased cerebrospinal fluid pressure on the blood flow and on the energy metabolism of the brain.' *Acta physiol. scand.*, Suppl. 339.

6—*Localized Treatments to the Brain*

Thomas J. Deeley

INTRODUCTION

In the treatment of many malignant lesions by radiotherapy, experience and repeated evaluation of the results of treatment have enabled us to formulate a policy of management. For many tumours we can state the optimum treatment conditions, the dose, method, fractionation, total overall treatment time, and so on; but this does not hold for many tumours of the central nervous system. Despite the many improvements that have occurred in the past few years, both in radiotherapy equipment and techniques and in neurosurgery, the results of the treatment of malignant tumours of the central nervous system have shown little, if any, improvement. The reports of treatment in the literature are somewhat confusing; whilst some radiotherapists give encouraging survival rates others have shown less enthusiasm. There may be many reasons for this, the selection of patients, the variations in radiation and surgical techniques used, the volume of tissue irradiated and the total dose given.

It is therefore difficult to give a dogmatic account of treatment at this site, although a few facts are known. Perhaps the most important is that we know that certain histological types of tumour are usually confined to a relatively localized area in the brain whilst others are known to seed throughout the cerebrospinal fluid pathway in a fair proportion of cases. Radiotherapy techniques can thus be divided into two groups, one where treatment is localized to the skull and the other where the whole cerebrospinal fluid pathway is included in the field of irradiation. This chapter will deal with localized treatments to the skull but will omit certain special sites; for example, the pituitary gland, which are dealt with in other chapters: it will thus deal mainly with the astrocytomas, oligodendrogliomas and meningiomas. These tumours form rather a 'mixed bag' extending from the slow-growing, relatively benign oligodendroglioma or well differentiated astrocytoma through varying grades of malignancy to what is one of the most malignant tumours in the body, the glioblastoma multiforme. They show varying degrees of radio-sensitivity and many are relatively radio-resistant; the dose of radiation that is given to them is determined by the tolerance of the surrounding normal brain tissue. The method of treatment given depends on the histology of the lesion but biopsy is not always practical and we must irradiate without this knowledge. One of our great problems is accurate tumour localization and whilst we are anxious to limit high doses to a relatively small area it may be at the risk of missing the tumour; we need, therefore, to examine critically our assessment of the volume of tissue to be irradiated. Different forms of radiation have been claimed to give better effects and investigations have been made of the value of radiotherapy combined with surgery or chemotherapeutic agents.

We will examine some of these points further and try to determine whether a policy of treatment can be formulated. It will be seen that consideration of one factor often leads us onto a consideration of another.

RADIATION EFFECTS ON THE NORMAL BRAIN TISSUES

For many years the misconception that nervous system tissues showed little response to irradiation led to the use of high tumour doses in the treatment of brain tumours. It is fortunate that the reports of brain damage have led us to review the possible late effects of radiation before we make indiscriminate use of megavoltage therapy with its higher depth dose and reduction of bone shielding effects. Successful irradiation of a brain tumour will result in some scarring; the effects on the normal tissues may be due to a direct effect on the glial tissues, on the neurons or on the supplying blood vessels. The tissues immediately surrounding a brain tumour, whilst not being involved by growth, may be far from normal and may show pathological changes as a result of the proximity of the tumour, especially changes in the blood vessels. Our information regarding the effects on normal brain in humans has been obtained where the brain has been included in the field of irradiation of lesions of the skull or scalp as, for example, the case of brain necrosis reported by Pennybacker and Russell (1948) after treatment for a rodent ulcer of the scalp. We have, in addition, obtained useful information from examination of animal tissues after irradiation.

Although sporadic reports in the literature had suggested that brain tissue could be damaged, other workers, for example, Pierce and colleagues (1945), has reported that doses as high as 10–15,000 roentgens could be given without deleterious effects. In 1948 Boden presented 10 cases of radiation-induced cervical myelitis and followed this in 1950 with a report of 7 cases of brain-stem damage. From these reports he was able to establish radiation tolerance curves applicable to nervous tissues. These curves plotted total dose in roentgens against duration of treatment in days, but Boden emphasized that there was also a third responsible factor, the volume of tissue irradiated. The dose that could be tolerated by brain tissue was inversely proportional to the volume of tissue irradiated. Thus, for large fields he suggested that the upper limit of tolerance was 3,500 roentgens in 17 days whereas for small fields treated over the same time a dose of 4,500 roentgens could be tolerated. Lindgren (1958) carefully analysed the literature and was able to produce two tolerance lines, one giving the lowest dosage level producing brain necrosis and a line above which there was a very high incidence of necrosis. If necrosis is to be avoided the dose must always be below the minimum recorded dose producing necrosis. If we are to achieve eradication of the tumour some risks need to be taken and this lower dose must be exceeded; there is no justification, however, in giving a dose of radiation which will exceed the highest of Lindgren's two curves and produce a high incidence of necrosis. Vaeth (1965), using more protracted overall treatment times than Boden, was able to show that it was possible under these conditions to exceed Boden's tolerance doses.

These effects may be altered by other factors; by the age of the patient, it seems probable that young children show a greater sensitivity than does the adult; in old age the associated vascular changes may also account for an increased sensitivity of tissues; the presence of pre-existing disease such as infarcts may increase the areas of gliosis; in addition it is possible that some parts of the brain may tolerate radiation better than others, and also that damage may occur in some areas which are relatively silent and do not produce much in the way of symptoms. Hypertension may be responsible for providing more changes (Asscher and Anson, 1962; Almquist and colleagues, 1964). It is possible that all these differences are, in fact, related to differences in the oxygen tension of the tissues of the brain altered by general and local conditions.

Rubin and Casarett (1968) in their excellent book *Clinical Radiation Pathology*, give a description of four clinical periods:

(1) Acute. During the course of treatment there may be an increase in the intracranial pressure with headache, lethargy, vomiting and papilloedema, and continuation of treatment may produce seizures. Depending on the location of the lesion there may be a progression of existing neurological findings.

(2) Sub-acute. The patient may remain well for 6–12 months after treatment and then develop a recurrence of symptoms; because the radiation changes are in the same site as the original tumour it is to be expected that damage will produce the same symptomatology. Differential diagnosis between damage and recurrence is thus extremely difficult; EEG and arteriography will often only reveal an abnormality; MacDonald, Green and Rubin (quoted by Rubin and Casarett) suggested that serial scanning after treatment may show alterations in uptake, necrotic areas losing the ability to take up isotopes and recurrent areas showing a greater activity. An increasing space occupying lesion is suggested by increasing papilloedema.

(3) Chronic. The slower the process of gliosis the more insidious is the onset of the symptoms, which may not occur for many years after treatment. These include poor cerebration, mental confusion, progressive deterioration to the vegetable state, sometimes associated with epileptic seizures and convulsions. The differential diagnosis is again difficult; and cerebrovascular accidents may be suspected; indeed, infarction or haemorrhage may occur in the damaged area causing an exacerbation of symptoms.

(4) Late. Rubin and Casarett use this term to cover the malignant changes, fibrosarcomata that may occur in the irradiated brain.

The differential diagnosis can be difficult in all these cases—so much depends on the site of the lesion, the age of the patient, the dose delivered, the extent of the original lesion, and the interval between irradiation and clinical signs of damage.

PATHOLOGICAL CHANGES

Full accounts of the pathological changes involved in irradiation of the brain are given by Rubin and Casarett (1968), by Zeman and Samorajski (1971), Pennybacker and Russell (1948), Bouchard (1966), and Lampert, Tom and Rider (1959). It is not intended to give an account here but only to point out that these changes vary tremendously in the reported literature and are probably the result of irradiation both on the nervous tissue and the vascular supply.

The nervous system is composed of a complex system of cells, which may be affected by the radiation; the neuron, although a single cell, may show differing reactions to radiation in its various parts, the axon is relatively resistant as are the dendrites, but relatively small doses may produce changes at the synopses; of the glial cells, the astrocytes are relatively radio-sensitive and the oligodendrocytes perhaps less so. In addition, there may be changes in the blood vessels and resultant changes in the tissues supplied by them. We are not concerned here with the changes of acute radiation necrosis seen in animals after very high doses of irradiation but with the delayed effects seen in patients some months after a course of radiation given to a tumour. Macroscopically the involved area of the brain is shrunken and cavitated, shows areas of necrosis predominately affecting the white matter and bleeding may have occurred into the cavities. Histological changes are varied and consist of a mixture of degeneration and reaction. Demyelination of the white matter occurs and may be temporary or irreversible depending on the degree of damage caused. Degenerative changes may be found in the blood vessels and these may produce secondary vascular lesions. It appears that radiation may cause effects both on the nervous tissue cells and on the vascular system.

HISTOLOGY OF THE TUMOUR AND RELATIVE RADIO-SENSITIVITY

The different histological types of tumours have been discussed in Chapter 2. The radio-sensitivity of these tumours varies tremendously from one histological type to another and even within the same group. Richmond (1959) pointed out that we should not regard tumours in this site as having a fixed order of malignancy; in fact, serial biopsies have shown that the slowly growing lesion may assume more malignant characteristics. Bouchard (1966) suggested that in addition to the physical factors the radio-sensitivity of brain tumours may be related to certain biological factors which were difficult to fathom and about which we knew very little; these could include such specialized effects as growth restraint and tumour regression by the action of degenerative processes induced by the irradiation of the brain tissues.

We can, however, get a general idea of the degree of radio-sensitivity of brain tumours from our experience of the response of these lesions to treatment. Medulloblastomas are particularly radio-sensitive; their propensity for dissemination throughout the cerebrospinal fluid would preclude radical treatment if it were not for this because they respond to the relatively low doses that can be given to such a large area. The same applies to ependymomas and ependyblastomas, neuro-epitheliomas, medulloblastomas and pinealomas. These tumours are known to disseminate widely throughout the cerebrospinal fluid pathway or have a possibility of spreading widely in a fair proportion of cases. Bouchard and Peirce (1960) found dissemination in medulloblastomas in 12 per cent of cases, Phillips, Sheline and Boldney (1964) found seedlings in 5 per cent of ependymomas, but Sagerman, Bagshaw and Hamberg (1965) found the incidence to be 46 per cent. These widely disseminated tumours responding to a relatively low dose are thus treated by wide field irradiation and are dealt with in Chapter 7.

Astrocytomas form a very broad group with regard to radio-sensitivity; histologically they extend from the relatively differentiated tumour of Grade I to the highly malignant tumour in Grade IV. (Kernohan and Sayre, 1952). The Grade IV lesions are usually referred to as glioblastoma multiforme and Taveras, Thompson and Pool (1962) have called the Grade III tumours 'astrocytomas with glioblastomatous changes'; this type of tumour is somewhat more slowly growing than the true glioblastoma. The same authors point out that this tumour may become more malignant with the passage of time and that variations of malignancy may occur throughout the tumour. It is usually accepted that radio-sensitivity is low in the glioblastomas and that the radiation necessary to eradicate these lesions will cause necrosis of the surrounding brain tissues. The more differentiated tumours in Grades I and II have been reported to be radio-resistant but there is considerable difference of opinion probably because these tumours are usually treated surgically and have a relatively good prognosis with this method of treatment. However, it has been shown that survival rates can be improved by post-operative radiotherapy (Bouchard and Peirce, 1960). The relatively slow-growing oligodendrogliomas are relatively benign tumours but they may recur locally after removal. Their sensitivity has varied in reports from resistant to showing sufficient radio-sensitivity as to make irradiation after surgery worthwhile (Shenkin, 1965; Sheline and colleagues, 1964). The non-gliomatous group of tumours all show varying degrees of radio-sensitivity.

Bouchard (1966) describes the histopathological effects of irradiation; after treatment histological examination shows that the effect which may be attributed to radiation can hardly be differentiated from variable degrees of necrosis, haemorrhage, and vascular changes which may be found occurring spontaneously in non-irradiated tumours. In other parts of the body these changes would

136

be ascribed to the irradiation, but because such changes have been observed without treatment (Nessa, 1938; Freid and Davidoff, 1951) we must be careful before we suggest that treatment has caused them; it is not unusual to find malignant cells in the necrotic area. Bouchard, reviewing the autopsy findings in 63 patients who had had intensive radiation therapy for a cerebral tumour found malignant cells in all; it is possible, though, that these cells may not have been viable. Pennybacker and Russell (1948) and Lindgren (1958) reported finding no malignant cells at autopsy in only one case of glioblastoma, two cases of glioblastoma and one glioma. There are thus very few cases where histological examination of material obtained at autopsy subsequent to irradiation has failed to reveal malignant tumour in the sections taken of the treated area.

Thus, in those tumours which are limited to the brain the response to irradiation is variable, is not directly related to histological type and whilst most lesions have been shown to be relatively radio-resistant some have shown a degree of sensitivity which would suggest that radiation could be used with a chance of success in the primary treatment of inoperable lesions and that post-operative treatment may yield a higher proportion of cures or longer palliation.

OPERABILITY

Histological examination will only be obtained if the lesion is operable and if the patient's general condition is suitable for this. The surgical techniques have been discussed in Chapter 4. If it is not possible to remove a lesion it is usual to obtain a piece of tissue for biopsy but in some sites this is not possible or is unduly hazardous. In these cases operation may be limited to procedures aimed at reducing the intracranial pressure. Biopsy may be contra-indicated in tumours of the mid-brain and pons, Bouchard and Peirce (1960) point out that the errors made in making a clinical diagnosis of tumour in these regions are small, the majority of tumours being gliomas. Thus, in this area it is quite possible and justifiable to give a radical course of radiotherapy without biopsy (Bouchard and Peirce, 1960; Sheline, Phillips and Boldrey, 1965; Whyte, Colby and Layton, 1969).

LOCALIZATION

The extent of the tumour determines the field sizes to be used, and consequently the volume of brain tissue to be irradiated, which in turn dictates the dose of radiation that can be given without causing necrosis. It is thus imporant to try and locate the extent of the tumour as accurately as possible and this has been discussed in previous chapters. But, even if a tumour can be accurately located does this define the limits of pathological spread and what area of apparently normal tissue must also be included in the field of irradiation? We have discussed the tumours in which spread is likely to occur throughout the whole cerebrospinal fluid pathway; the remaining lesions have a tendency to remain localized. Some tumours may be multicentric in origin; the well differentiated astrocytomas Grades I and II tend to remain localized, but the glioblastomas have a tendency to infiltrate within the brain substance and may involve the meninges.

Concannon, Kramer and Berry (1960) described an investigation to determine the value of radiation therapy for patients with intracranial gliomata: one group of patients received surgery and a matched group of patients received, in addition, a course of radiotherapy. Radiation techniques were based on two factors, the histology and the apparent extent of the tumour as shown by clinical radiographic and operative findings. Fields were selected to cover the tumour and the dose was varied from 5,000 roentgens in 6 to 7 weeks for large lesions to 7,000 roentgens for tumours less than 8 cm in diameter. Bull and Rovit, in 1957, had described an investigation of the results of localization in radiographic diagnosis of brain tumours, but Concannon, Kramer and Berry (1960) considered that while this was good for surgical use the extension of only a small part of the tumour outside the field of irradiation may lead to a failure of radiation therapy; they therefore used a modified method of classification. The radiographic findings were compared with the subsequent histological findings in 29 cases—in 14 per cent of cases the localization was excellent, it was good in 38 per cent and poor in 48 per cent. Twenty-one patients were treated by x-ray therapy and a comparison of field size and subsequent histology showed that the tumour had been adequately covered in 2 (10 per cent), the accuracy of coverage was questionable in 11 (52 per cent) and the tumour was missed in 8 (38 per cent). In these investigations they assumed that a zone of 1 cm of apparent normal tissue had to be included beyond the apparent limits of the lesion. No consideration was given in this investigation to possible microscopic infiltration beyond the tumour mass, the delineation being that seen on gross appearance. Of their 29 patients, 27 had malignant tumours graded III or IV. The authors concluded that large fields are necessary in the treatment of astrocytic gliomata grades III and IV, otherwise the treatment was unlikely to be effective because of inadequate tumour coverage. This posed the question of whether the tumour dose that could be achieved with large volume irradiation would be effective. In smaller differentiated tumours in grades I and II the smaller fields need to be very accurately applied, requiring exact localization and field positioning; again, it is likely that failure of tumour coverage may be a reason for poor results. As Kramer (1969) pointed out in a later article, the patients chosen for this investigation formed a selected group, who died soon after admission, with highly malignant tumours which may have been larger and more rapidly growing than those tumours in patients who survived longer periods.

Todd (1963) suggested two possibilities of treatment with these tumours: either (1) to accept that tumour localization is difficult and that it should be irradiated with a wide margin which means about one-quarter of the brain; this was the policy adopted by Richmond as early as 1949; or (2) considering that these tumours are relatively radio-resistant, to limit the volume to be treated and to give as high a tumour dose as is possible with safety. Todd compared two radiation techniques—small field, beam directed and quarter-brain technique—equivalent to under and over 500 cu cm. The one-year survival rate was 78 per cent for over 500 cu cm as compared with 40 per cent for under 500 cu cm. He considered that there were some factors which favoured a good prognosis and removed these patients from his analysis (these were those patients where there was possibility of surgical cure, those with a pre-treatment history of over three years, patients under 20 years of age, and cases of ependymoma and oligodendroglioma). The corrected figures for the two techniques were then 72 and 32 per cent. He suggested that margins of 2–3 cm should be taken around the apparent tumour.

From these reports it would appear that there is a great danger of not accurately localizing the tumour, with the result that malignant cells may be outside the volume raised to a cancericidal dose—a dose which may need to be high considering the relative radio-resistance of tumours at this site.

Discussion of the volume to be irradiated naturally leads to questions of the dose to be given; this will obviously be related to the damage caused to normal tissues rather than that needed to ablate that particular tumour; i.e. maximum tolerated dose rather than optimum dose. Todd suggested that for volumes of less than 500 cu cm a dose of 4,500 rads using 4 MeV could be tolerated over a treatment time of three weeks, 4,000 rads for volumes over 1,000 cu cm and 3,750 rads for the whole brain. Richmond (1959) had suggested a tumour dose of 4,000 rads in four weeks using his regional treatment plan.

Aristizibal and Caldwell (1971) investigated the time–dose–

volume relationships in 74 patients with glioblastoma multiforme, all but five of these patients had had a previous craniotomy either for biopsy or excision. The doses given were either 4,000, 4,500 or 5,600 rads given in from 20 to 22 treatments equivalent to 1,370, 1,470 and 1,700 rets respectively; for tumour doses of 1,400 to 1,700 rets there was little difference in survival—for less than 1,400 and more than 1,700 rets the results were worse. The same authors also investigated the use of split-dose techniques—giving 2,800 rads in 10 or 11 treatments, followed by three weeks' rest and then 2,800 rads in ten treatments (this gave an NSD of 1,730 rets but the treatment was later modified to give a lower dose of 1,600 rets). The patients treated by the split-dose technique fared less well than those by continuous conventional therapy; those treated to a ret dose 1,730 did particularly badly. The authors concluded that for lesions requiring 100–150 sq cm (using opposed lateral fields) the optimum dose was 1,500–1,600 rets. This paper is based on relatively small numbers of patients when they are divided into groups according to technique, dose and volume irradiated, but even these few results suggest that there is an optimum dose below and above which the results of radiation are worse. The split-dose technique may have been expected to give better results because it allowed the normal tissues to recover somewhat before completing radiation; however, the intervals used may not have been the best for glial tissues and it is suggested that these techniques are further evaluated with differing doses and rest periods.

At the present stage of our knowledge the dose given to the localized cerebral tumour is that which can be tolerated taking into account the volume, fractionation and overall treatment time. We have, as yet, very little knowledge on which we can attempt to correlate this to the histological type of lesion.

RADIATION TECHNIQUES

As Richmond has pointed out, there is little difficulty in obtaining an adequate tumour dose to the brain with orthovoltage therapy. The thin, membranous bone of the skull does not absorb sufficient radiation to reduce the dose more than a small amount. Jones (1960) reported the use of supervoltage x-ray therapy and considered that the radiation damage was reduced with this energy. To achieve the same biological effects Richmond (1959) increased the dose given, using orthovoltage therapy, by 10 per cent when using a telecobalt unit over the same period of time. Bouchard (1966) allowed an increase of 20 per cent over doses given with orthovoltage when using cobalt or 4 MeV x-rays but never exceeded a dose of 6,500 rads over 50 days, and Mitchell (1960) suggested an increase of 25 per cent with radiation in the 20–30 MeV range. Arnold, Bailey and Laughlin (1954) used a 23 MeV betatron and gave doses up to 6,500 rads in 30 days and 7,500 rads in 26–30 days; they concluded from their histological studies of operation or autopsy specimens that the finding were more intense than with orthovoltage therapy; the doses they gave were on the high side of tolerance curves and it is probably this and not the supervoltage therapy, *per se*, that may be accounting for the increased radiation effects.

Churchill-Davidson (1967) reported that the use of hyperbaric oxygen therapy gave disappointing results in eight cases of brain tumour; although the patients had good palliation, none of the tumours was sterilized. Lawrence and Tobias (1967) used the Bragg peak of the alpha particle beam to irradiate brain tumours. Although they were able to deliver adequate tumour doses with little effect on the normal tissues the authors point out that the big problem is that of localization of the tumour area. Zuppinger (1967) gave encouraging results with the use of high-speed electrons; the results, expressed as the proportion with no sign of tumour, were about twice as good as those with 30 MeV x-rays; the best results were obtained with glioblastoma. He suggests that brain tolerance is enhanced with electron therapy.

It is more convenient to use megavoltage therapy; the improved depth dose means that a better distribution can be obtained and there may be improved radiobiological effects, but the big limiting factor of any method of irradiation is the determination of the limits of the tumour.

Implantation of radioactive materials has been described by various people—Cushing (1932) implanted radium, Sachs (1954) radon seeds, and Talairach and colleagues (1955) gold grains. Buckley (1969) described the treatment of 30 patients who had excision and direct irradiation (mainly radium sources) followed by external irradiation and compared the results with excision alone or combined with external irradiation; although the immediate palliation was improved the ultimate survival was not influenced.

SURGERY AND RADIOTHERAPY—ALONE OR COMBINED?

It is important to compare the relative merits of surgery and radiotherapy in the management of cerebral tumours and to determine whether the results of surgery are improved by subsequent radiotherapy. This will be discussed for the main histological types.

Astrocytomas

Bouchard (1966) reviewed the results of treatment in supra-tentorial tumours, comparing his series with those previously reported by Levy and Elvidge (1956); taking all grade I and II cerebral astrocytomas the five-year survival rate of surgical removal alone was 26 per cent and with post-operative radiation Bouchard obtained a survival of 49 per cent. Both articles suggest that the results of surgery in supra-tentorial grade I and II astrocytomas are improved by subsequent radiotherapy. In infratentorial lesions of the same type Levy and Elvidge reported a survival of 76 pèr cent after surgery alone; for this site Bouchard suggests that it is not clear that post-operative radiation has extended the survival and that the primary treatment should be surgery.

Glioblastoma Multiforme

Bouchard reported that surgical decompression, followed by intensive irradiation, was the treatment of choice. Taveras (1962) advocated adequate surgical decompression, partial or total removal of the tumour followed by radiotherapy, and showed that at 12 months only 2 per cent were alive after partial resection alone, whereas 32 per cent were alive when this was followed by radiotherapy. The ultimate prognosis, however, was poor and Jones (1960) pointed out that although a proportion of these tumours were sensitive the response is usually transient. Zulch (1969) gave a cautious opinion of the use of radiotherapy in cerebral tumours but thought that it may be indicated in some cases of grade III and IV tumours; he suggested that this group needed further investigation. Stenberg and Moberg (1971) pointed out the difficulties always present in comparing the merits of surgery and surgery plus radiotherapy—it may be that a patient is referred for radiotherapy because the surgeon thinks the prognosis is poor or the operation is incomplete.

Oligodendroglioma

The results of surgery alone are quite good. Horak (1954) reported a five-year survival rate of 34 per cent and McCarty (1962) of 44 per cent. Sheline and colleagues (1964) reported a five-year survival of 31 per cent for surgery alone and 85 per cent for surgery and radiotherapy; the corresponding ten-year survival rates were 25 and 55 per cent. They thought that post-operative radiotherapy greatly improved the results, but Shenkin (1965) thought that as the time of recurrence was unpredictable and in some cases did not occur radiotherapy should be delayed until there was definite evidence or regrowth—in a small series treated in this way the results of subsequent radiotherapy were good.

It would appear that in the rapidly growing grade III and IV astrocytomas, post-operative therapy was always indicated, that it is probably indicated in grades I and II and in oligodendrogliomas, but it may be kept in reserve in this later group. The reported series are on relatively small groups of patients and obviously more investigations are needed.

CAN THE RESULTS OF TREATMENT BE IMPROVED WITH CHEMOTHERAPY?

There are few reports of the effects of chemotherapeutic agents. Llewellyn and Creech (1962) gave the results of perfusion of various agents and found no improvement. Bouchard (1966) thought that 'chemotherapy used systemically has failed so far to prove its value' but, transitory improvement may be found in the use of arterial or perfusion methods. Edland, Javid and Ansfield (1971) compared the results in a prospective randomized trial in proved cases of glioblastoma multiforme: 17 patients had post-operative high-dose supervoltage therapy, while a similar group of 15 patients had the same treatment plus concomitant systemic 5-fluorouracil chemotherapy. The respective average survival was $11 \cdot 7$ months and $11 \cdot 5$ months and they concluded that chemotherapy did not improve the results of treatment.

ASSESSMENT OF RESULTS OF TREATMENT

In assessing the results of any method of treatment we need to consider the proportion of survivors at a known period of time, the palliation achieved in those patients and in those who do not survive, the degree of morbidity produced as a result of treatment both immediately and at a later date, and the quality of life obtained in those patients who do survive. These assessments obviously need to be made at different periods of time, and although they are often considered separately there is a need to correlate them with each other.

Survival

This is, of course, a convenient end point; it is a positive observation and is an important method of assessing the result of a certain treatment.

143

Quality of Survival

This is related to time of survival and it is necessary to fix a standard of survival and to compare this at different periods of time. This assessment is subjective and demands an assessment of his condition and ability to resume work made by the patient and an interpretation of this by the clinician together with his own observations. We must remember that we are dealing with 'the brain' and disease of such a structure invariably imparts tremendous gravity to the patient and his immediate circle of family and friends; injury or disease to this site frequently implies that 'he will never be the same again' and that 'he must take things easy'. Although this response may be found in disease at many sites there is a particular foreboding when an 'essential organ' such as the brain, the eyes and the heart are involved. Attempts have been made to grade recovery after treatment; thus Bouchard (1966) used two grades: (*a*) good—active useful life; and (*b*) fair—partial disability. Deeley and Rice-Edwards (1968) assessed their patients as either being able to return to normal work or not; thus a failure to resume their normal activities was assessed as failure to respond to treatment.

When we are considering long-term survivors we may have difficulty in differentiating late recurrence from late irradiation effect.

Palliation

Here we meet a further problem, how much of the improvement can be attributed to the effects of the radiation and how much is due to the surgical decompression and total or partial removal of tumour? There is no doubt that both contribute to the palliation achieved; in some cases decompression produces dramatic effects but the patient may deteriorate again if radiotherapy is not given; radiotherapy alone may produce quite marked palliation, especially in the more anaplastic lesions.

Morbidity

The improvement obtained must be balanced against the untoward effects of radiotherapy; these will include immediate—somewhat transitory—effects and the more permanent effects coming on as a late sequel months or years after the treatment. There is, of course, the problem of the difficulty of making a differential diagnosis between recurrence and radiation effect, a problem exacerbated when we are dealing with a very slow-growing tumour such as an oligodendroglioma. Even when late effects are apparent and symptoms occur any assessment must take into account the number of

144

years symptom-free, the severity of the symptoms and the effect that these may have on living a normal life.

We have thus posed some problems in assessment, the only factual assessment being length of survival. In any comparative, prospective trial aimed at comparing two alternative methods of treatment, it is essential that not only survival but the other factors mentioned above are compared. This demands some attempt at a comparison using, if possible, a grading system to cover all possibilities of palliation, assessment of survival and morbidity. This is a difficult problem which has, so far, not been resolved but to carry out any controlled clinical trial it is necessary that our assessment of results of treatment is satisfactorily reduced to a mathematical level.

Recurrent Tumours

A tumour may recur after surgical removal and a full course of radiotherapy can then be given to the brain; indeed, as we have already seen, this is one method of management in the slow-growing tumours, such as the oligodendrogliomas, where there is a possibility of complete surgical removal. There is no problem in the case where tumour has been left behind after operation—radiation is given in a radical dose to the residual growth. Re-treatment of a recurrence after a previous radical course of radiation raises the serious problem of radiation damage. The factors which must be considered when contemplating re-treatment will be the previous dose given, the possibility of producing late radiation damage, and the possible palliation that may be achieved. Is the palliation that may be achieved worth taking the risk of further damage? If damage is likely to occur will the patient live long enough to develop this? As in repeated treatments at other sites in the body we may consider that palliation is desirable even with its attendant risks because it is unlikely that the patient will survive sufficient length of time to develop damage.

Radiation-induced Malignant Tumours

Recurrent symptoms may be due to radiation necrosis, re-growth of the tumour or to a new growth induced by the previous irradiation. There are now several reports of a fibrosarcoma developing in a previously irradiated brain—summaries of these reports are given by Bouchard (1966), Murphy (1967), Rubin and Casarett (1968), and Zülch (1969). The reported changes have occurred from 5 to 20 years after the initial radiation; the incidence of these tumours is low but must be borne in mind in the differential diagnosis of recurrent intracranial lesions and in assessing the results of treatment.

145

Other Localized Intracranial Tumours

This chapter would be incomplete without mention of other intracranial tumours which may be treated by localized fields.

Meningiomas

The majority of these tumours are benign and the primary treatment is surgery; they are only referred for radiotherapy when surgery has been incomplete because the tumour was adherent to vital structures or invading bone. Post-operative irradiation may also be indicated in these tumours which show sarcomatous changes. There has been considerable variation in the reports of the radio-sensitivity of meningiomas but it has been shown that radiation is worthwhile in those cases where it is known that tumour was left behind after operation.

Pinealomas

There has been considerable discussion about the origin of these tumours, Zimmerman, Netsky and Davidoff (1956) believed that they are teratomatous in origin and that they occur not only in the pineal body but in the surrounding tissues. The site of these lesions makes them unsuitable for operative techniques and they may be referred for radiotherapy without biopsy; however, if subsequent resolution does occur it cannot be associated directly with this pathology.

Vascular Tumours

The haemangiomas are not malignant, being collections of tortuous blood vessels which, if accessible, are treated by surgery. In the inaccessible tumour giving symptoms, such as repeated small haemorrhages, the use of x-ray therapy has been advocated by some workers (Bouchard, 1966). Haemangioblastomas and haemangio-endotheliomas are malignant lesions; treatment is usually surgical but radiotherapy is given if there is incomplete removal or the lesion is at a site which would make surgery hazardous.

Sarcomas

These may be of several types involving various connective tissues; because of this there are marked variations in radio-sensitivity and response to irradiation. Treatment would appear to be surgery in the first instance followed by radiotherapy (Kernohan and Wihlein, 1962).

Reticuloses

Various reticuloses have been reported in the brain, and it is thought that these may have arisen initially in the brain tissue—they are usually rapidly growing.

Metastases

These will be discussed separately in a further chapter. Only about half of the patients have single metastases in the brain and as it is not possible to distinguish these by normal investigative methods the whole brain has to be irradiated.

Radiation therapy may be used to treat those patients with cerebral lesions which are inoperable or in whom operation has left behind residual tumour. The dose of radiation given will depend on the tolerance of the tissues as with the gliomatous tumours.

CONCLUSION

We can now try to put together the points we have discussed, in an attempt to reach some conclusion about the irradiation of those tumours of the brain which can be treated by localized fields. We have discussed only those pathological types which would appear to grow slowly and remain localized; another chapter in this book deals with tumours which are known to disseminate throughout the cerebrospinal system.

The radio-sensitivity of cerebral tumours is a subject which has not been studied fully; the present policy of treatment is to irradiate to tissue tolerance—i.e. the tolerance of the surrounding normal tissues—rather than to the optimum dose necessary to ablate a particular tumour. We have evidence, in the radiotherapy of malignant disease at other sites, that some tumours do not need such high doses as it has been customary to give them. The tolerance dose is based on the known effects of irradiation on normal tissues; this, naturally, is affected by the fractionation and the overall treatment time and in addition by the volume of tissue to be irradiated. There has been a tendency because of the risk of radiation damage, to limit the size of the field but it has been shown quite conclusively that there is a great danger of missing certain tumours, especially those where the tumour infiltrates widely in tissues. If we could localize the tumour accurately we would also need to know what area of apparently normal tissue would need to be included in the field to be irradiated. The problem of localization has been dealt with in previous chapters in this book; great advances have been made but there is still room for considerable improvement. Until we can do this there appears to be little advantage in limiting the size of the irradiated area to that which will tolerate a relatively high dose.

From the evidence presented in the literature it seems that certain tumours are affected by radiation and indeed at certain sites radiotherapy alone will produce a proportion of cures. At other sites surgery alone is sufficient but we have evidence that at others the addition of post-operative irradiation will increase the proportion of cures. It is possible that the normal tissues of the brain will withstand less irradiation after radical surgery than they would normally. We need, therefore, to be sure that attempts at radical surgery are justified; it may be that only sufficient surgery to obtain material for histological examination, or to reduce the increased intracranial pressure, should be attempted and that in some cases it is better not to proceed to partial removal because of the subsequent increase of radiation damage.

We really know very little about the irradiation of cerebral tumours; we need to know much more about their radio-sensitivity, their modes of spread and infiltration, and as a result we will have a better idea of the size of fields to be employed. In radiotherapeutic practice at other sites in the body we have been helped by the use of controlled clinical trials. Can we obtain more information by their use in the treatment of brain tuomurs?; before we discuss these further we must consider what end points may be used for the assessment. Always the least controversial of these is survival; this is factual and there is no problem about measuring it. But, has the patient died from a recurrence or from the radiation effect? This can only be distinguished *post mortem*. When we come to consider morbidity we again meet the problem of whether there is recurrence, radiation damage or even a new growth. Various methods of assessing the value of subsequent life have been developed for other sites and what we need is universal acceptance of some such system for the central nervous system. Obviously we will need pathological proof of the findings at subsequent post-mortem examination.

As a result of considering the points made above possibly controlled clinical trials suggest themselves:

(1) A comparison of surgery with surgery and post-operative radiotherapy in group I and II astrocytomas.

(2) A comparison of immediate post-operative radiotherapy with radiotherapy delayed until such time as recurrent symptoms may develop in cases of oligodendrogliomas.

(3) A comparison of the results of radiation after removal of as much tumour as possible in one group, with removal of only sufficient tissue to obtain histological proof or to reduce the increased intracranial pressure in the second group in cases of glioblastoma multiforme.

(4) Variations of tumour dose given to differing histological types of tumours.

These are a few suggestions only; we must assure adequate tumour coverage, this will mean extension of the work reported earlier in the glioblastomas to cover other tumours at all sites, we must develop methods of localization which are confirmed by subsequent autopsy. The problems of the differential diagnosis of recurrent symptoms will need to be resolved by collating the symptoms with subsequent autopsy findings. The relative paucity of information on the radiation of cerebral tumours will need to be augmented by collecting all information available on a national, or even international, scale.

Improvements will only be made by very careful co-operative studies—carried out by neurologists, neurosurgeons, pathologists and radiotherapists. Although some useful information may be obtained from retrospective analyses this information will serve no more than to indicate the line of future prospective studies. There would appear to be definite possibilities of carrying out some controlled clinical trials at this site.

REFERENCES

Almquist, S., Dahlgren, S., Notter, G. and Sundbom, L. (1964). 'Brain necrosis after irradiation of the hypophysis in Cushing's disease.' *Acta radiol.*, **2**, 179.

Aristizibal, S. A. and Caldwell, W. L. (1971). 'Time–dose–volume relationships in the treatment of glioblastoma multiforme.' *Radiology*, **101**, 201.

Arnold, A., Bailey, P. and Laughlin, J. S. (1954). 'Effects of Betatron radiation on the brain of primates.' *Neurology*, **4**, 165.

Asscher, A. W. and Anson, S. G. (1962). 'Arterial hypertension and irradiation damage due to the nervous system.' *Lancet*, **2**, 1343.

Boden, G. (1948). 'Radiation myelitis of the cervical cord.' *Br. J. Radiol.*, **21**, 464.

— (1950). 'Radiation myelitis of the brain stem.' *J. Fac. Radiol.*, **2**, 79.

Bouchard, J. (1966). *Radiation Therapy of Tumours and Diseases of the Nervous System*. London; Henry Kimpton.

— and Peirce, C. B. (1960). 'Radiation therapy in the management of neoplasms of the central nervous system, with a special note in regard to children: twenty years experience, 1939–1958.' *Am. J. Roentgenol.*, **84**, 610.

Buckley, T. F. (1969). 'The direct irradiation of cerebal gliomata.' *Clin. Radiol.*, **20**, 219.

Bull, J. W. D. and Rovit, R. L. (1957). 'Radiographic localization of intracerebral gliomata.' *J. Fac. Radiol.*, **8**, 147.

Churchill-Davidson, I. (1967). 'Oxygen therapy—clinical experiences.' In *Modern Trends in Radiotherapy*, Ed. by T. J. Deeley and Constance A. P. Wood. London; Butterworths.

Concannon, J. P., Kramer, S. and Berry R. (1960). 'The extent of intra-cranial gliomata at autopsy and its relationship to techniques used in radiation therapy of brain tumours.' *Am. J. Roentgenol.*, **84**, 99.

Cushing, H. (1932). *Intracranial Tumours*. Springfield, Ill.; Thomas.

Deeley, T. J. and Rice-Edwards, J. M. (1968). 'Radiotherapy in the management of cerebral secondaries from bronchial carcinoma.' *Lancet*, **1**, 1209.

Edland, R. W., Javid, M. and Ansfield, F. J. (1971). 'Glioblastoma multiforme. An analysis of the results of post-operative radiotherapy alone versus radiotherapy and concomitant 5-Fluorouracil.' *Am. J. Roentgenol.*, **111**, 337.

Freid, J. R. and Davidoff, L. M. (1951). 'Roentgen therapy of primary neoplasms of the brain.' *Radiology*, **57**, 25.

Horak. G. (1954). 'Benign "favourable" types of brain tumour, end results (up to 20 years) with statistics of mortality and useful survival.' *New Engl. J. Med.*, **250**, 981.

Jones, A. (1960). 'Supervoltage x-ray therapy of intra-cranial tumours.' *Ann. R. Coll. Surg. Engl.*, **27**, 310.

Kernohan, J. W. and Sayre, G. P. (1952). *Tumours of the Central Nervous System*, Section X. Fasciles 35 and 37. Washington D.C., Armed Forces Institute of Pathology.

— and Wihlein, A. (1962). *Sarcoma of the Brain*. Springfield, Ill.; Thomas.

Kramer, S. (1969). 'Tumour extent as a determining factor in radiotherapy of glioblastomas.' *Acta Radiol.*, **8**, 111.

Lampert, P., Tom, M. I. and Rider, W. D. (1959). 'Disseminated demyelination of the brain following ^{60}Co (gamma) radiation.' *Archs Path.*, **69**, 322.

Lawrence, J. H. and Tobias, C. A. (1967). 'Heavy particles in therapy.' In *Modern Trends in Radiotherapy*, Ed. by T. J. Deeley and Constance A. P. Wood. London; Butterworths.

Levy, L. F. and Elvidge, A. R. (1956). 'Astrocytoma of the brain and spinal cord; a review of 176 cases 1940–1949.' *J. Neurosurg.*, **13**, 413.

Lindgren, M. (1958). 'On tolerance of brain tissue and sensitivity of brain tumours to irradiation.' *Acta radiol.*, Suppl. 170.

Llewellyn, R. C. and Creech, O. Jr. (1962). 'Perfusion for cerebral tumours.' In *The Biology and Treatment of Intra-cranial Tumours*, Ed. by W. S. Fields and P. C. Sharkey. Springfield, Ill.; Thomas.

MacCarty, C. S. (1962). 'Results of the surgical management of glial tumours of the brain.' In *The Biology and Treatment of Intra-cranial Tumours*, Ed. by W. S. Fields and P. C. Sharkey. Springfield, Ill.; Thomas.

Mitchell, J. S. (1960). *Studies in Radiotherapeutics*. Cambridge, Mass.; Harvard University Press.

Murphy, W. T. (1967). 'Cancer of the central nervous system.' In *Radiation Therapy*. Philadelphia; Saunders.

Nessa, C. B. (1938). 'Effect of treatment of brain tumors with roentgen rays.' *Radiology*, **31**, 670.

Pennybacker, J. and Russell, D. S. (1948). 'Necrosis of the brain due to radiation therapy; clinical and pathological observations.' *J. Neurol. Neurosurg. Psychiat.*, **11**, 183.

Phillips, T. L., Sheline, G. E. and Boldney, E. (1964). 'Tumours affecting central nervous system; ependymoma.' *Radiology*, **83**, 98.

Pierce, C. B., Cone, W. V., Eldvidge, A. E. and Tye, J. G. (1945). 'Roentgentherapy of primary neoplasms of the brain and brain stem.' *Radiology*, **45**, 247.

Richmond, J. Jackson (1949). 'Radiotherapy of cerebral tumours.' *J. Fac. Radiol.*, **1**, 23.

— (1959). 'Malignant tumours of the central nervous system.' In *Cancer*, Ed. by R. W. Raven. London; Butterworths.

Rubin, P. and Casarett, G. W. (1968). *Clinical Radiation Pathology*. Philadelphia; Saunders.

Sachs, E. (1954). 'The treatment of glioblastoma with radium.' *J. Neurosurg.*, **11**, 119.

Sagerman, R. H., Bagshaw, M. A. and Hanbery J. (1965). 'Considerations in the treatment of ependymoma.' *Radiology*, **84**, 401.

Sheline, G. E., Boldrey, E., Karlsberg, P. and Phillips, T. L. (1964). 'Therapeutic consideration in tumours affecting the central nervous system: oligodendrogliomas.' *Radiology*, **82**, 84.

— Phillips, T. L. and Boldrey, E. (1965). 'The therapy of unbiopsied brain tumours.' *Am. J. Roentgenol.*, **93**, 664.

Shenkin, H. A. (1965). 'The effect of roentgen-ray therapy on oligodendrogliomas of the brain.' *J. Neurosurg.*, **22**, 57.

Stenberg, B. and Moberg, A. (1971). 'Radiotherapy of intracerebral astrocytoma.' *Acta radiol.*, **10**, 27.

Talairach, J., Ruggiero, G., Aboulker, J. and David, M. (1955). *Br. J. Radiol.*, **28**, 62.

Taveras, J. M., Thompson, H. J. and Pool, J. L. (1962). 'Should we treat glioblastoma multiforme?' *Am. J. Roentgenol.*, **87**, 473.

Todd, I. D. H. (1963). 'Choice of volume in the x-ray treatment of supratentorial gliomas.' *Br. J. Radiol.*, **36**, 645.

Vaeth, J. (1965). 'Radiation induced myelitis.' In *Progress in Radiation Therapy*, Vol. III, Ed. by F. Buschke. New York; Grune & Stratton.

Whyte, T. R., Colby, M. Y. and Layton, D. D. (1969). 'Radiation therapy of brain-stem tumours.' *Radiology*, **93**, 413.

Zeman, W. and Samorajski, T. (1971). 'Effects of irradiation on nervous system.' In *Pathology of Irradiation*, Ed. by J. S. C. C. Berd. Baltimore; Williams & Wilkins.

Zimmerman, H. M., Netsky, M. G. and Davidoff, L. M. (1956). *Atlas of Tumours of the Nervous System*. Philadelphia; Lea & Febiger.

Zülch, K. J. (1969). 'Roentgen sensitivity of cerebral tumours and so-called late irradiation necrosis of the brain.' *Acta radiol.*, **8**, 92.
Zuppinger, A. (1967). 'Treatment by supervoltage machines—electron beam therapy.' In *Modern Trends in Radiotherapy—I*, Ed. by T. J. Deeley and Constance A. P. Wood. London; Butterworths.

7—Whole Central Nervous System Irradiation

J. M. Henk

In some malignant diseases of the central nervous system tumour cells may spread by way of the cerebrospinal fluid, to give rise to multiple seedling deposits in the ventricular system and in the arachnoid of the brain and spinal canal. Tumours which behave in this way are mainly relatively radio-sensitive, so that their treatment by irradiation of the whole cerebrospinal fluid space is a practical proposition. In 1925, Bailey and Cushing identified the medulloblastoma; they recognized that its cells were uniquely vulnerable to radiation and also noted metastases in the meninges of the spinal canal. They therefore advocated systematic irradiation of the brain and spinal axis in all cases, a practice which is now universally adopted as the standard treatment for this disease. Whole central nervous system irradiation was later applied to ependymoma and pinealoma; more recently it has been used extensively in the treatment and prophylaxis of meningeal leukaemia.

MEDULLOBLASTOMA

Pathology

The medulloblastoma is an uncommon tumour. Estimates of its incidence vary between 3·8 per cent (Zulch, 1965) and 7·1 per cent (Russell and Rubinstein, 1963) of all brain tumours. At least 80 per cent of medulloblastomas occur in children under the age of 15, in whom this tumour comprises approximately 20 per cent of all intracranial neoplasms; it is twice as common in boys as girls (Crue, 1958). Its histogenesis is the subject of much controversy. The most widely held view is that of an embryonal tumour arising from undifferentiated cells derived from the germinal bud of the cerebellum during foetal life, capable of differentiation into both neuronal and glial elements. Persistent foci of these primitive cells may be found in the posterior medullary velum in children and occasionally also in adults (Raaf and Kernohan, 1944). This theory is in keeping with the fact that the most common site of origin of the tumour is the roof of the fourth ventricle. Similar primitive cells are found in the external granular layer of the cerebellum, which normally disappears during early childhood, hence the occasional origin of the tumour within the cerebellar hemispheres. In older children and young adults the medulloblastoma in the cerebellar hemisphere often excites a considerable stromal reaction, so that connective tissue elements, especially abundant reticulin, are conspicuous on histological examination. A tumour with these characteristics has been thought by some to be of different origin and has been given the name of 'cerebellar arachnoid sarcoma'. However, it is now no longer regarded generally as a distinct entity but merely a variant of the medulloblastoma (Rubinstein and Northfield, 1964) and should be treated as such.

Medulloblastoma presents as a posterior fossa tumour. Its characteristic clinical features and natural history are superbly described by Cushing (1930). Spread of malignant cells into the cerebrospinal fluid occurs readily, so that multiple seedling arachnoidal and ventricular deposits are the rule. These are most often found in the spinal canal; presumable cells settle in the spine under the influence of gravity. They may also be found in the ventricular system and over the surface of the brain.

Blood-borne metastases have been reported more frequently in medulloblastoma than in any other primary cerebral tumour. The most frequent manifestation of blood-borne spread is that of multiple osteosclerotic skeletal secondaries (Black and Keats, 1964); there are now over 20 other separate reports of such spread confirmed at autopsy.

Treatment

There is no doubt that medulloblastoma is the most radio-sensitive of all cerebral neoplasms, and that whole central nervous system irradiation offers the only hope of a cure. The role of surgery is less clear. It is never possible to remove the tumour completely, and operative mortality is high, so that in 1936 Cutler, Sosman and Vaughan suggested that suspected medulloblastoma be treated by radiotherapy alone, avoiding any form of surgical procedure. They suggested a small local dose of radiation as a therapeutic test in the differential diagnosis of medulloblastoma from other posterior fossa tumours; if rapid improvement occurred the diagnosis was assumed to be medulloblastoma and radiotherapy continued; in the absence of such improvement exploration was undertaken. This policy was not widely accepted because most neurosurgeons and radiotherapists prefer to have a firm histological diagnosis before embarking on definitive treatment, there being other lesions which produce a similar clinical picture but which must be treated very differently, e.g. the cerebellar astrocytoma by radical surgery, the brain-stem glioma by local radiotherapy. Aspiration biopsy as a prelude to radiotherapy was proposed by Peirce and colleagues (1949), but is not without risk and has not gained wide acceptance, as a mortality of 3 out of 24 cases was reported by Berger and Elvidge (1963). The surgical procedure usually adopted is a posterior fossa craniotomy, with removal of as much of the tumour as possible. This both establishes a histological diagnosis and reduces intracranial pressure. The fewer the malignant cells present at the time of starting radiotherapy the greater the chance they will all be destroyed, so removal of the main bulk of the tumour should at least theoretically increase the chance of a radiotherapeutic success. The advantages of surgery seem far to outweigh the loss from operative mortality.

Radiotherapy should begin as soon after the operation as possible. In the very ill child with a large amount of tumour still present at the primary site it is advisable to begin with small doses confined to the posterior fossa, proceeding to whole central nervous system when the general condition improves. In a patient in reasonably good condition it is advisable to treat the whole volume from the outset.

The posterior fossa must receive a high dose, because the most usual cause of treatment failure is recurrence at the primary site (Bloom, Wallace and Henk, 1969). With supervoltage radiation a tumour dose of about 4,500 rads in five weeks, or 5,000 rads in seven weeks, is usually recommended. The remainder of the subarachnoid space must also be irradiated in an endeavour to eliminate any microscopic seedling deposits; for such 'prophylatic' irradiation 3,000 rads in five weeks using supervoltage (or equivalent dosage for different treatment times or qualities of radiation) is probably adequate. Viable malignant cells may be floating freely in the cerebrospinal fluid, so ideally the whole volume should be treated at each session.

The radiotherapy technique must be designed so that the desired dose is given to the central nervous system with minimal dosage to surrounding normal tissues, especially sensitive structures such as the lens of the eye and the thyroid gland. The basic principle is to irradiate the entire cerebrospinal fluid space, that is the whole brain, basal cisterns and spinal canal as low as the termination of the arachnoid at the second sacral segment. Regions sometimes under-dosed include the tips of the temporal lobes (Green and George, 1970) and the projections of arachnoid into the spinal foramina. To avoid such possibilities the lower border of the skull fields should be a line running through the supra-orbital ridge and the tip of the mastoid process, while spinal fields should always be wide enough to cover the whole vertebrae including the transverse processes.

Using orthovoltage the brain can be treated by lateral and posterior fields and the spine by multiple posterior fields (Bloom, Wallace and Henk, 1969). A more complex orthovoltage technique achieving better homogeneity of dose distribution has been described by Paterson and Farr (1953) who used a large spade-shaped posterior field at long f.s.d., including the skull and spine, the anterior part of the brain being treated originally by two anterior oblique ortho-voltage fields, and more recently by lateral wedged cobalt fields (Paterson, 1963). This technique has been further refined by Bottrill, Rogers and Hope-Stone (1965) using a specially constructed copper filter for the posterior field, achieving a uniform dose throughout the spinal canal. These orthovoltage techniques have the disadvantage of skin reaction, increased bone absorption, and an unduly long treatment time which for the spinal field may be as much as 30 minutes. In addition, it is almost impossible to avoid some dosage to both the eye and the thyroid gland. These problems can largely be overcome with supervoltage irradiation if the brain and cervical spine are treated by lateral fields and the remainder of the spine by a posterior field, although there is then a higher dose to the abdominal organs. A cobalt technique on these latter principles has been described by Chang, Housepian and Herbert (1969).

Protracted fractionation is essential in the treatment of a volume of tissue as large as that of the whole central nervous system. Brain-stem tolerance determines the posterior fossa dose, but the bone marrow is the critical normal tissue limiting the dose which can be given to the spine. It is standard practice to prescribe a tumour dose of 120–150 rads per day, and to 'rest' the patient from treatment if the white blood count falls below 2,000; in some cases it may be necessary to abandon treatment short of the intended total dosage if the count cannot be maintained above this level. More prolonged treatment with an initial dose per fraction of 50 rads, gradually increasing to 150 rads, minimizes the effect on bone marrow as judged by the rate of fall of the white blood count. However, it is not known whether such fractionation has a similar 'sparing' effect on the tumour cells to that on the marrow! Also, there is some evidence that stem cells migrate into irradiated marrow from non-irradiated areas; should this process occur continuously during a course of radiotherapy, the more protracted treatment with higher total dosage may be expected to cause the greater long-term exhaustion of the bone marrow. A great deal more must be learned about the cell kinetics of both the tumour and the normal bone marrow before optimum fractionation schemes can be designed.

Prognosis

Studies of survival rates after whole central nervous system irradiation show that the concept of medulloblastoma as an inevitably fatal disease is no longer tenable. McFarland and colleagues (1969) collected the data from 23 publications and concluded that 10 per cent of patients had lived 15 years or more from the time of first treatment. More recent series suggest that the survival rates have increased with the use of more homogeneous whole central nervous system irradiation, and now approximately one-third of patients completing their radiotherapy are completely cured of their disease (Table 1). The small series reported by Hope-Stone (1970) suggest that meticulous attention to technique may bring further improvement in results. Nevertheless many patients die before any treatment can be instituted, and operative mortality remains high. McFarland and colleagues (1969) analysed 18 publications with adequate data, and found a cumulative operative mortality of 24 per cent. Pearson (1971) estimates that at the present time in the Manchester region approximately one-third of all patients with medulloblastoma do not receive a full course of radiotherapy because of mortality and morbidity before and after operation. Considering all factors the current cure rate in Great Britain appears to be about 20 per cent.

TABLE 1

Survival of Patients with Medulloblastoma Treated by
Whole Central Nervous System Irradiation

Author	No. of patients treated	Five-year survival rate %
Paterson (1958)	27	41
Smith, Lampe and Kahn (1961)	8	62
Bouchard (1966)	62	32
Bloom, Wallace and Henk (1969)	58	38
Chang, Housepian and Herbert (1969)	6	50
Hope-Stone (1970)	13	77
Nöel and Méthot (1970)	13	46
Aron (1971)	22	40

Significant factors influencing prognosis of medulloblastoma are difficult to find. Paterson (1958), McFarland and colleagues (1969) and several others have all drawn attention to the higher survival rates in girls compared with boys. The age of the patient at presentation does not appear to affect the ultimate outcome, although the younger the patient the sooner will he die if treatment be unsuccessful. The outlook seems a little better for those patients in whom the tumour was not invading the brain stem, where a complete macroscopic removal was possible. Neither the length of history, nor the histological features of the tumour have been demonstrated to have any correlation with survival rate.

Some of the patients successfully treated have considerable residual disability, but the majority of survivors are able to live an active life and at least half have no apparent mental or physical sequelae (Bloom, Wallace and Henk, 1969).

Recurrence

The majority of recurrences of medulloblastoma occur within the first two years after treatment, but some may appear many years later. Collins (1955) defined a 'period of risk' for embryonal tumours equal to the age of the patient at presentation plus nine months. This concept assumes that the tumour beginning *in utero* becomes clinically manifest after a period of time determined by its growth rate which remains constant. If the malignant cells not destroyed by treatment maintain the same growth rate the tumour should attain a clinically recognizable size within the same period of time, i.e. age at presentation plus the nine months' gestation period. Recurrences are expected to occur before this period of risk has elapsed; the patient is assumed to be cured if he survives longer without clinical evidence of disease. Medulloblastoma appears to follow this rule with only occasional exceptions. There are very few histologically authenticated cases of recurrences occurring after a lapse of time longer than Collins' period of risk. It is advisable to consider an alternative diagnosis, for example a radiation-induced fibrosarcoma (*vide infra*), when symptoms suggestive of recurrence occur after the end of the period of risk.

Recurrence most commonly occurs first in the posterior fossa, but it may appear elsewhere in the central nervous system, and occasionally multiple deposits become clinically manifest at the same time. In patients in fairly good general condition in whom recurrent tumour is causing distressing symptoms, e.g. headache, dysphagia or root pain, palliative radiotherapy is often worthwhile. In such cases the treatment should be limited to the affected area and the dose given restricted to that which brings relief: 1,500 rads in two weeks is usually adequate. A higher dose with more radical intent can be given to any recurrence developing in a previously untreated or under-dosed area. Occasionally re-treatment can give a further period of good health lasting several years, especially in patients who have had a long disease-free interval before recurrence appears.

Recurrent tumour can sometimes be controlled for fairly long periods by the use of cytotoxic drugs. Intrathecal methotrexate has been used with some success; its value in medulloblastoma has been comprehensively discussed by Wilson (1970). Intravenous vincristine has been shown to be effective in causing regression of some recurrent medulloblastoma (Lassman, Pearce and Gang, 1965; Lampkin, Maurer and McBride, 1967). This drug is extremely toxic if given intrathecally, and so it must be administered systemically. It has the advantage of causing only minimal marrow depression so it can safely be combined with extensive radiation. Trials are now in progress in several centres to ascertain the value of vincristine when given pre-operatively and as long-term maintenance therapy after radiotherapy. The routine use of cytotoxic drugs in this manner has improved the prognosis considerably in other embryonic tumours, notably nephroblastoma, so the results of such trials are awaited with interest.

EPENDYMOMA

The ependymoma is another relatively uncommon tumour. Its incidence is less than 10 per cent of all intracranial gliomas. It is a tumour of childhood and early adult life. It can arise in any part of the brain, but in over half the cases it arises in the posterior fossa, most commonly in the floor of the fourth ventricle. It may also occur in the spinal cord, and in the cauda equina where it arises from the filum terminale. The histological appearance of this tumour varies from the benign to the highly malignant. Those of a more benign histological appearance are generally slow-growing with a long natural history but are not necessarily the most likely to be cured. The most malignant varieties of ependymoma which show tumour cells of embryonal type with increased mitotic activity are often termed 'ependymoblastoma' (Rubinstein, 1970).

The majority of ependymomata respond to radiotherapy, the routine use of which has been shown to improve the prognosis in those patients in whom complete surgical removal of the tumour

159

could not be achieved (Barone and Elvidge, 1970). The ependymo-blastoma responds especially well, and is probably the second most radio-sensitive primary intracranial tumour. The advisability of whole central nervous system irradiation in ependymoma is the subject of considerable controversy, arising from disagreement about the incidence of central nervous system metastases. It has been recognized for many years that the tumour can spread in the cerebrospinal fluid, giving rise to multiple arachnoid deposits, first described by Spiller (1907). There is a surprising difference in the incidence of this phenomenon between various reported series, not easily explained. For instance, Phillips, Sheline and Boldrey (1964) and Kricheff and colleagues (1964) found clinical evidence of seeding in only 2 out of 42, and 1 out of 72 cases, respectively, of intracranial ependymoma, and accordingly advised against whole central nervous system irradiation. On the other hand, Svein, Gates and Kernohan (1949) studied 19 autopsies of patients with intracranial ependymoma and found evidence of seeding in 6 out of 12 cases where the primary was in the fourth ventricle, but no evidence of seeding in 7 where the tumour arose supratentorially. Sagerman, Bagshaw and Hanbery (1965) found clinical evidence of seeding in 6 out of 11 cases; 7 were infra-tentorial of whom 5 seeded. These latter authors rightly point out that the highest incidence of seeding are reported in groups of patients seen and followed up by one group of physicians, where there is a high proportion of autopsy examinations in fatal cases, compared with the larger series in whom information was obtained mainly from hospital notes with very few autopsies available.

Ependymoma is most often treated by excision, followed by local radiotherapy in those cases where complete removal was not possible. The prognosis after such therapy is tolerably good—for example Bouchard (1966) reported a five-year survival rate of 70 per cent in 20 patients treated and advised against whole central nervous system irradiation. Nevertheless with increasingly effective radiation to the primary tumour clinical manifestations of metastases in the spinal canal are being seen more frequently, especially where the primary was situated in the fourth ventricle. I have personally seen five such cases. The fourth ventricular ependymoblastoma often resembles the medulloblastoma in its clinical features, behaviour and radio-sensitivity, and indeed may be confused with it histologically; it is best treated in a similar manner, that is, by irradiation to the posterior fossa to the maximum tolerable dosage and to the remainder of the cerebrospinal axis prophylactically. In all other types of ependymoma seeding is rare, so the radiation should be limited to the known extent of the tumour.

PINEALOMA

A variety of histological types of tumour occur in the pineal body. All are relatively rare. Two of them, namely the pinealoblastoma and the atypical teratoma, are very radio-sensitive, and may occasionally spread by way of the cerebrospinal fluid (Fowler, Alexander and Davis, 1956). However, a positive histological diagnosis is rarely obtained in patients with pineal tumours, biopsy being extremely dangerous (Davidoff, 1966; Cole, 1971). When a patient presents with clinical and radiological features of a pineal tumour the treatment of choice is a Torkildsen (1939) shunt followed by radiotherapy.

Spinal canal metastases occur in less than 10 per cent of all pineal tumours (Maier and Dejong, 1967). The radiotherapist is therefore usually confronted with a patient in whom no histological diagnosis has been made, with only a very small chance of cerebrospinal fluid spread. In such circumstances irradiation of the whole cerebrospinal axis is not justified. Radiotherapy should be localized to the tumour itself, using fairly generous fields to cover possible local infiltration. Long survival after such treatment is the rule; nearly all patients live at least five years.

MENINGEAL LEUKAEMIA

The most spectacular improvement in treatment of malignancy in the past few years has been seen in the field of acute lymphoblastic leukaemia. In children with this disease the use of multi-agent combination chemotherapy has radically altered the prognosis, so that survival rates of over 70 per cent at two years and over 20 per cent at five years may now be expected (Holland, 1970). Intensive combination therapy, followed by prolonged maintenance therapy, with cytotoxic drugs is now very successful at inducing and maintaining complete haematological remission. It has become apparent, however, that remission is frequently terminated by proliferation of leukaemic cells in 'sanctuary' areas of the body which are relatively inaccessible to cytotoxic agents administered systemically. Of such areas the central nervous system is by far the most important, as none of the drugs commonly used in the treatment of acute leukaemia will cross the blood–brain barrier in sufficient concentration to attain therapeutic levels in the cerebrospinal fluid. Leukaemic cells can enter the subarachnoid space, probably by diapedesis from small vessels crossing it (Thomas, 1965). There they proliferate to form infiltrates around the vessels entering the brain substance and also spread in the cerebrospinal fluid, where they can be identified in a lumbar puncture

161

specimen. Eventually symptoms of meningeal irritation and raised intracranial pressure appear.

In patients treated by systemic cytotoxic agents meningeal involvement develops in half the patients within one year of attaining haematological remission and is the most frequent cause of relapse (Aur and colleagues, 1971). Treatment by intrathecal injections of methotrexate relieves symptoms and signs, but recurrence inevitably appears within about four months. Small doses of radiotherapy to the whole central nervous system, to a total dosage of 500–1,000 rads, may also relieve symptoms temporarily. Much longer remission, permanent in some cases, can be achieved by initial intrathecal methotrexate, followed by radiotherapy in higher dosage. There is no doubt that for best results at least 2,500 rads must be given to the whole brain, but it is not clear whether such a large dose need be given to the spine with its smaller volume of nervous tissue. Spinal irradiation can lead to serious marrow depression in patients who have already received intensive cytotoxic drug therapy. A compromise regime commonly employed consists of 2,500 rads in three weeks to the whole brain, with 1,000 rads to the spinal canal during the third week.

Radiotherapy to the central nervous system is now being used 'prophylactically' as part of the initial therapy for acute lymphoblastic leukaemia, in an attempt to prevent the development of meningeal involvement. The treatment is given as soon as possible, usually within the first three months of therapy, after induction of remission with vincristine and prednisone, followed by a short term of intensive chemotherapy with antimetabolites and alkylating agents. The best results to date from such an approach are those of Aur and colleagues (1971) who have reported the use of irradiation to the whole brain to a dose of 2,400 rads in $2\frac{1}{2}$ weeks, at the same time giving methotrexate 12 mg/m^2 intrathecally twice weekly for five doses. Thirty patients treated by this regime attained remission and were followed up for at least two years; only three developed meningeal leukaemia. An alternative and probably equally effective method of prophylaxis of meningeal laukaemia is to treat both brain and spine to a tumour dose of 2,500 rads in four weeks, without exhibition of methotrexate. This avoids repeated lumbar punctures and possible central nervous system toxicity of methotrexate, but may be more marrow depressant and so limit subsequent chemotherapy.

Technique

Treatment fields should cover the whole subarachnoid space as for medulloblastoma. Deposits sometimes occur in the optic nerves so it is advisable to include the posterior half of the orbits in the cranial fields. Where the higher doses are to be given to the spinal canal it is advisable to treat the upper cervical spine by lateral fields in continuity with the cranial fields, preventing any appreciable exit dose to the lenses of the eyes and facilitating accurate 'junction' of spinal fields.

COMPLICATIONS OF RADIATION TREATMENT

Acute Effects

There are few immediate complications of whole central nervous system irradiation, apart from the effect on the bone marrow already discussed. Nausea, vomiting and skin reaction are rarely major problems. Epilation always occurs, but if supervoltage is used the hair usually re-grows within two to six months after completion of treatment.

Late Effects

The majority of patients are children, some of whom survive very many years, so great attention must be paid to possible long-term complications of radiotherapy, i.e. delayed damage to normal tissues and induced malignancy.

Central Nervous System

The effect of irradiation on the normal human brain is extremely difficult to study, so that tolerance levels are not easy to define. The most useful information is obtained from patients in whom parts of the central nervous system, not in themselves diseased, are irradiated in the course of treatment for a nearby extracranial neoplasm. Boden (1948) was able to define spinal cord tolerance from a series of patients in whom the cervical spine was irradiated in the course of treatment for head and neck carcinomata. He demonstrated that doses in excess of 3,500 rads in 17 days with orthovoltage radiation carried a high risk of damage. He later demonstrated that the tolerance of the brain stem was similar to that of the cervical cord (Boden, 1950). All Boden's patients were treated in a period of 17 days. Using Strandquist's (1944) formula relating tolerance of normal skin to treatment time he estimated tolerance levels for times up to eight weeks. However, Vaeth (1965) has produced data to suggest that for treatment times of six weeks or longer the tolerance of the cervical spinal cord is greater than that predicted by Boden. He found that 6,000 rads in seven weeks with 1 MeV radiation was well tolerated. Lindgren (1958) published data for 17 cases of necrosis of brain

163

tissue that was considered free of tumour, and plotted time–dose curves in a manner similar to that of Boden. These suggested that the tolerance level of the cerebral hemisphere is about 10 per cent higher than that of the brain stem and spinal cord. This is in accordance with findings in monkeys by Clemente and Holst (1954) who irradiated the heads of monkeys and found much greater destruction of neurons in the brain stem compared with the cerebrum and the cerebellum. In patients treated for paranasal sinus and nasopharyngeal carcinoma, brain-stem damage is an occasional complication but the temporal lobes are rarely damaged despite usually receiving larger doses of radiation. There does, therefore, seem to be quite conclusive evidence that the brain stem is the most vulnerable to radiation of all the intracranial tissues.

In the above studies 'tolerance' is defined as the dose of irradiation which carries a negligible risk of gross brain necrosis. To avoid this complication the maximum dose to the brain stem from supervoltage irradiation should not exceed 4,500 rads in five weeks, or 5,000 rads in seven weeks, assuming five fractions per week. These dose levels are not normally exceeded in the course of whole central nervous system irradiation for medulloblastoma or ependymoblastoma, so that necrosis is unlikely, and has not been described. However, one cannot be so certain about the possibility of more subtle neurological damage which may lead to mild or moderate degrees of functional impairment in long-term survivors, especially when the irradiation is given to young children. Physiological changes can certainly be demonstrated after very small doses. For example, Zeleny (1956) demonstrated inhibition of conditioned reflexes in rats after whole brain irradiation with 200 rads. There is also apprehension about the possible interference with development of the central nervous system when very young children are subjected to whole-brain irradiation, but there seems little risk of this since neurons do not undergo mitosis after the seventh foetal month, and myelination is complete in most regions of the brain by the age of two. Evidence on both these latter risks in man is scanty, and can only be obtained from long-term follow up of successfully treated patients. Such studies in children under the age of 15 irradiated for brain tumours have been presented by Bouchard (1966) and Bloom, Wallace and Henk (1969). In these series the majority of survivors were living active useful lives. Where there was neurological deficit this could be attributed to the damage resulting from the original tumour and its associated hydrocephalus. Behaviour problems were fairly common but were most likely due to psychological difficulties resulting from a prolonged illness and parents who had been given a gloomy prognosis. There are numerous examples among those who have reached adult life who are able to earn their living at a skilled occupation.

There is no evidence to date in man that irradiation of the whole central nervous system to the dosage recommended in this chapter leads to any subsequent neurological or intellectual impairment. Bouchard points out that his 'post-irradiation brain tumour patients treated during infancy and childhood have grown physically and developed mentally as well as any other group of comparable size might have done if picked at random in the general population'.

Other Normal Tissues

The lens of the eye receives doses of between 700 and 1,200 rads with most orthovoltage techniques, at which level the occasional cataract may be expected (Merriam and Focht, 1957). Irradiation of the spine produces some disturbance of growth, but the spinal epiphyses are treated uniformly so scoliosis does not usually occur. However, there may be slight reduction in stature, the limbs appearing disproportionately long when the patient reaches adult life.

Endocrine development in long-term survivors is normal. There is no foundation for the widely held belief that irradiation of the pituitary in childhood may lead to hypopituitarism. Bouchard (1966) presented the results of follow-up of 119 children treated by radiotherapy for intracranial tumours five years or more previously, and found no cases of pituitary deficiency. The occasional case of pituitary insufficiency after irradiation has been reported but the doses given were far in excess of those used for the treatment of cerebral tumours.

From orthovoltage techniques the dose to the ovaries is approximately 120 rads and to the scrotum approximately 75 rads. Therefore, there may possibly be some genetic hazard and risk of sterility. Nevertheless female patients menstruate normally and there are now numerous reports of patients becoming mothers or fathers to normal offspring many years after treatment in childhood.

Malignancy

Radiation is known to be carcinogenic to the thyroid, especially in young children. When the cervical spine is treated by a single posterior field the thyroid gland receives between 1,000 and 2,000 rads according to the energy used. This dose level in children may be expected to induce the occasional thyroid carcinoma, and indeed several cases have been reported following radiotherapy to the whole central nervous system (Raventos and Duszynski, 1963; Andrews and Kerr, 1965). Fortunately most radiation-induced tumours of the thyroid are of the well-differentiated papillary type with a good prognosis after surgical removal (Hempelman and colleagues, 1967).

Radiation-induced fibrosarcoma of the brain is a rare phenomenon but one which should not be overlooked. This tumour usually occurs after an interval of not less than six years following irradiation. It probably arises from the dura in the irradiated field and infiltrates brain tissue. It is seen most often after radiotherapy for benign tumours, especially chromophobe adenoma of the pituitary, not surprisingly since prolonged survival following treatment of these conditions is the rule. However, two cases have been reported following whole central nervous system irradiation for medulloblastoma (Noetzli and Malamud, 1962; Waltz and Brownell, 1966). Successful surgical extirpation of a fibrosarcoma may be possible, so it is always advisable to consider this diagnosis when signs of a further intra-cranial tumour appear a number of years after treatment for medulloblastoma.

Malignant tumours in other tissues are seen occasionally. For example, osteosarcoma of the skull has been reported by Berg, Landberg and Lindgren (1966). Hope-Stone (1970) reported a case of a basal-cell carcinoma of the scalp in a 20-year-old woman, 13 years after radiotherapy.

SUMMARY

Radiotherapy to the whole central nervous system is mandatory in medulloblastoma, where cure without radiation damage is possible in about 20 per cent of cases. Similar treatment is advised for fourth ventricular ependymoblastoma, but not for other ependymomata or for pineal tumours. Irradiation of the brain and spinal canal to a moderate dosage is effective for both treatment and prophylaxis of meningeal involvement in acute leukaemia. The majority of patients undergoing whole central nervous system radiotherapy are children, so late radiation sequelae are occasionally seen, but are insignificant in comparison with the gravity of the disease for which the treatment is given.

REFERENCES

Andrews, D. S. and Kerr, I. F. (1965). 'Carcinoma of the thyroid following irradiation for medulloblastoma.' *Clin. Radiol.*, **16**, 282.

Aron, B. S. (1971). 'Medulloblastoma in children, 22 years' experience with radiation therapy.' *Am. J. Dis. Child.*, **121**, 314.

REFERENCES

Aur, R. J. A., Simone, J., Hustu, H. O., Walters, T., Borella, L., Pratt, C. and Pinkel, D. (1971). 'Central nervous system therapy and combination chemotherapy of childhood lymphocytic leukaemia.' *Blood*, **37**, 272.

Bailey, P. and Cushing, H. (1925). 'Medulloblastoma cerebelli, common type of mid-cerebellar glioma of childhood.' *Archs Neurol. Psychiat.*, **14**, 192.

Barone, B. M. and Elvidge, A. R. (1970). 'Ependymomas, a clinical survey.' *J. Neurosurg.*, **33**, 428.

Berg, N. O., Landberg, T. and Lindgren, M. (1966). 'Osteonecrosis and sarcoma following irradiation of intracerebral tumours.' *Acta radiol.*, **4**, 417.

Berger, E. C. and Elvidge, A. R. (1963). 'Medulloblastoma and cerebellar sarcomas: clinical survey.' *J. Neurosurg.*, **20**, 139.

Black, S. P. and Keats, T. E. (1964). 'Generalized osteosclerosis secondary to metastatic medulloblastoma of cerebellum.' *Radiology*, **82**, 395.

Bloom, H. J. G., Wallace, E. N. K. and Henk, J. M. (1969). 'The treatment and prognosis of medulloblastoma in children.' *Am. J. Roentgenol.*, **105**, 43.

Boden, G. (1948). 'Radiation myelitis of cervical spinal cord.' *Br. J. Radiol.*, **21**, 464.

— (1950). 'Radiation myelitis of brain stem.' *J. Fac. Radiol.*, **1**, 79.

Bottrill, D. O., Rogers, R. T. and Hope-Stone, H. F. (1965). 'A composite filter technique and special patient jig for the treatment of the whole brain and spinal cord.' *Br. J. Radiol.*, **38**, 122.

Bouchard, J. (1966). *Radiation Therapy of Tumours and Diseases of the Nervous System*. London; Kimpton.

Chang, C. H., Housepian, E. N. and Herbert, C. (1969). 'An operative staging system and a megavoltage radiotherapeutic technique for cerebellar medulloblastoma.' *Radiology*, **93**, 1351.

Clemente, C. D. and Holst, E. A. (1954). 'Pathological changes in neurons, neuroglia and blood-brain barrier induced by x-irradiation of heads of monkeys.' *Archs Neurol. Psychiat.*, **71**, 66.

Cole, H. (1971). 'Tumours in the region of the pineal.' *Clin. Radiol.*, **22**, 110.

Collins, V. P. (1955). 'Wilms' tumour: its behavior and prognosis.' *J. Louisiana med. Soc.*, **107**, 474.

Crue, B. L. (1958). *Medulloblastoma*. Springfield, Ill.; Thomas.

Cushing, H. (1930). 'Experiences with the cerebellar medulloblastoma; a critical review.' *Acta path. microbiol.*, **7**, 1.

Cutler, E. C., Sosman, M. C. and Vaughan, W. W. (1936). 'Place of radiation in treatment of cerebellar medulloblastoma: report of 20 cases.' *Am. J. Roentgenol.*, **35**, 429.

Davidoff, L. M. (1966). 'Some considerations in the therapy of pineal tumours.' *Proceedings of the Virchow Society of New York*, **25**, 92.

Fowler, F. D., Alexander, E. and Davis, C. H. (1956). 'Pinealoma with metastases in central nervous system: rationale of treatment.' *J. Neurosurg.*, **13**, 271.

167

Green, M. and George, F. (1970). 'Total brain therapy: technical considerations.' *Radiology*, **96**, 429.

Hempelman, L. H., Pifer, J. W., Burke, G. J., Terry, R. and Ames, W. R. (1967). 'Neoplasms in persons treated with x-rays in infancy for thymic enlargement: report of third follow-up survey.' *J. Natn. Cancer Inst.*, **38**, 317.

Holland, J. F. (1970). 'Hopes for tomorrow versus realities of today: Therapy and prognosis in acute lymphocytic leukaemia in childhood.' *Pediatrics*, **45**, 191.

Hope-Stone, H. F. (1970). 'Results of treatment of medulloblastomas.' *J. Neurosurg.*, **32**, 83.

Kricheff, I. I., Becker, M., Schneck, S. A. and Taveras, J. M. (1964). 'Intracranial ependymomas, factors influencing prognosis.' *J. Neurosurg.*, **21**, 7.

Lampkin, B. C., Maurer, A. M. and McBride, B. H. (1967). 'Response of medulloblastoma to vincristine sulfate. A case report.' *Pediatrics*, **39**, 761.

Lassman, L. P., Pearce, G. W. and Gang, J. (1966). 'Effect of vincristine sulphate on intracranial gliomata of children.' *Br. J. Surg.*, **53**, 774.

Lindgren, M. (1958). 'On tolerance of brain tissue and sensitivity of brain tumours to irradiation.' *Acta radiol.*, Suppl. 170.

Maier, J. G. and Dejong, D. (1967). 'Pineal body tumours.' *Am. J. Roentgenol.*, **99**, 826.

McFarland, D. R., Horwitz, H., Saenger, E. L. and Bahr, G. K. (1969). 'Medulloblastoma—a review of prognosis and survival.' *Br. J. Radiol.*, **42**, 198.

Merriam, G. R. Jnr. and Focht, E. F. (1957). 'Clinical study of radiation cataracts and relationship to dose.' *Am. J. Roentgenol.*, **77**, 759.

Nöel, J. and Méthot, Y. (1970). 'La radiothérapie du médulloblastome: dix ans expérience.' *Union Med. Can.*, **99**, 1848.

Noetzli, M. and Malamud, N. (1962). 'Post-irradiation fibrosarcoma of the brain.' *Cancer*, **15**, 617.

Paterson, E. (1958). 'Malignant tumours of childhood.' *J. Fac. Radiol.*, **9**, 170.

— and Farr, R. F. (1953). 'Cerebellar medulloblastoma: treatment by irradiation of whole central nervous system.' *Acta radiol.*, **39**, 323.

Paterson, R. D. (1963). *The Treatment of Malignant Disease by Radiotherapy*, 2nd ed. London; Edward Arnold.

Pearson, D. (1971). Personal Communication.

Peirce, C. B., Cone, W. V., Bouchard, J. and Lewis, R. C. (1949). 'Medulloblastoma: non-operative management with roentgen therapy after aspiration biopsy.' *Radiology*, **52**, 621.

Phillips, T. L., Sheline, G. E. and Boldrey, E. (1964). 'Tumours affecting central nervous system: ependymomas.' *Radiology*, **83**, 98.

Raaf, J. and Kernohan, J. W. (1944). 'Relation of abnormal collections of cells in posterior medullary velum of cerebellum to origin of medulloblastoma.' *Archs Neurol. Psychiat.*, **52**, 163.

Raventos, A. and Duszynski, D. O. (1963). 'Thyroid cancer following irradiation for medulloblastoma.' *Am. J. Roentgenol.*, **89**, 175.

Rubinstein, L. J. (1970). 'The definition of the ependymoblastoma.' *Archs Path.*, **90**, 35.

— and Northfield, D. W. (1964). 'Medulloblastoma and so-called "arachnoidal cerebellar sarcoma".' *Brain*, **87**, 379.

Russell, D. S. and Rubinstein, L. J. (1963). *Pathology of Tumours of the Nervous System*, 2nd ed. London; Edward Arnold.

Sagerman, R. H., Bagshaw, M. A. and Hanbery, J. (1965). 'Considerations in the treatment of ependymoma.' *Radiology*, **84**, 401.

Smith, R. A., Lampe, I. and Kahn, E. A. (1961). 'Prognosis of medulloblastoma in children.' *J. Neurosurg.*, **18**, 91.

Spiller, W. G. (1907). 'Gliomatosis of the pia and metastases of glioma.' *J. nerv. ment. Dis.*, **34**, 297.

Strandquist, M. (1944). 'Studien über die kumulative Wirkung der Röntgenstrahlen bei Fractionierung.' *Acta radiol.*, Suppl. 55.

Svein, H. J., Gates, E. M. and Kernohan, J. W. (1949). 'Spinal subarachnoid implantation associated with ependymoma.' *Archs Neurol. Psychiat.*, **62**, 847.

Thomas, L. B. (1965). 'Pathology of leukaemia in the brain and meninges.' *Cancer Res.*, **25**, 1555.

Torkildsen, A. (1939). 'A new palliative operation in cases of inoperable occlusion of the sylvian aqueduct.' *Acta chir.*, **82**, 117.

Vaeth, J. (1965). 'Radiation-induced myelitis.' In *Progress in Radiation Therapy*, Vol. 3, pp. 16–26, Ed. by F. Buschke. New York; Grune & Stratton.

Waltz, T. A. and Brownell, B. (1966). 'Sarcoma: possible late result of effective radiation therapy for pituitary adenoma: report of two cases.' *J. Neurosurg.*, **24**, 901.

Wilson, C. B. (1970). 'Medulloblastoma: current views regarding the tumour and its treatment.' *Oncology*, **24**, 273.

Zeleny, V. (1956). 'The influence of local x-irradiation on functional processes in the central nervous system.' In *Progress in Radiology*, pp. 403–409, Ed. by J. S. Mitchell, B. E. Holmes and C. C. Smith. Edinburgh; Oliver & Boyd.

Zulch, K. J. (1965). *Brain Tumours*. London; Heinemann.

8—Radio-sensitization of Brain Tumours

Takao Hoshino

INTRODUCTION

Neuroectodermal tumours, which comprise more than 40 per cent of all brain tumours, are not, with the exceptions of pinealomas, medulloblastomas and ependymomas, very susceptible to radiotherapy. However, since no other beneficial form of therapy has been available, radiotherapy has been used extensively in their treatment. Recently, in the fields of radiobiology and nuclear physics, two important advances were made that will change the results of radiotherapy on such tumours. Briefly, the former field has provided the biological basis for our learning how to increase the susceptibility of tumour cells to radiation, and the latter field has introduced stronger, more powerful rays such as high energy x-rays, neutron, proton and phi meson rays as therapeutic agents. In this chapter, I will describe a therapeutic plan designed to increase the radio-sensitivity of malignant brain tumours, based on these new radiobiological contributions. A brief review of some basic facts about chemical radiosensitization is included.

The effects and the mechanisms of action of many radio-sensitizing compounds (for example, oxygen, alkylating agents, purine and pyrimidine analogues, hydroxyurea and other anti-metabolites) have been extensively analysed, and some of these agents have been used clinically (Bagshaw, 1963; Doggett, Bagshaw and Kaplan, 1969). An agent that is a good radio-sensitizer at the molecular or cellular level is not, however, always appropriate for clinical use. Its systemic effects, its toxicity *in vivo*, and its fate as well as the anatomical and biological characteristics of the tumour, are important factors to be considered.

The most important requirement of a radio-sensitizing agent for clinical use is that it sensitize the tumour alone, not the normal tissue that surrounds the tumour. If the radio-sensitizer does enhance the susceptibility of both tumour and normal tissue, the degree of sensitization should be markedly greater within the tumour. Many of the chemical sensitizers used to treat systemic malignant tumours are relatively non-specific with respect to brain tumours and hence of limited clinical value in this area.

The second requirement of a radio-sensitizer is that it have limited side effects. The side effects of any one agent are modified by the choice of route by which it is administered. Since intra-tumorous injection is difficult within the brain other routes of administration must be chosen. Besides the systemic route, there are the intra-arterial and intra-thecal routes, both of which theoretically yield a high concentration of the drug within the central nervous system. However, the results of most treatment via these routes have not differed remarkably from those achieved by systemic administration. Because of this, and because of the complexity of technique and the possible morbidity involved (Wilson and Hoshino, 1969) these routes of administration have been utilized less and less frequently, but the present study indicates that the intra-arterial route still merits attention.

The ideal radio-sensitizer, then, is one with a strong affinity for the tumour alone and with few side effects. BUdR (5-bromo-2′ deoxyuridine) is one agent that satisfies these requirements for brain tumour radiotherapy. The remainder of this chapter is devoted primarily to a discussion of radio-sensitization of brain tumours with BUdR, since the other radio-sensitizing agents such as hyperbaric oxygen, alkylating agents and anti-metabolites are already discussed in other chapters of this series, and since they do not have a specific sensitizing effect on brain tumours.

RELEVANT BIOLOGICAL PROPERTIES OF BUdR AND RELATED PYRIMIDINE ANALOGUES

Bromouridine (BUdR) is a halogenated pyrimidine analogue (the methyl radical in the pyrimidine is replaced by bromine—(*Figure 1*) that can be incorporated into cellular DNA as a substitute for thymidine. In other words, BUdR can be taken up by cells preparing for mitosis. This is probably because the methyl radical (thymidine) and the bromine (BUdR) in the fifth position on the pyrimidine ring are almost identical with respect to the radius of Van Der Walls (Szybalski, 1962). How this makes the cell radio-sensitive is not known.

A similar radio-sensitizing action is found in other pyrimidine analogues such as IUdR (5-iodo-2'deoxyuridine) (Erikson and Szybalski, 1963) and in halogenated deoxycytidine BCdR (5-bromo-2'deoxycytidine) and ICdR (5-iodo-2'deoxycytidine) which are de-aminated intracellularly to BUdR and IUdR, respectively, and then incorporated into DNA (Kriss and Revesez, 1962; Kriss and colleagues, 1963–1964). A different activity is that of 5-fluoro-2'deoxy-uridine (FUdR) and irs precursor, 5-fluorouracil (5-FU), which do not act as thymidine analogues but as powerful and selective inhibitors of the enzyme thymidilate synthetase. By this mechanism, they block the conversion of uridylate to thymidilate and thus inhibit the synthesis of DNA (Cohen and colleagues, 1958; Danneberg, Montag and Heidelberger, 1958; Hartmann and Heidelberger, 1961).

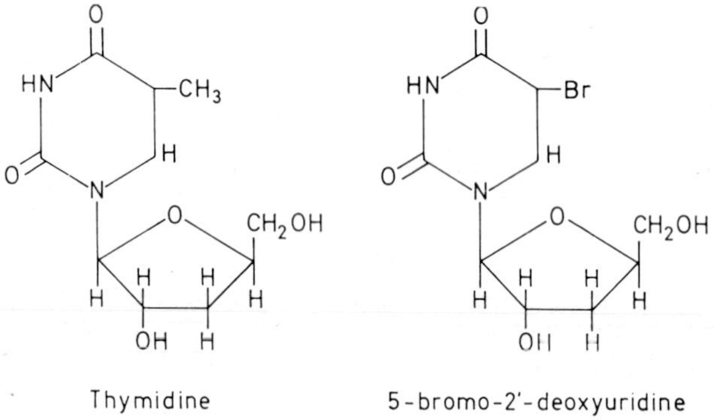

Thymidine   5-bromo-2'-deoxyuridine

Figure 1

BUdR and BCdR have almost equal radio-sensitizing ability and liquid solubility (the sodium salt form of BUdR (Takeda Chemicals Industry—Osaka, Japan) now available has a solubility of 20 per cent at 20°C and that of BCdR is similar), but BUdR is more readily available and less toxic. IUdR and ICdR are somewhat less water soluble and somewhat more toxic than BUdR.

The basic studies in the radio-sensitizing abilities of BUdR were done by Djordjeric and Szybalski (1960), Kaplan, Smith and Tomlin (1962), and Erickson and Szybalski (1963). Their studies showed that BUdR, at the doses they used, produced no cellular toxicity while increasing radio-sensitivity by a factor of two to three. Mohler and Elkind (1963) found that the increased cellular radio-sensitivity induced by BUdR was reversible, so that further cell replication occurred when the BUdR was no longer given. This fact aroused keen interest from the standpoint of radiotherapy. Since one dominant characteristic of malignant tumours is unrestricted proliferation, these tumours would predictably incorporate large amounts of BUdR and become radio-sensitized. If the surrounding normal tissue were also proliferating, selective sensitization of the tumour would not occur, but unless the normal tissue were irradiated it would not be damaged and would return to normal radio-sensitivity after several mitoses.

Another significant characteristic of BUdR is its systemic dehalogenation. Kriss and Revesez (1962) and Kriss and colleagues (1963) reported that when Br^{82}-tagged BUdR was given intravenously in both human and rat the radioactivity of the serum rose quickly and remained at a plateau. However, when resin, which attaches bromine, was added to the serum, the radioactivity of the serum dropped precipitously and remained quite low, indicating that a dehalogenation process had occurred. Isolated perfusion studies in rats demonstrated that the liver is the principal site of this dehalogenation. By continuous monitoring expired C^{14} degraded from C^{14}-labelled halogenated pyrimidines, Kriss and colleagues (1964) confirmed this site in man.

It is therefore clear that if a halogenated pyrimidine analogue is to be used as a differential radio-sensitizer in the clinical radiotherapy of neoplastic disease, it must be infused intra-arterially directly through the tumour circulation since its intravenous administration would result more in its destruction by the liver than in its incorporation into tumour cell DNA. In the treatment of brain tumours, this rapid degradation of BUdR is an advantage because BUdR is broken down after it passes through the tumour before its side effects become too severe.

In vitro, the amount of BUdR incorporated into DNA has been found to be proportional to the amount of BUdR in the medium, and this amount in turn determines the susceptibility of the cells to irradiation. However, since the cell can synthesize all the necessary nucleotides to duplicate its DNA, it may not actively incorporate an exogenous thymidine analogue. If this *de novo* synthesis of thymidine is inhibited, however, by the presence of small amounts (1/10—1/100 of the therapeutic dose) of an anti-metabolite such as methotrexate, 5-FU or FUdR, the cells will be forced to incorporate the available thymidine analogue in order to synthesize DNA. This has been widely confirmed in *in vitro* and *in vivo* systems (Cohen and colleagues 1958; Sano, Hoshimo and Nagai, 1968; Brown and colleagues, 1971; Tanaka and Takahashi, 1970).

173

THE CLINICAL APPLICATION OF BUdR TO BRAIN TUMOURS

Rationale

The clinical application of BUdR as an adjuvant to radiotherapy of neoplastic disease has been proposed by many workers. However, as expressed by Andrews (1968), the potential usefulness in general human cancer radiotherapy of inducing an increase in cancer radiosensitivity by selective incorporation of a halogenated pyrimidine is severely limited by these specific factors:

(1) Rapid degradation of these drugs by the liver.

(2) Lack of tumour specificity with respect to BUdR incorporation into cellular DNA.

(3) Damage to proximal normal tissue.

(4) Degree of incorporation required for significant radiosensitization.

(5) Prolonged administration.

Since DNA synthesis in the tumour cells take place at random, the duration that BUdR must be kept in the circulation must exceed the duration required for all viable tumour cells to pass through the phase of DNA synthesis.

Bagshaw and colleagues (1967) and Bagshaw and Doggett (1969) first used BUdR clinically to radio-sensitize tumours in the head and neck, since prolonged arterial infusion and macroscopic observation of the effects were possible. In 19 patients selected randomly, they placed a catheter in the external carotid artery which fed the tumour and administered 500 mg of BUdR per day for six weeks. Radiation therapy was started four days after the infusion had been started. Regional control of tumour growth was achieved in 33 per cent of these patients, which is slightly less than the 38 per cent observed in patients who received only radiation therapy. In addition, an increased tissue reaction to irradiation occurred in the vascular bed of the artery through which the BUdR was administered and elipation and severe ulceration of the skin occurred in the irradiated area. From this, it could be concluded that BUdR might perhaps be more safely used against brain tumours (especially gliomas) for the following reasons:

(1) Most brain tumours, even the most malignant ones such as glioblastoma multiforme, are solitary and rarely metastasize. Thus, BUdR would be directed toward the totality of a malignant threat.

(2) The surrounding nerve cells, having no mitotic ability, would not incorporate BUdR into their DNA, and would also probably be protected from BUdR by the normal blood–brain barrier.

174

(3) Not only is prolonged intra-arterial infusion feasible, but also there are few tissues in the vascular beds of the internal carotid or vertebral arteries that are actively proliferating.

Thus malignant brain tumours have been selected for clinical investigation since 1965 (Sano, Hoshimo and Nagai, 1968; Hoshino, Nagai and Sano, 1967; Hoshino and Sano, 1969; Hoshino and colleagues, 1970).

Method

The method that we have used in Japan was published in detail in 1968 by Sano, Hoshino and Nagai. It consists of (a) intra-arterial infusion of BUdR, which will make the tumour cells radio-sensitive, together with an anti-metabolite, which will enhance the BUdR incorporation into DNA, and (b) fractionated radiotherapy.

First, the pathological diagnosis is made and as much tumour as possible is removed. Then, if the tumour is located in the cerebral hemisphere, a siliconized polyethylene tube is inserted into the internal carotid artery from the common carotid artery, and the continuous infusion is carried out by means of a small pump. For infratentorial tumours or tumours fed by the posterior cerebral ateries, the catheter is placed in the vertebral artery. This is rather difficult, but usually the catheter can be passed from the right internal thoracic artery across the right subclavian artery, to the right vertebral artery since the opening of the right internal thoracic artery usually faces the opening of the right vertebral artery.

This cannulation should be done one or two weeks after craniotomy once the brain swelling related to the operation has decreased. Infusion therapy is started immediately after cannulation and continued for 24 hours a day. (At first, the infusion consisted of 600–1,000 mg/day of BUdR with 0·5 to 1 mg/day of methotrexate dissolved in 250 ml of saline. The same amount of sodium salt of BUdR used today can be dissolved in 5 ml of saline, and is infused by a small spring-powered pump which the patient carries with him. The bag containing the solution is refilled every third or fourth day.)

After one to two weeks of infusion, a six-week course of radiation therapy is begun with a total tumour dose of around 6,000 rads.

If decompressive craniotomy must be done (in patients whose tumours were only partially removed) to accommodate the brain swelling that occurs when radiation is begun, it should be done before the infusion is begun, since an interruption of radiation therapy during this regimen may result in loss of benefit to the patient.

Because the duration of the period of continuous infusion is so

critical to this therapy, three to four weeks of infusion have been proposed for each patient with glioblastoma to take into account the
assumed generation time of the tumour cells. However, we encourage
efforts to infuse for a five- to six-week period since no serious side
effects have been found with BUdR at the doses used.

Thus, ideally, a patient has infusion therapy alone for one or two
weeks, then another four- or five-week infusion concomitant with
radiation therapy, then by a one- or two-week period with radiation
therapy alone.

Results

Major neurosurgical clinics in Japan are using this regimen with
minor modifications. By the end of 1969, 203 patients had been
treated by intracarotid (181) or by intravertebral (22) infusion of
BUdR (IIIrd Conference on BUdR). The tumours involved were:
135 highly malignant gliomas (glioblastoma—112; oligodendroblastoma—7; ependymoblastoma—7; medulloblastoma—5; retino-
blastoma—2; pineoblastoma—2); 44 moderately malignant gliomas
(astrocytoma—29; oligodendroglioma—8; ependymoma—7), and 24
malignant brain tumours such as sarcomas. The total amount of
BUdR administered to each patient averaged 25,000 mg—80 per cent
of the patients were given amounts ranging from 10,000 to 40,000 mg;
6 per cent were given over 40,000 mg without any serious side effects.
The average duration of the continuous infusion was five weeks;
67 per cent of the patients were infused for more than four weeks.

The evaluation of the effects of any therapy for malignant brain
tumours is difficult because there is no valid method for precisely
measuring tumour response as long as the patient is alive. For
example, improvement in neurological signs and symptoms is our
best method at present, but this is affected by the location and size of
the tumour as well as status of the neurological deficits present before
therapy. Of those treated satisfactorily with the regimen described
here, 76 per cent demonstrated evidence of tumour regression—i.e.
neurological improvement over the pre-treatment status. The final
evaluation of this therapy, however, should be based on patient
survival, and not enough time has passed to make this possible.
Table 1 shows the follow-up data reported by Sano and colleagues
(1972) on 48 patients with highly malignant gliomas (glioblastoma—
33; oligodendroblastoma—7; ependymoblastoma—5; medulloblastoma—3). Efforts to treat such tumours by total operative removal or by administration of chemotherapeutic agents with or
without radiation therapy have resulted in extremely few cures. In
most large series, such as those reported by Frankel and German

(1958), Jelsma and Bucy (1967) and Lay and colleagues (1962), patients harbouring glioblastomas had a median post-operative survival of six months and few survived beyond 18 months; 16 of the 48 patients reported by Sano and colleagues survived for more than 18 months. However, their patients were selected, in the sense that the technical problems of prolonged intra-arterial infusion limited it mainly to hemispheric brain tumours at the beginning.

TABLE 1

Follow-up of Patients with Malignant Hemispheric Gliomas*
Treated with Bromouridine, Methotrexate and Radiation

Length of follow-up* (months)	Number of patients		
	Alive (14)	Dead (34)†	Total (48)
0–6	1	7	8
7–12	4	4	8
13–18	2	5	7
19–24	0	2	2
25–30	1	5	6
30–36	3	0	3
More	3	2	5

* Glioblastomas, malignant astrocytomas, malignant oligodendrogliomas and ependymomas.
† Nine died before treatment was completed (February, 1971, Tokyo).

The side effects of this form of therapy are related to: (a) drug administration; (b) the prolonged infusion technique; and (c) radiotherapy. Only the first two are relevant to the present discussion.

Even though BUdR is destroyed very quickly by the liver, the accumulative side effects of the portion that enters the general circulation included: moderate depilation of the forehead, delayed onychomadesis of the fingernails, and desquamation of the palmar skin. All these changes were reversible.

Onychomadesis is of particular interest. It became noticeable two to three months after completion of therapy and was more common in the fingernails than in the toenails. It appeared on all ten nails simultaneously, and consisted of a white, thickened bar across each nail which was probably established in the nail matrix during the period of infusion therapy. The affected nails were replaced by normal new ones during the next four to six months.

Severe leukopenia and disturbed liver function were observed only in patients receiving both BUdR and an anti-metabolite. These symptoms resolved when the anti-metabolite was discontinued.

The major complications resulting from this technique of long-term, continuous intra-arterial infusion were: arterial occlusion (18 cases) during or after the therapy, most cases being asymptomatic; local infection at the site of cannulation (3 cases); sepsis developed from abscess at the site of cannulation (3 cases); and cerebral infarction (3 cases). Although 26 instances of morbidity in 200 patients is a low morbidity rate, efforts should be made to eliminate the above complications since the success of treatment depends upon an uneventful long-term infusion period.

Further Considerations

Since BUdR is relatively non-toxic, it is a promising sensitizer for brain tumour radiotherapy. However, many problems besides the purely technical ones must be solved before the optimum treatment regimen can be established. The two most important problems are: (1) how to get all of the tumour cells to incorporate a thymidine analogue into their DNA; and (2) how to determine the amount of thymidine analogue required within cellular DNA for maximum radio-sensitivity.

Population kinetics on brain tumours have not provided a complete answer to the first question. The early work done in this area revealed that at any given time only a very small fraction of cells (less than 1 per cent) are synthesizing DNA even in malignant gliomas with a relatively long (one month) cell cycle time. This suggested that a long-term infusion (one month) would be required to let all tumour cells incorporate BUdR (Johnson and colleagues, 1960; Chigasaki, 1963). A more recent study (Kury and Carter, 1965; Hoshino and colleagues, 1972) indicated that an average of 5–10 per cent of cells in viable areas of malignant gliomas, including glioblastomas, are actively synthesizing DNA at any specified moment. This finding implies that the chance of incorporating BUdR into DNA is higher than had been assumed. In addition, other accumulated data suggest that the average cell cycle time is on the order of one week (Kury and Carter, 1965; Tym (1969) rather than one month. Still, the heterogenic biological behaviour of tumour cells, a common phenomenon in solid tumours in general, does not permit all of them to incorporate BUdR within so short a time. For example, BUdR will not be incorporated by the cells in necrotic or necrobiotic areas within a tumour that do not actively participate in DNA synthesis or by the cells residing outside the proliferating pool, and these cells will not be sensitized during a limited period of BUdR infusion. As was pointed out by Suit (1966), the overall sensitivity of the tumour will be decreased by this radio-resistant, residual, thymidine analogue-free cell population. It is possible that the increased death rate of sensitized proliferating cells may cause those resting cells to start propagating and therefore to incorporate BUdR, but this has not been confirmed by direct experimentation. Since cure of brain tumours can only occur if the cells in both the proliferating and the non-proliferating compartments are killed, the chances of this form of therapy effecting such a cure, even with further modification of drug choices and radiation schedules, is slight at present.

The second problem, that of determining the optimum dose of a radio-sensitizing agent, is obviously laborious in humans. The best way to study this problem is in animal tumour models, which can be made to simulate the clinical situation. Brown and colleagues (1971) examined the radio-sensitizing effects of BCdR delivered intra-arterially to KHT sarcomas implanted in the thighs of syngeneic C3H mice treated with fractionated x-irradiation. Approximately 5 per cent of all thymines in the tumour replaced with BCdR when 1 mg/day of BCdR was infused continuously for one to nine days. This suggests that some portion of thymine in nuclear DNA cannot be replaced by BUdR; 100 μg of 5-FU and 150 μg of FUdR enhanced this replacement to 7·6 per cent and 18 per cent respectively, but, interestingly, did not significantly alter the sensitivity of the tumour to irradiation. Thus, continuous infusion of BCdR during the fractionated regimen sensitized the tumours to irradiation by a dose modification factor of 1·30, whereas sensitization of the tumour with both BCdR and FUdR infusion showed the dose modification factor of 1·32.

Dose modification factor =

$$\frac{\text{Radiation dose (without sensitizer) to produce observed response}}{\text{Actual dose received (with sensitizer)}}$$

It is of clinical interest that the sensitization produced by the BCdR infusion was achieved even though only approximately 5 per cent of those thymidine molecules in the DNA of the proliferating cells were replaced by BUdR molecules.

Goffinet and colleagues (1972) tried prolonged intra-carotid infusion of 1 mg of BCdR (40 mg/kg) with 0·025 mg (10 γ/kg) of FUdR a day through a catheter for 10 days with concomitant fractionated irradiations of 300 rads each in intracerebrally implanted SK-26 mouse glioma. Non-irradiated tumour-bearing mice survived for 28 days regardless of whether they had received infusions of BCdR. The irradiated mice which received either BCdR or BCdR + FUdR had survival times of 55 and 57 days respectively. Thus, the addition of FUdR did not lengthen survival time, and by extension, did not increase the radio-sensitivity of the cells over the effect of BCdR alone.

The lack of increased radio-sensitivity even when 5-FU or FUdR was shown to increase the incorporation of BCdR or BUdR into the tumour cell DNA can be explained by the following assumptions:

(1) The elimination of breadth of the shoulder in the radiation dose response curve is more important than the final slope of the single-dose cell survival curve in determining the response of a cell population to a multifraction course of irradiation.

(2) The degree of sensitization of the tumour could have been limited by the proportion of the cells that had been through DNA synthesis during the infusion period between fractions of radiation therapy rather than by the magnitude of the sensitization.

SUMMARY

Among various chemical radio-sensitizing agents, the group of halogenated pyrimidines is promising as an adjuvant to radiotherapy of malignant brain tumours. Bromouridine (BUdR, 5-bromo-2′ deoxyuridine), a member of this group, has been chosen for extensive clinical trials for the following reasons:

(1) BUdR is incorporated into the DNA of dividing cells in place of thymidine.

(2) BUdR is degraded rapidly by the liver, and with feasible intra-arterial infusion it can selectively radio-sensitize brain tumour cells, since surrounding nerve cells have no mitotic activity and are also protected by an intact blood–brain barrier.

(3) The toxic side effects of BUdR are minor.

BUdR has been used clinically in the following manner: It is infused continuously through the carotid or vertebral artery for five to six weeks concomitantly with a six-week course of radiation therapy begun two weeks after the start of the BUdR infusion.

These preliminary investigations indicate that BUdR does improve the radio-sensitivity of gliomas. Although this particular form of treatment may not be definitive, it deserves further study both clinic-ally and experimentally so that methods giving the greatest hope of cure to patients with malignant brain tumours can be developed.

ACKNOWLEDGEMENT

This work is supported in part by US Public Health Service Training Grant No. NS55593, and by NIH Cancer Center Grant No. CA. 11249–01.

REFERENCES

Andrews, J. R. (1968). 'The halogenated pyrimidines and inherent radio-sensitivity.' In *The Radiobiology of Human Cancer Radiotherapy*, pp. 194–199. Philadelphia; Saunders.

Bagshaw, M. A. (1963). 'Approaches for combined radiation and chemo-therapy.' *Laval méd.*, **34**, 124.

— and Doggett, R. L. S. (1969). 'A clinical study of chemical radiosensitization.' In *Frontiers in Radiation Therapy and Oncology*, Vol. 4, pp. 164–173. New York; Karger.

— — Smith, K. C., Kaplan, H. S. and Nelsen, T. S. (1967). 'Intra-arterial 5-bromodeoxyuridine and x-ray therapy.' *Am. J. Roentgenol.*, **99**, 886.

Brown, J. M., Goffinet, D. R., Cleaver, J. E. and Kallman, R. F. (1971). 'Preferential radiosensitization of mouse sarcoma relative to normal skin by chronic intra-arterial infusion of halogenated pyrimidine analogs.' *J. natn. Cancer Inst.*, **47**, 75.

Chigasaki, H. (1963). 'Studies on the DNA synthesis function of glial cells by means of ^{3}H-thymidine microautography.' *Brain Nerve, Tokyo*, **15**, 767.

Cohen, S. S., Flaks, J. G., Barner, H. D., Loeb, M. R. and Lichtenstein J. (1958). 'The mode of action of 5-fluorouracil and its derivatives.' *Proc. natn. Acad. Sci.*, **44**, 1004.

Danneberg, P. B., Montag, B. J. and Heidelberger, C. (1958). 'Studies on fluorinated pyrimidines. IV. Effects on nucleic acid metabolism in vivo.' *Cancer Res.*, **18**, 329.

Djordjevic, B. and Szybalski, W. (1960). 'Genetics of human cell lines. III. Incorporation of 5-bromo and 5-iododeoxy uridine into the deoxyribo-nucleic acid of human cells and its effect on radiation sensitivity.' *J. expl. Med.*, **112**, 509.

Doggett, R. L., Bagshaw, M. A. and Kaplan, H. S. (1967). 'Combined therapy using chemotherapeutic agents and radiotherapy.' In *Modern Trends in Radiotherapy—1*, pp. 107–131, Ed. by T. J. Deeley and Constance A. P. Wood. London; Butterworths.

Erickson, R. L. and Szybalski, W. (1963). 'Molecular radiobiology of human cell lines. V. Comparative radiosensitizing properties of 5-halodeoxycytidines and 5-halodeoxyuridines.' *Radiat. Res.*, **20**, 252.

Frankel, S. A. and German, W. J. (1958). 'Glioblastoma multiforme—review of 219 cases with regard to natural history, pathology, diagnostic methods, and treatment.' *J. Neurosurg.*, **15**, 489.

Goffinet, D. R., Brown, J. M., Bagshaw, M. A. and Kaplan, H. S. (1972). 'Prolonged carotid arterial radiosensitizer infusion and radiation therapy of mouse glioma.' *Am. J. Roentgenol.*, **114**, 7.

Hartmann, K. U. and Heidelberger, C. (1961). 'Studies on fluorinated pyrimidines. XIII. Inhibition of thymidine synthetase.' *J. Biol. Chem.*, **236**, 3006.

Hoshino, T. and Sano, K. (1969). 'Radiosensitization of malignant brain tumors with bromouridine (thymidine analogue).' *Acta radiol.*, **8**, 15.

— Nagai, M. and Sano, K. (1967). 'Application of bromouridine in radiotherapy of malignant brain tumors.' *Nippon acta neuroradiol.*, **8**, 36.

— — Sato, F., Sano, K. and Watari, T. (1970). 'Bromouridine (BUdR) as a radiosensitizing agent of malignant brain tumors.' In *Radiation Protection and Sensitization*, pp. 491–497, Ed. by Moroson and Quintiliani. London; Taylor and Francis.

— Barker, M., Wilson, C. B., Boldrey, E. B. and Fewer, D. (1972). 'Cell kinetics of human gliomas.' *J. Neurosurg.*, **37**, 15.

Jelsma, R. and Bucy, P. C. (1967). 'The treatment of glioblastoma multiforme of the brain.' *J. Neurosurg.*, **27**, 388.

Johnson, H. A., Haymaker, W. E., Rubini, J. R., Fliedner, T. M., Bond, V. P., Cronkite, E. P. and Hughes, W. L. (1960). 'A radioautographic study of a human brain and glioblastoma multiforme after the in vivo uptake of tritiated thymidine.' *Cancer*, **13**, 636.

Kaplan, H. S., Smith, K. C. and Tomlin, P. A. (1962). 'Effect of halogenated pyrimidines on radiosensitivity of E. coli.' *Radiat. Res.*, **16**, 98.

Kriss, J. P. and Revesez, L. (1962). 'The distribution and fate of bromodeoxyuridine and bromodeoxycytidine, in the mouse and rat.' *Cancer Res.*, **22**, 254.

— Maruyama, Y., Tung, L. A., Bond, S. B. and Revesez, L. (1963). 'The fate of 5-bromodeoxyuridine, 5-bromodeoxycytidine and 5-iododeoxycytidine in man.' *Cancer Res.*, **23**, 260.

— Shaw, R. K., Loevinger, R. and Edmunds, N. (1964). 'Measurements of the in vivo degradation of carbon 14-labelled thymidine and its halogenated analogues in man by continuous monitoring of expired carbon-14 carbon dioxide.' *Nature, Lond.*, **202**, 1021.

Kury, G. and Carter, H. W. (1965). 'Autoradiographic study of human nervous system tumors.' *Archs Path.*, **80**, 38.

Ley, A., Ley, A. Jnr., Guitart, J. M. and Oliveras, C. (1962). 'Surgical management of intracranial gliomas.' *J. Neurosurg.*, **19**, 365.

Mohler, W. C. and Elkind, M. M. (1963). 'Radiation response of mammalian cells grown in culture: III. Modification of x-ray survival of Chinese hamster cells by 5-bromodeoxyuridine.' *Expl Cell Res.*, **30**, 481.

Sano, K., Hoshino, T. and Nagai, M. (1968). 'Radiosensitization of brain tumor cells with a thymidine analogue (bromouridine).' *J. Neurosurg.*, **28**, 530.

— Nagai, M., Arai, T. and Hoshino, T. (1972). 'Follow up results of BAR therapy of malignant brain tumors.' In *Present Limits of Neurosurgery*, pp. 71–75. Prague; Avicenum.

REFERENCES

Suit, H. D. (1966). 'Theoretical evaluation of a limitation in the use of pyrimidine analogs in radiation therapy.' *Radiology*, **87**, 1065.

Szybalski, W. (1962). 'Properties and application of halogenated deoxyribonucleic acid.' In *The Molecular Basis of Neoplasia*. Baltimore; Williams and Wilkins.

Tanaka, Y. and Takahashi, M. (1970). 'Clinical studies of intra-arterial infusion of 5-bromodeoxyuridine plus 5-fluorouracil and radiation.' In *Radiation Protection and Sensitization*, Ed. by Moroson and Quintiliani. London; Taylor and Francis.

Third Conference on BUdR—Radiation Therapy of Brain Tumours. Tokyo, December 23, 1969.

Tym, R. (1969). 'Distribution of cell doubling times in in vivo human cerebral tumors.' *Surg. Forum*, **445**.

Wilson, C. B. and Hoshino, T. (1969). 'Current trends in the chemotherapy of brain tumors with special reference to glioblastomas.' *J. Neurosurg.*, **31**, 589.

9—Chordomas

Theodore L. Phillips and Harry Newman

INTRODUCTION

The chordoma is a relatively rare but very debilitating tumour which exhibits a long history and is extremely resistant to many forms of treatment. Although it is rare, more than 500 cases were reported and reviewed by Utne and Pugh in 1955. Although it is apparently benign in many instances, metastases have been reported in an average of 10 per cent of the cases. The fact that the tumour can arise from any portion of the cranial cavity and the spinal column in which the primitive notochord was located leads to a protean list of initial manifestations and ultimate disabilities. The inaccessible location of these tumours has made them incurable by radical surgery in most cases. Thus the role of radiotherapy is an extremely important one. It is imperative that the optimum approach be used in combining surgery and radiotherapy in the first treatment attempt. This paper will be a review of the natural history, diagnosis, treatment and prognosis of chordomas with an emphasis on their radiotherapeutic management.

HISTORICAL BACKGROUND

The discovery of the nature of the notochord remnants and their relationship to the tumour later known as chordoma is summarized well by Windeyer (1959) and by Wright (1967). Luschka and Virchow separately described small jell-like protrusions in the skull from the region of the clivus in 1857. They were named by Virchow 'Ecchondrosis physaliphora'. Although Virchow originally considered these to be degenerative lesions in the spheno-occipital synchondrosis, Muller in 1858 suggested that these were residual remnants of the foetal notochord. His view was controversial until Ribbert in 1895 firmly established that these lesions did arise from the foetal noto-chord. He based his conclusions on experiments conducted in rabbits with the intervertebral disc. He was the first to apply the term chor-doma to tumours arising from the residual notochord tissue.

Benign residual heterotopic notochordal remnants are rare but are occasionally found if sought at autopsy with an incidence of 0·5 to 2 per cent.

Although occasional cases of what appeared to be chordomas were described in the 1800s, it was rarely reported until the 1900s when Stuart reported the first case in Britain. At that time only 26 cases were found in the world's literature. This number has gradually increased so that the review of Utne and Pugh in 1955 revealed 505 cases. A significant number have been added since that time and, although no exact tally exists, it is likely that over 1,000 cases could be found.

EMBRYOLOGICAL AND AETIOLOGICAL FACTORS

The sites of origin of chordomas in man are closely associated with the location of the remnants of the foetal notochord. In the embryo this structure extends from the spheno-occipital junction to the coccyx. At its upper end it approaches the inner surface of the sphenoid bone and as it passes caudally it comes close to the pharyn-geal surface of the occipital bone. During the fifth week of foetal development the notochord becomes enclosed within the bodies of the primitive vertebrae, the body of the sphenoid and the inter-vertebral discs. The notochord usually disappears as an entity with the exception of its participation in the formation of the nucleus pulposus of the intervertebral discs.

During the complex events which occur in the cranial, occipital and sacral regions it is possible for small derivatives of the disinte-grating notochord to become separated and form atrophic remnants. Wright (1967) feels that this process, which is associated with de-generation and increased activity, may lead to the presence of residual primitive tissue which can be found in cadavers as the previously mentioned notochordal remnants. The topographical distribution of these remnants corresponds to the primary sites for occurrence of chordoma. Chordomas rarely arise in the nucleus pulposus but usually arise from within these remnants. Some authors have attempted to identify trauma as a common initiating factor, particu-larly Utne and Pugh in 1955. They claimed a history of trauma in 40 per cent of their patients. It is also interesting to note that the high incidence of this tumour in males and the frequent location in the sacral region could also be associated with a traumatic aetiological factor. Obviously it is difficult to prove the relationship between precedent trauma and a tumour and impossible to demonstrate that it is, in fact, causative.

LOCATION AND INCIDENCE

Chordomas have been described along the entire track of the original notochord. They are most common in the sacro-coccygeal region with approximately 45 per cent of the tumours arising there, 39 per cent in the cranial region and 16 per cent in the vertebral

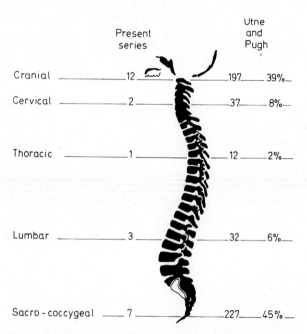

Figure 1. Distribution of cases by site in the present group of cases, left, and in the review of 505 cases by Utne and Pugh (1955), right. The relative increase in the cranial cases in our series is probably due to the fact that UCSF is a brain tumour referral centre

region. The distribution found in the large series of Utne and Pugh is compared with cases from the University of California and the California Tumor Registry presented in this paper and shown in *Figure 1*. The sacro-coccygeal lesions have predominated in all the large series. The predominance of cranial lesions in this group from California is probably due to the nature of referral to the University of California Medical Center of neurological cases. The rarity of this tumour is exemplified by the observation that, between 1937 and 1970, 13 chordomas have been found at the University of California Medical Center in San Francisco. During that time 27,000 malignant tumours were registered in the Tumor Registry. Between 1942 and 1970, 728 brain neoplasms were recorded by the Tumor Registry; of these 10 were considered malignant chordomas originating within the skull. The California Tumor Registry reports 11 cases of malignant chordoma out of 268,940 cases of cancer reported between 1942 and 1969. These figures are obviously only approximations since the fact that there is confusion as to the malignancy of chordoma may lead to under-reporting. However, an intensive search of all cross-indexed references of tumours was conducted to yield the 13 cases from the University of California Medical Center at San Francisco.

In addition to emphasizing the usual site of origin of these tumours, it should be mentioned that they are capable of metastasis. The incidence of metastasis varies widely in the series but the average incidence is stated as 10 per cent by Littman in 1953. Metastases are observed in most organs. The lymph nodes, liver and lungs are felt to be most common but skin, muscle and brain have also been involved.

AGE AND SEX DISTRIBUTIONS

In the great majority of reported groups of chordoma cases there has been a predominance of males. In the report of Utne and Pugh (1955) there were 68 per cent males and 32 per cent females. In that series the average age was 47 years. There is a tendency for the average age to be about ten years younger in the cranial cases than in the spinal or sacro-coccygeal cases. In the Utne and Pugh series the average was 37 years for cranial, 48 for spinal and 51 for sacro-coccygeal. Although Wright (1967) indicates that a number of smaller series have an almost equal male to female ratio, this is not true in other series such as that of Mabrey (1935), Higinbotham and colleagues (1967) and that of Kamrin, Potanos and Pool (1964). Although these also show a similar age distribution with a tendency for younger cases in the cranial lesions, the age of onset ranges from as low as 3 years to as late as 79 years. In the cases from the University of California at San Francisco and the California Tumor Registry (Table 1), there were 15 male and 9 female patients. The average age was 48 years with a range of 9–80 years.

187

It should be noted that occasional cases of multifocal origin of chordoma have been reported. One is documented by Anderson and Meyers (1968) and one was seen in the California Tumor Registry series. This 41-year-old female presented with a twelve year history of cranial symptoms and was found to have a sphenoid chordoma treated by means of a craniotomy. Five months later lumbar symptoms were evident and a laminectomy was performed at the level L-3, at which time a second chordoma was found.

TABLE 1

Summary of University of California at San Francisco
and Tumor Registry Cases

Site:	skull	12
	cervical	2
	thoracic	1
	lumbar	3
	sacro-coccygeal	7
		—
	Total	25 (one patient had a lesion at two sites)
Sex:	15 male	
	9 female	
Age:	9 to 80. The average was 48 years	
Average duration before treatment:	26 months	
Survival:	Longest—126 months	
	All but 1 of the 18 died with tumour	
	5 patients are alive, 1 was lost	
	Of the 5 alive, 4 had clivus lesions apparently under control for 28 to 126 months with a combination of surgery and radiotherapy; 1 had a sacro-coccygeal lesion and went for 43 months with a tumour with a combination of surgery and radiation	

PATHOLOGY

The microscopic pathology has been particularly well described by Dahlin and MacCarty (1952). They described the ordinary chordoma as a lobulated, fairly well encapsulated and partially translucent mucoid tumour. The lobules are often large, grossly visible and measure up to 2 or 3 cm in diameter. The lobule size ranges down to that below those that are grossly detectable. Such small lobules can be found beyond the apparent gross capsule of the tumour. The tumour may contain several or multiple calcified masses and numerous haemorrhagic areas which convert the translucent lobules into currant-jelly-like masses. There may be cystic areas filled with fluid. The tumour often extends, expands and destroys bone with poorly defined margins. The growing tumour usually pushes soft tissues ahead of it and destroys by pressure. Grossly the lesion may be confused with mucin-producing adenocarcinomas and chondromas. Sacro-coccygeal lesions may reach a size of 16 cm or greater, those in the cranial region are usually much smaller because of the early production of symptoms.

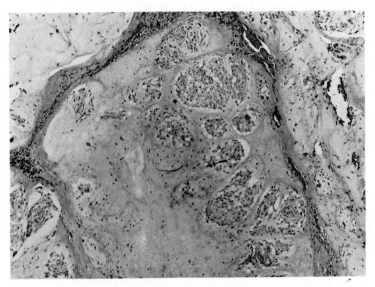

Figure 2. The physaliferous cells are organized into lobules within a myxo-cartilaginous stroma (H. & E. × 24)

Microscopically the tumours have a classic appearance. This appearance is demonstrated at low power in *Figure 2* from one of the University of California, San Francisco, cases. Such a lobular arrangement of tumour cells as demonstrated in *Figure 2* is a constant finding in at least some areas of all of the tumours studied by Dahlin and MacCarty. Intracellular mucus in the form of cytoplasmic vacuoles is observed in almost every case. Areas of large so-called physaliphorous cells are seen in many areas, as shown in *Figure 3*. The tumour cells are often arranged in cords in a background of mucus. In such areas the cytoplasm often forms a syncytium with disappearance of the cell membranes. Extracellular mucus is present in almost every case and is strongly positive with mucicarmine stain in some instances although this is not a specific test. These tumours may be differentiated from chondromas and chondrosarcomas because of the intracellular vacuoles. Mucus-producing adenocarcinomas of the rectum may also be confused at times. Histological evidence of malignancy is not uncommon in chordomas. In Dahlin's material, 20 of his 59 cases showed definite anaplasia and in 21 mitotic figures were noted.

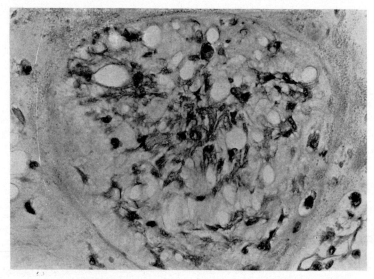

Figure 3. The characteristic physaliferous cells with the distinctive vacuolated cytoplasm are demonstrated (H. & E. × 240)

CLINICAL FEATURES

The intracranial or spheno-occipital chordomas usually present with symptoms of approximately one year in duration. The most frequent symptom is headache of a generalized nature or a visual disturbance. Patients most often complain of bilateral or unilateral visual impairment or diplopia. Some patients show visual field defects as indicated by Kamrin, Potanos and Pool (1964) and by Dahlin and MacCarty (1952). Less common symptoms are dysphagia, endocrine dysfunctions, ptosis and hearing loss. The most frequent neurological change is involvement of the sixth nerve and involvement of other structures at the base of the brain. Since the tumours rise from the region of the spheno-occipital synchondrosis they may extend anterosuperiorly to involve principally the area of the pituitary and optic chiasm. They may remain in the midline and press on the pons, medulla and cranial nerves or extend into the floor of the middle fossa.

Posterior extension may involve the glossopharyngeal, vagus, hypoglossal and spinal accessory nerves. Inferior extension may present as a mass in the nasopharynx with bleeding and obstruction.

Cervical, thoracic and lumbar chordomas usually present in a fashion similar to other neoplasms of the vertebral body. The most common initial findings are signs of compression of the spinal cord or nerve roots with pain or weakness. In the cervical region the mass may present laterally and be palpable in the neck. The lesion often destroys a portion of the bodies of the vertebral column. It often spares the intervertebral discs but not necessarily. It is important to note that the neurological symptoms may either be radicular or spinal cord in origin. Long track signs may be evident.

The lesions in the sacro-coccygeal region usually present with pain in the immediate sacro-coccygeal area. In many patients it may radiate along the course of one or both sciatic nerves. Constipation is also quite frequent as is impairment in the function of the bladder and anal sphincters. In almost every case a rectal examination reveals a palpable retro-rectal mass beneath the rectal mucosa. As the tumours enlarge they spread upward through the sacrum and may present posteriorly in the buttock and inferiorly medial to the femur.

ROENTGENOGRAPHIC FINDINGS

The roentgenographic changes noted in chordoma are not specific for this tumour but may be highly suggestive. Sennett (1953) and Utne and Pugh (1955) emphasized the roentgenographic findings. The major changes are those of bone involvement and those due to the soft tissue mass. The tumour is usually destructive of bone with involvement of the clivus, sella turcica, sphenoid and petrous bone in the cranial lesions. There is evident vertebral destruction and in some cases increased density noted in the spinal lesions. The sacro-coccygeal lesions show destruction of the sacrum, a scalloped margin, marked trabeculation and expansion of the sacrum.

The soft tissue mass is noted by both direct and indirect evidence. It may be seen directly when it protrudes into the pharynx or nasopharynx and when it forces the rectum forward in the sacro-coccygeal region. Vertebral lesions may displace the trachea or the aorta. Indirect evidence includes displacement of the ventricular system as demonstrated by pneumoencephalogram and by the displacement of the intracranial vessels on angiogram. Myelography may demonstrate the outlines of a mass as it impinges on the column of contrast material.

A number of these roentgenographic features are demonstrated in *Figures 4* to *10* from the University of California at San Francisco material. In all of our new cases either bone destruction or soft tissue

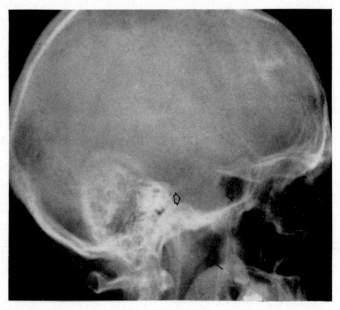

Figure 4. Lateral view of the skull shows destructive process involving the sella turcica and basisphenoid. The tumour has extended downwards into the nasopharynx (closed arrow)

masses were evident, or both. The majority of these illustrations indicate the indirect evidence which is available through the more sophisticated pneumoencephalographic, arteriographic and myelographic techniques.

The major problems in differential diagnosis of chordomas are provided by tuberculous lesions, chondrosarcomas and chondromas, solitary myelomas and lytic metastases from various primary sites. Obviously biopsy proof of the nature of the lesion is required, particularly in view of the very difficult kind of therapy required for chordomas. Although needle biopsy is sometimes successful, large sections obtained at open biopsy are preferable.

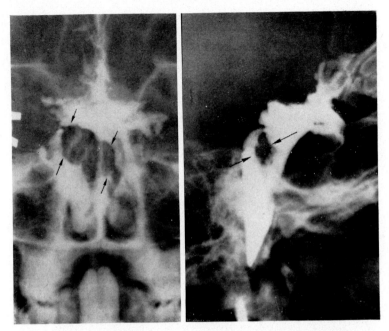

Figure 5. Frontal and lateral views of a myelogram reveal a well-defined mass in the region of the clivus extending laterally

TREATMENT

Surgery

Surgical treatment plays a major role in the management of chordomas, as is emphasized by all reports, including those of Higinbotham and colleagues (1967) and that of Rosenquist and Saltzman (1959), Rissanen and Holsti (1967) and Windeyer (1959). Although the tumour tends to expand and grow locally and to metastasize with only a 10 per cent incidence, it is not an ideal candidate for surgical resection. The almost universal failure of surgery to cure these lesions is due to their location and their insidious mode of spread. All the reported series show excellent palliation by repeated surgical resections of the tumour with intervals of several years often occurring between resections. It has only been in the sacro-coccygeal region, however, that radical surgery has achieved a significant number of permanent controls. This has been reported by Dahlin and MacCarty (1952). They advocate resection of several vertebral bodies above the gross tumour with preservation of the upper sacral nerves.

193

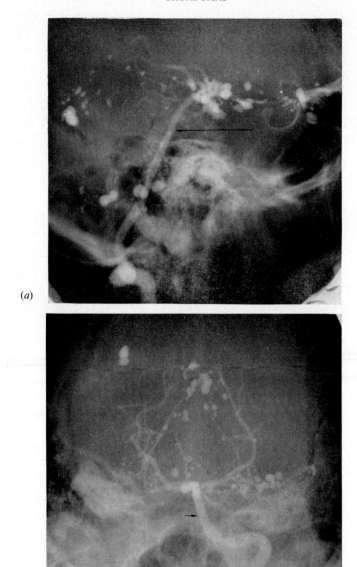

(a)

(b)

Figure 6. (a) A vertebral arteriogram in the lateral projection demonstrates posterior displacement of the basilar artery by a clivus chordoma (note destruction of the clivus). (b) Antero-posterior projection demonstrates lateral displacement of the basilar artery

194

A significant advance was achieved when Stevenson and colleagues (1966) developed a direct approach to the clivus by means of the submental approach, using a large anterior neck incision and approaching the clivus through the posterior pharyngeal region,

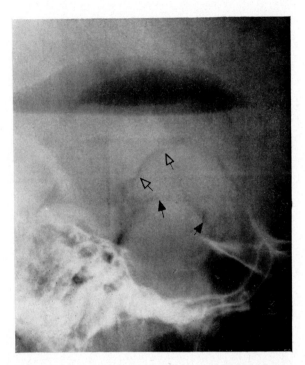

Figure 7. Pneumoencephalogram in the upright lateral view reveals superior displacement of the third ventricle by an extensive chordoma (open arrows). Note the upward displacement of the suprasellar cistern (closed arrows)

removing the odontoid, the arch of the atlas and a portion of the clivus. Through this approach they were able grossly to resect a mass which had failed to respond to radiation therapy and which was causing severe compression of the brain stem in a 20-year-old man. All the larger reviews, including that of Kamrin, Potanos and Pool (1964), Mabrey (1935), Utne and Pugh (1955), Dahlin and Mac-Carty (1952) and Wright (1967) indicate that as radical a surgical excision as possible should be performed in all cases.

Radiation Therapy

For a significant time chordomas were thought resistant to radiation treatment. Sennett in 1953 reported on eight patients treated with radiation therapy. He felt that the treatment was useful but only as a palliative measure in which complete surgical removal was

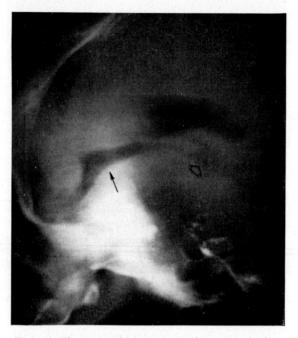

Figure 8. There is marked superior and posterior displacement of the fourth ventricle (closed arrow) and superior displacement of the third ventricle (open arrow) by the mass lesion arising from the clivus. Note the stretching of the aqueduct of Sylvius

not possible. The report of Windeyer (1959) was much more encouraging, in that he reported on two cases that had gone over four years without evidence of recurrence following high dose radiation therapy. Also in 1959 Rosenquist and Saltzman reported on radiotherapy alone in seven patients. They reported very satisfactory alleviation of pain, considerable decrease in tumour size in all but one patient but no permanent control in any patients. A similar conclusion is reached by Higinbotham and colleagues (1967).

Rissanen and Holsti (1967) report on seven patients in whom rather marked remission occurred in three cases. They also described an interesting patient with lung metastases. It was possible to observe

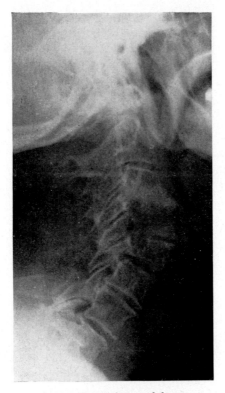

Figure 9. Lateral view of the cervical spine shows destruction of C.4 associated with involvement of the adjacent vertebral bodies by the tumour

the growth of this lesion for over a year and a doubling time of 3·3 months was measured.

The whole question of radiation dose and the control of chordomas has recently been reviewed by Pearlman and Friedman (1970). They report 15 of their own patients and review all the reported irradiated cases in whom it was possible to obtain the time and dose

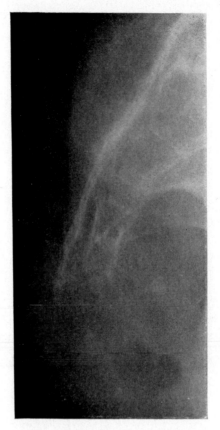

Figure 10. There is marked destruction of the distal sacrum and coccyx by the chordoma

information. They plotted 54 cases in whom the dose and the overall time was known. We have taken this material and added our own cases with the results shown in *Figure 11*. All these cases had sub-total removal or biopsy alone. Only one case achieved control for over five years with 5,000 rads or less. All the others occurred at higher doses. All the data available in the literature has been summarized by Pearlman and Friedman. They also included cases in which the overall time was not known. Patients receiving 4,000 rads or less showed a 6 per cent five-year success rate. The results were 20 per cent for 4,000 to 6,000 rads, 26 per cent for 6,000 to 8,000 rads, and 80 per cent for over 8,000 rads. The number of cases was small for this group with 8 of the 11 having control for more than five years.

These figures emphasize the rather marked radio-resistance of the chordoma and the need for very high local doses. It is only possible to deliver these doses to the entire tumour with good margins when

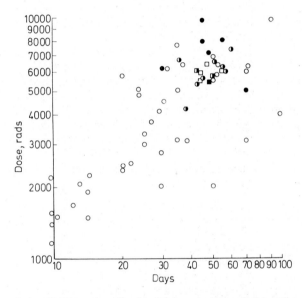

Figure 11. Time–dose plot for chordoma patients. Solid circles represent patients with the tumour controlled over five years, from the review of Pearlman and Friedman (1970). Similar cases from our material are shown by closed squares. In a similar fashion half open circles and squares indicate cases controlled for three to five years. Open circles and squares are failures

the tumour is located away from the spinal cord or brain stem. Thus the lesions in which a dose with a high probability of achieving control is possible are limited to those in the lower sacrum, buttock, etc. The information certainly emphasizes the need for very careful treatment planning and the achievement of as high a dose as possible. Megavoltage beams are essential, as is careful tumour localization, simulation and treatment planning. Because of the rather indefinite borders of all these tumours it is essential to give rather wide margins about the radiographically evident tumour. This, of course, further complicates the problem of delivering a sufficient dose.

199

Combination Therapy

Because a complete radical surgical resection is only possible in occasional chordomas and because massive radiotherapy is required for permanent control, it would seem likely that a more organized and planned combined approach would be beneficial for these patients. Such an approach is proving successful in soft tissue sarcomas. This approach involves as radical as possible a local resection of the tumour mass. The objective of this surgery should be to reduce the number of tumour cells and the amount of residual tumour to a very low level. This is often followed as soon as healing has occurred by radical radiotherapy with wide margins and with a dose as high as possible within the limits of tolerance of the region. Such an approach has not been widely practised. In general all of the past cases, including those in our own group presented here, have had either very minimal surgery and moderate radiotherapy or have had more radical surgery and radiation later when failure is apparent. It is likely that a planned combined approach would give better results but is not by any means proven.

PROGNOSIS AND COURSE OF THE DISEASE

The chordoma is commonly a slow growing, partially encapsulated tumour silently expanding over a period of years to a considerable size before the symptoms appear. Mabrey (1935) documents intervals between first symptoms and first treatment of from 4 to 24 months. In the University of California and California Tumor Registry material summarized in Tables 1, 2 and 3, the average duration before treatment was 26 months, with the shortest being one month and the longest 12 years. Thus it is difficult to measure the effects of treatment on survival in these patients. In the combined University of California San Francisco and California Tumor Registry cases the longest survival is 126 months after treatment. Of the total of 24 patients, 18 were dead, 17 with tumour the cause of demise; 1 patient was lost and 5 were alive; 1 of the 5 had a sacro-coccygeal lesion that was active, the other 4 had clivus lesions apparently under control for 28–126 months with a combination of surgery and radiation therapy.

Kamrin, Potanos and Pool (1964) reported average survival times of 43 months for cranial, seven years for cervical, four years for lumbar and three years for the sacro-coccygeal lesions; 8 of their 30 patients lived over five years. A number of these had active disease, however, and Higinbotham and colleagues (1967) emphasized the small number of patients who go over five years with no evidence of active tumour. This level was 8·7 per cent in their material.

The course of 13 patients treated at the University of California San Francisco is summarized in Table 2. All but 4 of these patients

TABLE 2

University of California at San Francisco Chordoma Cases

Case No.	Site	Age	Sex	Duration	Survival*	Treatment†
1	Skull	34	M	36 months	28 months A.W.	Radiation 5600/31/50
2	Skull	31	F	24 months	66 months A.W.	Surgery, 5400/35/49 surgery
3	Skull	19	M	9 months	23 months D.T.	Radiation 5000/?/? surgery
4	Skull	50	M	24 months	25 months A.W.	Radiation 6000/24/43
5	Skull	9	M	12 months	14 months D.T.	Radiation 5400/30/44
6	Skull	30	M	24 months	126 months A.W.	Radiation 6000/31/56
7	Skull	46	M	48 months	0 months D.T.	None—autopsy
8	Skull	41	M	30 months	78 months D.T.	Surgery, chemo-therapy
9	Skull	31	M	22 months	1 month D.T.	None
10	Skull	17	F	5 months	42 months D.T.	Radiation 6000/?/? surgery
11	Cervical	31	M	3 months	24 months D.T.	Surgery and radiation 6400/34/47
12	Sacro-coccygeal	60	F	24 months	37 months lost	Surgery X 2
13	Sacro-coccygeal	67	M	11 months	43 months A.W.	Surgery and radiation 5900/30/44

* A.W. = alive and well; A.T. = alive with tumour; D.T. = dead with tumour.
† Radiation = dose/fraction/overall time.

received radiation therapy. Their age, sex, site of disease and duration of symptoms prior to treatment is shown in Table 2. The longest survivals and the patients now free of tumour have occurred in patients with clival lesions treated with combinations of surgery and radiation and, in one case, re-operation. The longest survivor had only a biopsy followed by 6,000 rads.

The California Tumor Registry cases have all expired due to the tumour. The radiation dosage information is not available in these cases, but 6 of the 11 had radiation therapy as part of their management. The longest survival in this group was 54 months. Although the University of California San Francisco participates in this Tumor Registry, duplicate cases were removed and presented under the University of California at San Francisco material.

TABLE 3
California Tumor Registry Chordoma Cases

Case No.	Site	Age	Sex	Duration	Survival*	Treatment†
1	Skull/lumbar	41	F	12 years	15 months	Surgery
2	Skull	19	M	3 years	22 months	Radiation and surgery
3	Cervical	71	F	2 years	14 months	Unknown
4	Thoracic	49	M	1 year	32 months	Surgery and radiation
5	Lumbar	65	M	1 year	19 months	Surgery and radiation
6	Lumbar	76	F	3 years	31 months	Surgery and radiation
7	Sacro-coccygeal	46	M	1 month	19 months	Surgery
8	Sacro-coccygeal	70	M	2 months	0	None—autopsy
9	Sacro-coccygeal	80	F	4 years	26 months	Surgery
10	Sacro-coccygeal	65	F	8 months	54 months	Surgery and radiation
11	Sacro-coccygeal	65	F	4 months	7 months	Radiation

* All patients died of tumour except No. 9 who died of a cerebrovascular accident.
† Radiation doses not known.

CONCLUSIONS

Chordoma is an extremely interesting tumour of apparent embryological origin. It is in general slow growing, metastasizes late in only about 10 per cent of the patients and grows mainly by local infiltration and expansion. Because of its location, predominantly in the sacro-coccygeal region and the base of the skull, it is rarely completely resectable.

The few cases in which apparent permanent control of chordomas have been achieved are those in which either radical surgery with complete extirpation with wide margins was performed or those cases receiving a very high radiation dose, usually above 8,000 rads.

202

Because of the difficulty in delivering such doses, it is suggested that an optimum treatment course might involve a resection of all gross tumour or a subtotal resection followed by very radical radiotherapy using megavoltage techniques with careful localization, simulation and treatment planning.

ACKNOWLEDGEMENTS

This work was supported in part by the United States Public Health Service, National Cancer Institute through individual Training Fellowship No. 1 FO3 CA 52938–01.

REFERENCES

Anderson, W. B. and Meyers, H. I. (1968). 'Multicentric chordoma.' *Cancer*, 21, 126.
Dahlin, D. C. and MacCarty, C. S. (1952). 'Chordoma.' *Cancer*, 5, 1170.
Higinbotham, N. L., Phillips, R. F., Farr, H. W. and Hustu, H. O. (1967). 'Chordoma.' *Cancer*, 20, 1841.
Kamrin, R. P., Potanos, J. N. and Pool, J. L. (1964). 'An evaluation of the diagnosis and treatment of chordoma.' *J. Neurol. Neurosurg. Psychiat.*, 27, 157.
Littman, L. (1953). 'Sacro-coccygeal chordoma.' *Ann. Surg.*, 137, 80.
Mabrey, R. E. (1935). 'Chordoma: a study of 150 cases.' *Am. J. Cancer*, 25, 501.
Pearlman, A. W. and Friedman, M. (1970). 'Radical radiation therapy of chordoma.' *Am. J. Roentgenol.*, 108, 333.
Rissanen, P. M. and Holsti, L. R. (1967). 'Sacrococcygeal chordomas and their treatment.' *Radiol. clin. Biol.*, 36, 153.
Rosenquist, H. and Saltzman, G. F. (1959). 'Sacrococcygeal and vertebral chordomas and their treatment.' *Acta radiol.*, 52, 177.
Sennett, E. J. (1953). 'Chordoma, its roentgen diagnostic aspects and its response to roentgen therapy.' *Am. J. Roentgenol.*, 69, 613.
Stevenson, G. C., Stoney, R. J., Perkins, R. K. and Adams, J. E. (1966). 'A transclival approach to the ventral surface of the brain stem for removal of a clivus chordoma.' *J. Neurosurg.*, 24, 544.
Utne, J. R. and Pugh, D. G. (1955). 'The roentgenologic aspects of chordoma.' *Am. J. Roentgenol.*, 74, 593.
Windeyer, B. W. (1959). 'Chordoma.' *Proc. R. Soc. Med.*, 52, 1088.
Wright, D. (1967). 'Nasopharyngeal and cervical chordoma—some aspects of their development and treatment.' *J. Lar. Otol.*, 81, 1337.

10—Radiation Therapy in the Management of Craniopharyngiomas

Simon Kramer

INTRODUCTION

Craniopharyngiomas constitute a challenging group of tumours for the radiation therapist. Although universally benign histologically, their usual position within the head, lying immediately superior to the sella and often extending anteriorly, superiorly and posteriorly, makes surgical extirpation difficult, hazardous and often impossible. The curative value of radiation therapy and its relative safety in the treatment of these tumours has been reported repeatedly during the last decade (Kramer, McKissock and Concannon, 1961; Kramer, Southard and Mansfield, 1968; Svien, 1965; Leksell, Backlund and Johansson, 1967), although these facts are not yet universally recognized by our neurosurgical colleagues.

Craniopharyngiomas arise from residual cell masses, resembling squamous epithelium, which are found in the infundibulo-hypophyseal region, as described by Erdheim (1904). They may occur at any age and are relatively rare tumours, accounting for little more than 2 per cent of all intracranial neoplasms (Svolos, 1969). However, approximately 30 per cent of these tumours occur in childhood before the age of 15, and in this age group these tumours are the third most common intracranial tumour after the gliomatous tumours and the medulloblastomas. Matson (1969) estimates the incidence to be 9 per cent of all intracranial tumours in children and mentions various other estimates from 5 to 13 per cent. This tumour is thought to be slightly more frequent in males than in females.

MICROSCOPIC APPEARANCE

Three histological types are commonly recognized, as described by Bailey (1933): adamantinomas, simple squamous epitheliomas, and Rathke's cleft cysts. These have been described in the literature (Critchley and Ironside, 1926; Frazier and Alpers, 1931, 1934; Leddy and Marshall, 1951). From a practical point of view, the histological classification is not important, since clinically the behaviour of all craniopharyngiomas is similar, as are their tendency to recurrence after incomplete removal and their response to radiation therapy.

SIGNS AND SYMPTOMS

The signs and symptoms of this tumour depend on the age of the patient and on the structures which become involved as the tumour expands. Full descriptions of the signs and symptoms and the endocrinological problems have been given in the literature (Matson, 1969; Matson and Crigler, 1969; Svolos, 1969) and will be referred to here only as they affect the management by radiation therapy. It should be noted that there seems to be a markedly different growth pattern in children and in adults. In children, the growth appears to be relatively rapid and the length of the history is considerably shorter than in adults. In children, the tumour rapidly obstructs the foramen of Monro, and almost invariably the first signs are those of increased intracranial pressure due to this obstruction. A secondary symptom in children, endocrine dysfunction, is noted, referable to pituitary or hypothalamic involvement. Whereas in children involvement of the visual pathway often occurs, it is rarely the first evidence of this tumour. In adults, almost without fail, the visual disturbances usually come first, although a relatively mild degree of panhypopituitarism may also be present. Almost invariably in adults the history is a very gradual one and may extend over many years.

The importance of the endocrinological disturbances has been stressed by Matson (1969) and Matson and Crigler (1969). Recognition of a relatively subclinical degree of pituitary hypofunction is most important since substitution therapy has to be given during the period of surgical manipulation, even when there is no gross clinical disturbance. It is equally important to recognize the possibility of subclinical hypofunction during the course of radiation therapy, and it is particularly important to recognize the need for additional substitutional therapy if infection or some other complication occurs during the course of radiation therapy. Endocrinological investigation should be as complete as possible before any diagnostic or surgical procedures are performed in order to obtain a baseline. Unfortunately, the patient is often not seen by the radiation therapist until after diagnosis has been obtained by craniotomy, and under those circumstances there is usually a profound endocrinological disturbance, particularly if there has been an attempted radical extirpation of the tumour. Under those circumstances empirical management has to be employed to restore the endocrinological balance of the patient as far as possible. Late endocrinological deficits are always the result of either the tumour or the surgical intervention. Radiation therapy, even in the relatively high doses employed for craniopharyngioma, has never, in our experience, produced a pituitary or hypothalamic deficit. Indeed, we have found it impossible to influence normal pituitary or hypothalamic function by doses of radiation in the therapeutic range.

DIAGNOSTIC PROCEDURES

The importance of endocrinological investigation has already been mentioned. Part of the general examination to establish a baseline

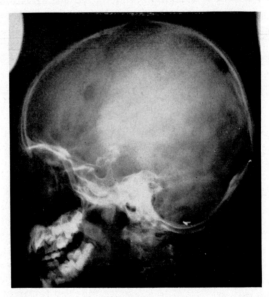

Figure 1. Typical suprasellar calcification in a 6½-year-old child

should include x-rays to establish the bone age. Carotid arteriography, electroencephalography, and radio-nuclear brain scanning usually form part of the work-up but are more useful in the adult than in the child. Plain films of the skull may show suprasellar or intrasellar calcification, abnormalities of the bony sella turcica or evidence of increased intracranial pressure. Calcification, usually suprasellar, but occasionally intrasellar, is almost invariably found in plain skull x-rays of children with this tumour. Only 1 of our 18 children has failed to show such calcification. In adults it is a good deal less common and is present in only approximately 50 per cent

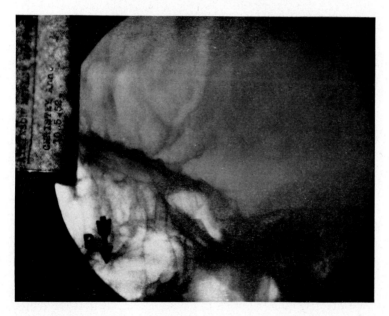

Figure 2. (a) Intrasellar calcification in an 8½-year-old child

of cases; in our series, it was present in 13 of 25 patients. The calcification may show solid masses, or a calcified rim of a craniopharyngiomatous cyst may be outlined. In either case, one must not assume that the calcification indicates the size or extent of the tumour. *Figure 1* shows the typical suprasellar calcification in a 6½-year-old child (M.G.) who is now alive and well after more than 20 years since his treatment. *Figure 2a* shows an intrasellar calcification in an 8½-

207

year-old patient (A.C.). A ventriculogram (*Figure 2b*) shows massive dilatation of both lateral ventricles, indicating that the tumour is much larger than the calcification and extends upwards to obstruct the foramen of Monro. This child is alive and well 20 years after completion of radiation therapy.

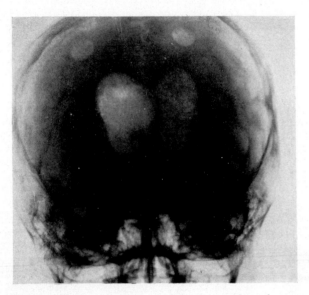

Figure 2. (b) A ventriculogram of the same patient, showing massive dilatation of both lateral ventricles, indicating that the tumour is much larger than the calcification and extends upward to obstruct the foramen of Monro

Air contrast studies, either by ventriculogram or encephalogram, are absolutely essential, both to delineate the extent of the tumour and to show its anterior, posterior and superior extension. This knowledge is useful for the surgeon in planning his operative attack and is essential for the radiation therapist to define the volume to be irradiated.

DIFFERENTIAL DIAGNOSIS

While the diagnosis is usually fairly clear-cut in the child, other intra-cranial masses must be considered. Thus, we have seen a glioma on the floor of the third ventricle showing calcification; and, on one occasion, a chromophobe adenoma in a child simulated the appearances of a craniopharyngioma, apart from the lack of calcification. In the adult, a chromophobe adenoma of the pituitary may have an appearance similar to that of a craniopharyngioma, but the visual field disturbances are usually more symmetrical. A tuberculum sellae meningioma must also be considered, but endocrine disorders are rare and there is rarely any change in the sella turcica.

The distinction between a chromophobe adenoma with extrasellar extension, and a craniopharyngioma without calcification, may be impossible to make clinically. This is one reason why we believe that chromophobe adenomas should be biopsied to establish the diagnosis, since the treatment of a craniopharyngioma calls for considerably higher doses of radiation than that of a chromophobe adenoma. Other tumours to be considered in the differential diagnosis are tuberculum sellae meningiomas and chordomas.

TREATMENT

Until the advent of corticosteroids in the 1950s, total removal of a craniopharyngioma was extremely hazardous and carried a mortality of approximately 40 per cent (Cushing, 1932; Love and Marshall, 1950; Hirsch, 1959; Gordy, Peet and Khan, 1949; Olivecrona, 1966). Even the surviving patients were badly damaged and few useful survivals have been reported (Cushing, 1932; Horrax, 1954; Gordy, Peet and Khan, 1949; Svolos, 1969). Since modern supportive treatment has become available, the mortality has been markedly reduced but, even so, extension of the tumour into the pituitary fossa and the hypothalamic region makes total removal virtually impossible; and even when this has been attempted or thought to have been carried out, the recurrence rate is unacceptably high. Matson (1969) and Matson and Crigler (1969), however, have persisted in advocating attempt at total removal of even extensive craniopharyngiomas. In their series, the mortality has been relatively low, but the postoperative damage to pituitary function has been extensive in every case. They stress the fact that great attention has to be paid to the endocrinological disturbances in the immediate post-operative period, and that continued surveillance is necessary to adjust and maintain endocrine balance. Other neurosurgeons (Svien, 1965) recommend total removal only if this can be easily accomplished, but recognize the value of radiation therapy post-operatively.

Radiation therapy was first advocated by Carpenter, Chamberlin and Frazier (1937). They describe four patients, aged 10 to 14, treated by various dosage schemes, who had remained well for periods of 20 to 39 months after their radiation. Unfortunately, no late follow-ups are available on these cases. Since that time treatment by external beam therapy has been mentioned sporadically (Love and Marshall, 1950; Hirsch, 1959).

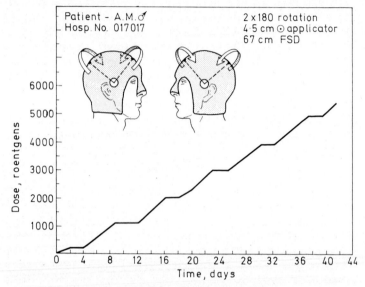

Figure 3. Method of treatment by two paths of rotation of 180 degrees, with details of dose and time of treatment. (Reproduced from Kramer, McKissock and Concannon (1961) by courtesy of the Editor of Journal of Neurosurgery)

A number of authors have introduced radioactive liquid such as Au^{192} or P^{32} into the craniopharyngiomatous cyst in an effort to suppress liquid formation (Bond, Richards and Turner, 1965; Leksell, Backlund and Johansson, 1967). While this has appeared to be quite successful, we rejected this method after due consideration, because we were impressed with the solid portions of these tumours so often found at a distance from the cyst, which would not receive adequate irradiation from the radioactive material introduced into the cyst to suppress growth permanently.

The first study of the value of radiation therapy was undertaken by us in 1952, and first reported in 1961 (Kramer, McKissock and Concannon, 1961) with later results reported in 1968 (Kramer, Southard and Mansfield, 1968). Our material consisted of ten con-

secutive cases treated between 1952 and 1954 and, since very long-
term follow-ups are available on these patients, they are reported
here in some detail. At that time it seemed to us that relatively high
doses of radiation would be required to be effective in a tumour that
was histologically benign and consisted of essentially well-ordered
squamous epithelium. We therefore undertook to perform the minimum surgery consistent with establishing the diagnosis and to
decompress the cystic portions so often present in these tumours.
Post-operatively radiation therapy was given with 2 MeV x-rays
irradiating the minimum size volume, as indicated by the radiological
and surgical procedures. We utilized one of two techniques, either
two 180 degree arcs (*Figure 3*) or 360 degree rotation on an inclined

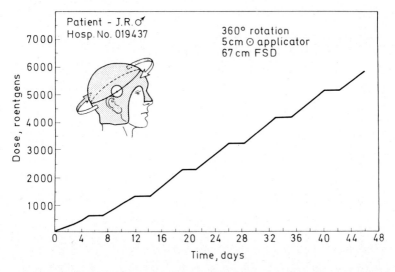

*Figure 4. Method of treatment by rotation of 360 degrees, with details of dose and
time of treatment. (Reproduced from Kramer, McKissock and Concannon (1961)
by courtesy of the Editor of* Journal of Neurosurgery)

horizontal plane running from the frontal through the suboccipital
region (*Figure 4*). Patients were treated with stationary equipment
and on a rotating platform. The tumour dose we chose was to be
7,000 rads in seven weeks for adult patients, and 5,500 rads in six
weeks for patients up to 14 years of age. The clinical, radiological
and pathological findings are given in Table 1, and the details of
surgical and radiation treatment in Table 2. A typical isodose distribution by a 360 degree rotational field and a field of 6 cm in

211

TABLE 1

First Series: Clinical, Roentgenological and Pathological Findings (1952–1954)

Case	Age, years	Sex	Presenting signs and symptoms	Duration	Roentgenological findings		Pathology	
					Calcification	Contrast	Gross	Histology
Children								
M.G.	6½	M	Intracranial hypertension, retarded growth	2½ years	+	+	Cystic	Cholesterol crystals in cystic fluid
A.C.	8½	F	Intracranial hypertension, diabetes insipidus	3 months	+	+	Cystic and solid	Cholesterol crystals in cystic fluid
A.M.	14	M	Failing vision, bitemporal hemianopsia, delayed puberty	6 months	+	+	Cystic	Cholesterol crystals in cystic fluid
J.R.	11	M	Failing vision, intracranial hypertension, bitemporal hemianopsia	6 years	+	+	Solid	Craniopharyngioma
K.G.	9	M	Intracranial hypertension, somnolence	2 months	+	+	Cystic and solid	Cholesterol crystals in cystic fluid
J.McA.	11	M	Failing vision, panhypopituitarism	5 years	O	+	Cystic and solid	Craniopharyngioma
Adults								
R.M.	35	F	Failing vision	2 years	O	+	Cystic and solid	Craniopharyngioma
L.B.	41	M	Failing vision, bitemporal hemianopsia	3 months	O	+	Cystic and solid	Cholesterol crystals in cystic fluid
A.H.	49	M	Failing vision, bitemporal hemianopsia	8 years	+	+	—	—
A.S.	59	M	Failing vision, bitemporal hemianopsia	25 years	O	+	Cystic and solid	Craniopharyngioma

diameter is given in *Figure 5*. It will be seen that the central portion
of the brain receives approximately 20 per cent or more of the chosen
target volume dose.

TABLE 2
First Series: Surgical Treatment and Radiation Therapy
(1952–1954)

Case	Age, years	Surgical treatment	Radiation therapy (2 MeV, HVL 11 mm Pb, FSD 67 cm, 2 × 180° or 360° rotation)
Children			
M.G.	6½	Ventricular drainage, cyst aspiration, burr-hole, Tor-kildsen operation	6 cm circle 5,600 rads in 44 days
A.C.	8½	Cyst aspiration, burr-hole, Torkildsen operation	4·5 cm circle 5,000 rads in 37 days
A.M.	14	Cyst aspiration, burr-hole	4·5 cm circle 5,400 rads in 41 days
J.R.	11	Attempted cyst aspiration, burr-hole	5 cm circle 5,700 rads in 46 days
K.G.	9	Cyst aspiration, burr-hole	4·5 cm circle 5,575 rads in 42 days
J.McA.	11	Cyst aspiration, burr-hole	5 cm circle 6,550 rads in 57 days
Adults			
R.M.	35	Right frontal craniotomy, aspiration and biopsy	4·5 cm circle 6,075 rads in 39 days
L.B.	41	Right frontal craniotomy, aspiration	6 cm circle 5,580 rads in 51 days
A.H.	49	—	6 cm circle 7,000 rads in 47 days
A.S.	59	Right frontal craniotomy, aspiration and biopsy	6 cm circle 6,950 rads in 39 days

It must be appreciated that 20 years ago a good deal less was
known about the delicate balance of the neurohypophysial axis, nor
were corticosteroids available on a routine basis. However, since
surgical intervention was kept to a minimum, no problems arose
with any acute hormonal imbalances in these patients post-operatively, and all patients completed their radiation therapy without
complications. Only one of these ten patients has developed an

additional endocrinological deficit, namely diabetes insipidus, since the onset of the combined therapy.

The long-term results are of interest. Of the four adults, one is surviving and is well, apart from bronchitis, 20 years after the initial surgery and radiation therapy. It is of some interest to know

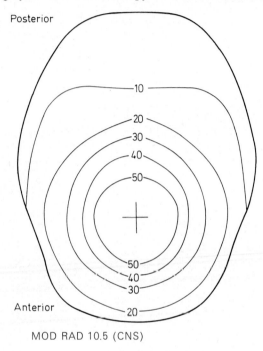

MOD RAD 10.5 (CNS)

Figure 5. A typical isodose distribution by a 360 degree rotational field and a field of 6 cm in diameter

that she had complained of headaches, as well as failing vision, and was kept under psychiatric care for two years before the correct diagnosis was established. Two other adults died of unrelated disease, one in his tenth post-treatment year, the other in his fourteenth post-treatment year. The fourth adult died of a coronary occlusion two years after his treatment, without evidence of recurrence.

The survival of the six children is perhaps of the greatest interest, since recurrence normally takes place most quickly in the younger patient and the question has been raised of the danger of high-dosage radiation therapy to the brain in the developing child. Table 3 gives

214

TABLE 3
First Series: Long-term Results (1952–1954)

Case	Age at onset, years	Date of treatment	Dose	Survival, years	Height	Weight, lb	Occupation	Leisure activities	Re-placement therapy or residual disability
M.G.	$6\frac{1}{2}$	March 1952	5,600 rads in 44 days	20	5 ft. 4 in.	140	Electrician	Home life	Pitressin
A.C.	$8\frac{1}{2}$	June 1952	5,000 rads in 37 days	20	4 ft. 10 in.	105	Dental nurse	Horseback riding, driving	None
A.M.	14	July 1952	5,400 rads in 41 days	20	5 ft. 9 in.	160	Accountant	—	Testosterone
K.G.	9	Sept. 1952	5,500 rads in 42 days	20	5 ft. 8 in.	196	Ph.D., biology	University fencing team	None
J.R.	11	June 1953	5,700 rads in 46 days	19	5 ft. 10 in.	193	Pharmacist	Scouts, church work, 'active social life'	Impaired vision OD
J.McA.	11	Nov. 1953	6,500 rads in 57 days	19	5 ft. 9 in.	155	Storekeeper	'Enjoys a full life'	Thyroid extract

215

details of these six children's present status. All have reached adult life and all are working full-time. One (A.M.) has just been married, and none of them show evidence of any damage resulting from the radiation therapy. *Figure 6* is a composite of these six children, 16 to 17 years after their treatment. These long-time survivals clearly indicate that radiation is effective for craniopharyngiomas and that it is safe, provided the suggested doses are not exceeded and surgical damage is kept to a minimum.

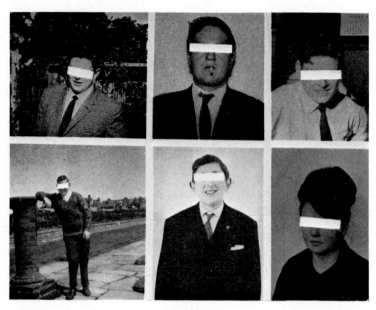

Figure 6. Appearance of six children from the first series of patients, 16 to 17 years after radiation treatment. (Reproduced from Kramer, Southard and Mansfield (1968) by courtesy of the Editor of American Journal of Roentgenology)

Since 1958, with the availability of moving-beam supervoltage equipment, we have changed our technique and use one of two methods. The one employs a 220 degree arc situated in the coronal plane as shown in *Figure 7*. This technique gives an area of high dose, lying somewhat above the axis of rotation, and this must be taken into consideration in the planning. This method is particularly useful when a relatively small volume is irradiated. Since we rotate our equipment in a vertical plane in order to obtain the appropriate coronal plane in the patient's skull, it is necessary for the patient's head to be either flexed or extended quite sharply, and this can be facilitated by raising the patient onto a wedge-shaped support. Where the plane cannot be obtained because of a short neck or where the tumour is large, a rotational technique is less advantageous; and an isocentric technique, using two lateral wedges and a superior open

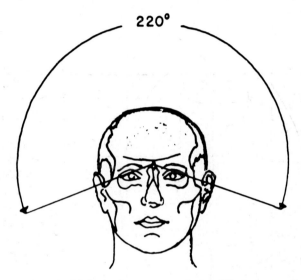

Figure 7. Method of treatment using a 220 degree arc situated in the coronal plane. (Reproduced from Kramer (1969) by courtesy of the Editor of Annals of the New York Academy of Sciences)

field is employed, as shown in *Figure 8.* As far as the tumour dose is concerned, we have, in the past, seen no need to decrease the dose below the value initially decided upon, since we have seen only one patient with an overt necrosis of the brain. However, with the three-field technique, a larger volume is irradiated homogeneously; and under these circumstances, it may well be wise to decrease the target volume dose to 6,500 rads so as to avoid a higher dose to any sizable volume in the brain. All treatment in both series has been given on the basis of five fractions per week. In the three-field technique, either two or, preferably, all three fields are irradiated each day.

Between 1958 and 1971 we have treated an additional 33 patients with craniopharyngiomas at the Thomas Jefferson University Hospital—12 children and 21 adults. The results have been reported previously in part (Kramer, Southard and Mansfield, 1968). In most of these patients the combined treatment was not as carefully planned as in the first series, since many times the neurosurgeon attempted a complete removal of the tumour, but abandoned the attempt and referred the patient to us for radiation therapy. Eight patients (two children and six adults) were referred only after a recurrence had taken place 6 weeks to $6\frac{1}{2}$ years after the initial surgical attempt.

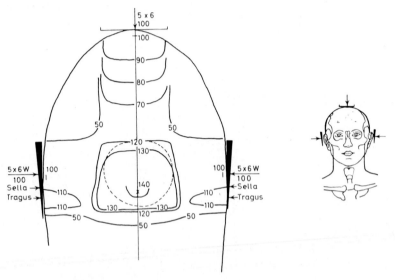

Figure 8. Isocentric three-field technique, using two lateral wedges and a superior open field

Consequently, many of these patients have considerably greater neurological and endocrinological deficits than the first series. It should be noted that of the additional 12 children, we definitely failed to control the tumour in one recurrent case. This patient had a huge recurrence, known to be present for three years before referral for radiation therapy. He improved after radiation therapy, but the disease progressed later, and he died four years after treatment. A second child did well for two years and eight months after radiation therapy and then suffered a head injury with sudden blindness; a craniotomy was performed, where residual tumour was seen, but no histological proof was obtained. The child died post-operatively and is considered to have died of disease. The other ten children in the second series are alive, and only one child has marked growth retardation, although she is mentally bright. This child has just been placed on growth hormone treatment, and is beginning to respond.

Of the adults in the second series, 13 survived and 8 have died. Of the latter, 2 have died of unrelated diseases, 3 following a second operative intervention thought necessary because of deterioration during or immediately following the course of radiation therapy. Two patients' deaths were possibly related to the treatment. One of them developed recurrent aseptic meningitis and at autopsy was found to have areas of necrosis, which may or may not have been related to treatment. The other patient, with a huge tumour filling the third and both lateral ventricles, died a year after treatment and post mortem was found to have not only a huge residual tumour, but also some areas of necrosis which could have been due either to pressure or to radiation therapy. One last patient is worthy of further comment. This was a 46-year-old woman with a relatively large craniopharyngioma in whom total removal was attempted. The attempt was abandoned when, at operation, it was discovered that the tumour was adherent to the base of the skull, and a considerable amount of tumour was left behind. Post-operatively she was totally obtunded and we were unable to use our rotational technique. Most of the treatment was given through lateral opposed fields. Her total tumour dose was 7,000 rads to the target volume in seven weeks. She recovered partially towards the end of her treatment and the last 1,700 rads were given by our usual rotational technique. However, her organo-mental syndrome persisted and she required custodial care in a nursing home. Eight months after the onset of radiation therapy she was admitted to the hospital in a coma and died three days later. On post-mortem examination, an area of acute softening was found in the right hemisphere in the fronto-parietal region. There was almost total occlusion of the right internal carotid and middle cerebral arteries. While the surgical intervention, which had also taken place on the right side, probably contributed to the brain damage, we must assume that the tissue dose of approximately 7,500 rads received in the area of necrosis was primarily responsible for the subsequent damage. This again demonstrated the importance of limiting the irradiated volume and considering the integrity of the blood supply to the irradiated volume. Incidentally, no evidence of residual tumour was found post mortem in this patient.

Our total experience of craniopharyngiomas is reported in Tables 4 to 6. Because the disease process is so different in children and adults, these are first reported separately, namely in children (Table 4), and in adults (Table 5). The total experience is shown in Table 6. It indicates that the results obtained by combination of surgery and radiotherapy are probably the best possible for these tumours.

Our experience indicates that there is probably never a need to attempt a radical removal of the craniopharyngioma, a procedure which increases the operative risk and certainly leads to considerably greater neurological and endocrinological morbidity. It should certainly never be attempted where there is the slightest doubt that it can be attempted safely. The best results will be obtained when

TABLE 4
Thomas Jefferson University Hospital—
Craniopharyngiomas in Children 1972

Total	18 (2 recurrent cases)			
Survival	At Risk	AsD	Dead	
>10 years	9	7	2	(1 recurrent case, DčD at 5 years; 1 new case, DčD 3 years 8 months)
> 5 years	14	12	2	
> 2 years	16	14	2	
< 2 years	18	16	2	

AsD: alive without disease.   DčD: dead with disease.

TABLE 5
Thomas Jefferson University Hospital—
Craniopharyngiomas in Adults 1972

Total	25 (6 recurrent cases)			
Survival	At Risk	AsD	Dead	
>10 years	10	6	4	(2 unrelated disease 1 post-operative 1 necrosis)
5 years	14	8	6	(4 unrelated disease 1 post-operative 1 necrosis)
3 years	18	9	9	(4 unrelated disease 2 post-operative 1 necrosis 2 possibly treatment-related)
< 3 years	25	14	11	(5 unrelated disease 3 post-operative 1 necrosis 2 possibly treatment-related)

AsD: alive without disease.

220

surgery is limited to obliteration of the cyst and possible removal of
that portion of the tumour that is easily accessible. Even when a
radical removal of the tumour has been accomplished with apparent
success, the danger of recurrence is extremely high, and even these
patients should invariably be given post-operative radiation (although perhaps in these patients a dose of 5,500 rads in $5\frac{1}{2}$ weeks
would be adequate).

TABLE 6

Thomas Jefferson University Hospital—
Craniopharyngiomas: Total Experience, 1972

Total	43	(8 recurrent cases)
Surviving 1–20 years	30	
Dead	13	(5 unrelated disease 2 recurrence 2 possibly treatment- related 3 post-operative 1 necrosis)

In patients with appreciable residual tumour and those in whom
only minimal surgery has been performed, a dose of 5,500 rads in 6
weeks is safe in the younger children, and a dose of 6,500 in $6\frac{1}{2}$ weeks
should be delivered to adults. It should be emphasized that close
collaboration between the neurosurgeon, endocrinologist and the
radiation therapist is necessary not only in the diagnosis and treatment planning of the management of a particular patient, but also in
the supportive therapy which is needed in the pre- and post-operative
period, and the period during and after radiation therapy. Many of
these patients have considerable endocrinological deficits, and a baseline must always be established before treatment is undertaken
unless the increased intracranial pressure presents an emergency.
Even then, endocrinological studies should be performed as soon as
possible after the surgical intervention and at intervals during and
after radiation therapy. Finally, it should be noted that absence or
marked depression of the growth hormone either immediately before
or after treatment does not necessarily mean that the young child will
become a dwarf. As pointed out by Kenny and colleagues (1968),
some of these children appear to be able to recoup sufficient growth
hormone activity, in some as-yet-unexplained way, to allow them to
proceed to normal growth. Here again, it should be noted that of the
six children treated 10–20 years ago, only one is of short stature,
while the others are of normal height. In each case, of course, an

individual decision has to be made as to what supportive hormone therapy is to be given, and this decision will depend not only on the availability of the hormones but also on the state of development of the child, and the deficit which has to be made up.

SUMMARY

Radiation therapy has been shown to be effective in the curative treatment of craniopharyngiomas. The best results have been obtained when surgical intervention has been limited to biopsy and cyst evacuation. Relatively high doses are needed for the control of these tumours. With precision techniques to keep the irradiated volume as small as possible, morbidity has been kept to a minimum. No endocrine disturbances have been observed as a result of the radiation therapy.

REFERENCES

Bailey, P. (1933). *Intracranial Tumors*, pp. 113–137. Springfield, Ill.; Thomas.

Bond, W. H., Richards, D. and Turner, E. (1965). 'Experiences with radioactive gold in treatment of craniopharyngioma.' *J. Neurol. Neurosurg. Psychiat.*, **28**, 30.

Carpenter, R. V., Chamberlin, G. W. and Frazier, C. H. (1937). 'The treatment of hypophyseal stalk tumors by evacuation and irradiation.' *Am. J. Roentgenol.*, **38**, 162.

Critchley, M. and Ironside, R. N. (1926). 'The pituitary adamantinoma.' *Brain*, **49**, 437.

Cushing, H. (1932). *Intracranial Tumors: Notes Upon a Series of 2000 Verified Cases with Surgical–Mortality Percentages Pertaining Thereto*, pp. 93–98. Springfield, Ill.; Thomas.

Erdheim, J. (1904). Über Hypophysengangsgeschwülste und Hirncholesteatome.' *Sitzungsberichte der Akademie der Wissenschaft, Wien*, **113**, 537.

Frazier, C. H. and Alpers, B. J. (1931). 'Adamantinomas of the craniopharyngeal duct.' *Archs Neurol.*, **26**, 905.

— — (1934). 'Tumors of Rathke's cleft.' *Archs Neurol.*, **32**, 973.

Gordy, P. D., Peet, M. M. and Kahn, E. A. (1949). 'The surgery of the craniopharyngiomas.' *J. Neurosurg.*, **6**, 503.

Hirsch, O. (1959). 'Symptomatology and treatment of the hypophyseal duct tumors (craniopharyngiomas).' *Confinia Neurol. (Basel)*, **19**, 153.

Horrax, G. (1954). 'Benign (favorable) types of brain tumor. The end results (up to twenty years) with statistics of mortality and useful survival.' *New Engl. J. Med.*, **250**, 981.

REFERENCES

Kenny, F. M., Iturzaeta, N. F., Mintz, D., Drash, A., Garces, L. Y., Susen, A. and Askari, H. A. (1968). 'Iatrogenic hypopituitarism in craniopharyngioma: unexplained catch-up growth in three children.' *J. Pediat.*, **72**, 766.

Kramer, S. (1969). 'Radiation therapy in the management of brain tumors in children.' *Ann. N.Y. Acad. Sci.*, **159**, 571.

— McKissock, W. and Concannon, J. P. (1961). 'Craniopharyngiomas. Treatment by combined surgery and radiation therapy.' *J. Neurosurg.*, **18**, 217.

— Southard, M. and Mansfield, C. M. (1968). 'Radiotherapy in the management of craniopharyngiomas: further experiences and late results.' *Am. J. Roentgenol.*, **103**, 44.

Leddy, E. T. and Marshall, T. M. (1951). 'Roentgen therapy of pituitary adamantinomas (craniopharyngiomas).' *Radiology*, **56**, 384.

Leksell, L., Backlund, E. O. and Johansson, L. (1967). 'Treatment of craniopharyngiomas.' *Acta chir. scand.*, **133**, 345.

Love, J. G. and Marshall, T. M. (1950). 'Craniopharyngiomas.' *Surgery Gynec. Obstet.*, **90**, 591.

Matson, D. D. (1969). *Neurosurgery of Infancy and Childhood*, pp. 544–574. Springfield, Ill.; Thomas.

— and Crigler, J. F., Jnr. (1969). 'Management of craniopharyngiomas in childhood.' *J. Neurosurg.*, **30**, 377.

Olivecrona, H. (1966). 'The craniopharyngiomas.' In *Handbuch der Neurochirurgie*, Vol. IV, p. 4. Heidelberg; Springer.

Svien, H. J. (1965). 'Surgical experiences with craniopharyngiomas.' *J. Neurosurg.*, **23**, 148.

Svolos, D. G. (1969). 'Craniopharyngiomas.' *Acta chir. scand.*, Suppl. 403.

11—Radiotherapy of Pituitary Tumours

Martin B. Levene

INTRODUCTION

The majority of tumours arising in the hypophysis and its immediate environs are histologically benign but nevertheless offer a challenge to successful treatment because of their relative inaccessibility and their proximity to other vital structures. Both surgical and radiotherapeutic modalities of treatment date back to the first decade of the present century. The trans-sphenoidal approach to the pituitary was pioneered by Schloffer in 1906 while, in the same year, Horsley reported on the intracranial route. Shortly thereafter Gramegna treated the first pituitary adenoma with radiation therapy in May, 1907, using an intraoral glass applicator to achieve temporary improvement in a 45-year-old female acromegalic. In the same year, Béclère successfully treated a 16-year-old girl with gigantism employing a five field technique. The patient responded to treatment with both an improvement in vision and subsidence of headaches and was reported to be alive and well 15 years later. The trans-sphenoidal approach was improved by Hirsch (1910) who successfully developed an endonasal route. Hirsch (1921) also pioneered in the brachytherapy of pituitary tumours employing a radium capsule with the sphenoid sinus for this purpose. The combined use of surgery and radiation therapy has had its advocates since the disclosure of Henderson (1939) that in Cushing's series post-operative radiotherapy raised the recurrence-free rate from 42 to 74 per cent for surgically treated chromophobe adenomas.

In 1946, Wilson proposed the use of fast protons for radiation therapy and noted that by using the Bragg peak region of the absorption curve it would be possible 'to treat a volume as small as 1·0 cc anywhere in the body and to give that volume several times the dose of any neighboring tissue'. Acting on this suggestion, Tobias, Anger and Lawrence (1952) reported the results of animal studies with beams of deuterons and alpha particles produced in the Berkley 184 inch cyclotron and in 1954 the first human patients were treated with a 340 MeV proton beam from this same machine with the object of pituitary ablation for palliation of metastatic breast cancer (Mc-Combs, 1957). In subsequent years, the use of heavy particle therapy has been extended to ablation of the pituitary in diabetic retinopathy and to the treatment of pituitary adenomas in acromegaly (Lawrence and colleagues, 1970 b) and Cushing's disease (Lawrence and colleagues, 1971).

A fourth approach to the treatment of pituitary adenomas and the ablation of the normal pituitary is interstitial implantation therapy utilizing a variety of radioactive materials ranging from radon in 1920 (Quick, 1920) to yttrium-90 (Rasmussen, Harper and Kennedy, 1953), gold-198 (Talairach and colleagues, 1956), and radioactive chromic phosphate (Rothenberg and colleagues, 1955) in the 1950s. The trans-nasal and trans-sphenoidal route to the hypophysis is generally used. Stereotaxic apparatus may be relied upon for the accurate positioning of the radioactive material (Jadresic and colleagues, 1965).

DIFFERENTIAL DIAGNOSIS

Since most new growths arising in the hypophysis are histologically benign, they manifest their presence by expansile growth producing pressure on adjacent structures, including the anterior lobe of the pituitary, with subsequent reduction in the production of hormones by this endocrine gland or by the autogenous production of one or more of these same hormones in excess of the body's requirements. Other pressure phenomena include visual disturbances due to the proximity of the optic chiasm, classically in the form of a bitemporal hemianopsia but often departing from this, headache, and rarely hypothalamic disturbances, including diabetes insipidus and drowsiness.

It is common practice to make the diagnosis of pituitary adenoma on clinical grounds and proceed with radiation therapy without histological confirmation. However, the relative ease with which a trans-sphenoidal biopsy may be obtained makes it possible to document the true nature of a lesion (Zervas, 1969). It well may eventually become routine to obtain histology for all lesions of the hypophysis.

There are a number of conditions which simulate one or more

aspects of signs and symptoms of pituitary adenoma and which must be considered in the differential diagnosis. In recent years, attention has been given to the 'empty sella syndrome'. The 'empty sella' describes a condition in which intrasellar air is demonstrated on pneumoencephalography with the pituitary gland compressed to form a small rim of tissue at the bottom of the sella (Kaufman, 1968). Enlargement of the sella turcica is a frequent accompaniment of this condition together with thinning of the dorsum sellae. Visual symptoms and optic signs suggesting pressure on the optic nerves may be present. Endocrine studies by Caplan and Dobben (1969) on six patients with this syndrome showed the presence of endocrine dysfunction of pituitary origin. It thus becomes imperative to perform pneumoencephalography on all patients with enlarged sellae prior to treatment, not only to determine the presence of suprasellar extension of adenomata but to exclude the 'empty sella syndrome'.

Other lesions which may cause enlargement of the sella turcica as well as bitemporal hemianopsia include meningioma of the tuberculum sellae, craniopharyngioma, oxycephaly (Grundy, Goree and Jimenez, 1970) and dilatation of the third ventricle. Craniopharyngioma may be quite difficult to differentiate from pituitary adenoma in the absence of calcification as occurs in approximately 25 per cent. However, changes produced in the sella turcica are more likely to be seen in the posterior clinoids with less tendency to expansion from within (Miskin, 1970). Meningioma may be differentiated by the presence of hyperostosis in adjacent bone. Gliomas of the optic chiasm produce loss of vision without alteration of pituitary function. They are commonly seen in children and are quite rare in adults. Aneurysm of the internal carotid artery produces a homonymous hemianopsia together with palsies of the third, fourth and sixth cranial nerves.

There are several radiological investigations which are of importance in the evaluation of lesions in and around the sella turcica. Sosman (1949) indicated that the plain lateral film disclosed changes in the sella in 93 per cent of patients with chromophobe adenoma and in 80 per cent of patients with acromegaly. However McLachlan, Wright and Doyle (1970) have found that tomographic assessment of the pituitary fossa will detect change in over 98 per cent of acromegalics. Pneumoencephalography is probably the most useful examination in determining the nature and extent of these lesions. Occasionally one may wish to combine tomography with the PEG to better delineate the third ventricle. Where the pneumoencephalogram has proved to be normal, angiography should be considered to detect possible aneurysm.

226

PITUITARY ADENOMAS

The incidence of pituitary adenomas has been variously reported to range between 7 per cent (Zulch, 1957) and 18 per cent (Henderson, 1939). The higher figure is that of Cushing's series and may well be elevated by his special interest in pituitary adenomas. Some 70–80 per cent of adenomata are of the chromophobe type and the bulk of the remainder are eosinophilic. A recent study by McCormick and Halmi (1971) suggests that most chromophobe adenomas can be demonstrated to contain chromophilic granules when fixed and stained with appropriate techniques. Eosinophilic adenomas are generally present in patients with acromegaly and gigantism, reflecting the overproduction of growth hormone by this type of adenoma. Chromophobe adenomas were once thought to be lacking in hormone production but it is now recognized that they are occasionally associated with Cushing's disease (Lindholm, Rasmussen and Korsgaard, 1969). The small and uncommon basophil adenoma is also occasionally found in this illness.

CHROMOPHOBE ADENOMAS

The growth potential of this tumour is easily underestimated. They are commonly quite large and may extend in any direction. As described by Wolman (1966), 'the extension could be upwards into the hypothalamus and third ventricle, forwards into or between the frontal lobes or through the optic foramen into the orbit, laterally into the cavernous sinus or middle cranial fossa, or backwards into the intrapeduncular fossa. These tumours could also extend downwards through the eroded bone of the floor of the pituitary fossa into the sphenoidal air sinus'.

Visual disturbances predominate as the presenting symptom. They generally begin as upper bitemporal quadrant defects and progress to a complete bitemporal hemianopsia. If the adenoma erodes through the lateral wall of the sella turcica and compresses the optic radiation, a homonymous hemianopsia may result. Diplopia is seen if the third, fourth or sixth cranial nerves are involved. Headache is also a prominent symptom and probably the second most common presenting complaint. Other symptoms relate to suppression of pituitary hormonal production and include easy fatiguability, diminished libido, amenorrhoea, soft, dry, pale skin, increased body weight with subcutaneous accumulation of fat over the hips and breasts and thinned hair with a soft silky texture. Less frequently one encounters polyuria and polydipsia, seizures, rhinorrhoea, visual hallucinations and hemiparesis (Chang and Pool, 1967).

The options available in the treatment of chromophobe adenomas include surgical removal, irradiation, or a combination of both. Advocates of surgery cite the need for a histological diagnosis, the danger of further optic injury during radiation therapy prior to relief of pressure and the hazards of late radiation damage. They also point to the poor response to radiation occurring in the 15 to 20 per cent of the adenomas which are cystic. The stereotaxic trans-sphenoidal biopsy technique of Zervas (1969) provides the desired histological information and evacuates the fluid contents of the cystic adenoma if such is present, partially overcoming these objections, while avoiding the major disadvantages of surgery which include a significant operative morbidity and mortality. Stern and Batzdorf (1970) have collected mortality figures from 20 major published series. These figures range between 0 and 35 per cent with a median value of 11·2 per cent. As noted earlier, the recurrence rate after surgical excision can be significantly reduced by post-operative irradiation (Henderson, 1939). Even those centres which regard radiation therapy as the modality of choice recognize certain indications for prior surgery. These include marked visual impairment especially with encroachment on the macula, rapidly advancing optic atrophy, more than moderately advanced visual loss, or a clinical picture leading one to doubt the diagnosis of pituitary adenoma.

Probably because of the benign histology associated with pituitary adenomas, treatment schedules during the years prior to the 1940s called for multiple courses comprised of repeated small radiation exposures. The frequency of these courses was dictated by the patient's symptoms. Kerr in 1948 published a series of cases treated by a relatively large dose delivered in a single intensive course, and called attention to the superiority of this technique. A retrospective analysis of 301 patients treated at the Presbyterian Hospital and the Neurological Institute of New York was reported in 1966 (Chang and Pool, 1967). This study divided patients with chromophobe adenomas into three groups by treatment technique. In the first group, patients received multiple courses of small-dose radiation with courses repeated at four- to eight-week intervals. The second group received multiple courses with 30 to 40 per cent higher doses in each course than the first group with the courses repeated at shorter intervals. The third group received a single course with high total dose as is generally carried out at present. Responses to treatment were evaluated in terms of improvement of vision. In the low-dose multiple course group a successful response was noted in 35 per

cent while the medium-dose multiple course group showed a successful response in 50 per cent. The best response rate was noted in the
high-dose single course group where a successful response was
obtained in 65 per cent. The authors concluded that the response is
dose dependent within the dose range used but cautioned against
attempting to extrapolate the data to imply that further increase in
dose will produce a still better response.

The figure 4,000 to 5,000 rads in four to five weeks appears to be
the accepted dose in most centres reporting results of treatment in
recent years (Kramer, 1968; Hayes, Davis and Raventos, 1971;
Carlson and Marsh, 1971).

The re-treatment of recurrences following radiation therapy is
generally dealt with surgically when feasible but the question of
further radiation therapy sooner or later is inevitably raised. Since
the original course of treatment often approaches what is believed
to be normal tissue tolerance, re-treatment can only be approached
with trepidation. Sheline (1971) offers some measure of reassurance
in his report of eight patients re-treated after previous combined
surgery and radiation therapy. Three patients had originally received doses less than 3,000 rads. The others had doses ranging
between 3,200 rads in 51 days to 4,700 rads in 35 days. Re-treatment
took place 3–12 years after original therapy and consisted of doses of
3,500 rads in 35 days to 4,600 rads in 39 days. Five patients under-
went surgery as well. Six of the eight patients improved. There was
no evidence of radiation damage with follow-up periods of 3–9 years.

EOSINOPHILIC ADENOMAS

These adenomas are generally associated with an overproduction of
growth hormone and the resulting alterations in body function and
growth largely characterize their presence. When they occur before
closure of the epiphyses, gigantism results. After puberty, growth
takes place largely in the hands, feet and facial bones, producing
acromegaly. The onset of the disease is insidious with the patient
gradually developing a fairly characteristic appearance with prog-
nathism, thick, leathery skin, enlarged hands and feet and coarse
facial features. Menstrual irregularities in the female are characterized by menorrhagia in the early stages and amenorrhoea in the later
stages. Similarly in the male, sexual hyperactivity may be present
early with diminished libido or impotence occurring as the illness
progresses. Other symptoms include headache, arthritic pains and
visual disturbances. Since eosinophilic adenomas tend to be considerably smaller than chromophobe adenomas, extension beyond

the limits of the sella turcica with consequent compression of the optic nerves is seen less than half the time.

In the past, it was believed that acromegaly is a disease which remains active for a number of years but eventually achieves a state where it is 'burned-out' or inactive. In the absence of visual disturbances, evidence of activity of the disease was sought as an indication for treatment. However, more recent investigations indicate that most untreated cases of acromegaly remain active (Greenwood and colleagues, 1965; Roth and colleagues, 1967). While the correlation between the severity of acromegaly and the plasma growth hormone levels is poor, its elevation above normal level should be used as one of the confirmatory signs of acromegaly. Wright and colleagues (1969) have found a highly significant correlation between the maximum lateral area of the sella turcica and the mean serum growth hormone level during a glucose tolerance test, which they feel suggests that growth hormone secretion is proportional to the size of the pituitary tumour.

If one accepts the premise that nearly all untreated acromegalics have continued activity of their disease, it follows that all such patients require treatment. Only left to be decided is the nature of such treatment. This is at present a somewhat controversial subject, not so much the customary controversy between radiation therapy and surgery but rather the modality of radiation therapy, i.e. conventional megavoltage therapy utilizing a photon beam or heavy particle therapy.

The advocates of heavy particle therapy point to what they consider the limited success of conventional photon beam therapy in both relieving the signs and symptoms of the disease and in prolonging life expectancy. It is their belief that heavy particle therapy utilizing a well collimated, precisely localized, non-divergent beam can safely deliver radiation doses high enough 'to inhibit or destroy the abnormal activity or the acidophilic cells without damage to surrounding structures or to the normal cells of the gland' (Lawrence and colleagues, 1970 b).

Several recent assessments of the efficacy of conventional radiation therapy in acromegaly (Roth, Gordon and Kirkland, 1970; Lawrence, Pinsky and Goldfine, 1971) demonstrate fall in growth hormone serum or plasma concentrations in all treated patients with reversal of acral changes, and marked improvement in glucose and insulin tolerance in several. In one series, Lawrence and her co-workers document a return to normal or very near normal levels of basal serum growth hormone levels in 21 of 27 (77 per cent) acromegalics treated by cobalt-60 or 2 MeV x-ray irradiation. Roth, Gordon and

Kirkland (1970) found a dose of 4,000 rads (time unspecified) delivered with 2 MeV radiation 'nearly always reduces plasma growth hormone within 1 to 2 years and usually produces a substantial further fall within 3 to 4 years'. These results strongly suggest that conventional photon therapy is capable of playing an important role in the therapy of acromegaly.

There is little argument about the efficacy of heavy-particle therapy in acromegaly. Lawrence and colleagues (1970 a) found that plasma growth hormone levels were reduced to below 10 ng/ml in all but 10 of 131 acromegalics treated with heavy particles together with a return to normal of other metabolic abnormalities as measured by glucose tolerance and insulin tolerance. Kliman and Kjellberg (1971) found plasma growth hormone levels reduced to 5 ng/ml or lower in 29 of 62 (47 per cent) patients with acromegaly treated with proton irradiation utilizing the Bragg peak.

The acceptance of heavy-particle therapy as a primary mode of therapy for acromegaly appears to depend on two factors, availability and one's judgement as to the acceptability of associated complications. Availability is dependent on an accelerator capable of producing high energy, heavy particles. Three such units are in medical use in the world today. These are cyclotrons located in Uppsala, Sweden, Berkeley, California, and Cambridge, Massachusetts. Lawrence and colleagues (1970 a) have compiled a list of 13 additional cyclotrons with energies of 100 MeV protons or higher which they suggest could be used therapeutically.

The complications of heavy-particle therapy are primarily ocular although other neurological deficits are reported. Kjellberg and Kliman (1971) have observed oculomotor palsies in 37 of 128 acromegalic patients (29 per cent) treated with high energy protons. As might be anticipated, the palsies were more common in those who had received prior treatment with x-ray photons or protons. Dawson and Dingman (1970) found that eight of nine patients who received proton therapy utilizing the Bragg peak technique developed complications. These included three oculomotor palsies, a severe bitemporal hemianopsia, and four cases of vertigo, as well as a patient with possible uncinate seizures. The complication rate reported by Lawrence and colleagues (1970 a) is lower. Three of six patients treated with heavy-particles following x-ray therapy developed ocular problems (two transient diplopia, one quadrant cut) but since this group eliminated patients with prior therapy in 1961 they have noted an overall complication rate of 3·5 per cent. They also eliminated from consideration for treatment patients with significant suprasellar extension who are referred instead for surgical management.

231

It should be noted that both of these centres depart from conventional fractionation schemes in employing heavy particles. At Berkeley, it has been customary to utilize six fractions delivered over an interval of 12 days (Lawrence and colleagues, 1970 a). At Cambridge, the entire dose has been administered in a single fraction (Kjellberg and colleagues, 1968). Since charged heavy particles do not appear to differ appreciably from other low LET radiations with respect to biological effect, one is forced to speculate that greater protraction of the period of treatment might be of value in lessening complications.

The complications associated with properly planned, well administered conventional megavoltage photon therapy are negligible. Such reports appear in the literature (Almquist and colleagues, 1964; Richmond, 1958) at infrequent intervals and consist primarily of brain necrosis occurring in patients treated with seemingly safe doses although in some re-treatment with high cumulative doses is involved (Peck and McGovern, 1966). The sites of damage are most commonly the hypothalamus and temporal lobes, the latter because of the propensity to treat the hypophysis through two opposing lateral portals.

The response of pituitary adenomas to irradiation appears to be dose related. It is quite likely that the same response can be obtained with conventional megavoltage x-ray photons as with heavy particles, provided one is willing to accept the complications which higher doses will bring. Considering the success that Kramer, Southard and Mansfield (1968) have had in delivering doses of 7,000 rads in seven weeks to the hypophyseal region, it is conceivable that with precise technique, using small carefully localized portals, and a well collimated beam, rigid immobilization and rotation in both the coronal and sagittal planes, the results of heavy particle therapy in acromegaly can be achieved with x-ray photons. At present, however, dosage in most centres is similar to that employed for treating chromophobe adenomas.

CUSHING'S SYNDROME

This syndrome occurs in response to hyperadrenocorticism from a variety of causes. Tumours of the adrenal cortex, both benign and malignant, adrenocortical hyperplasia and less frequently pituitary adenomas may represent the underlying aetiology. Secretion of an ACTH-like substance by carcinomas of the ovary, lung, thymus, pancreas and thyroid may also produce the syndrome. In 1958, Nelson and others called attention to the appearance of pituitary adenomas in patients who had previously undergone bilateral adrenalectomy for hyperadrenocorticism. These patients are characterized by the development of marked skin pigmentation and by extremely high circulating corticotrophin levels (Nelson, Meakin and Thorn, 1960). The adenomas are comprised mainly of chromophobe cells. It has been speculated that the adenomas are present prior to adrenalectomy and that their growth is enhanced by the ablative procedure. Such tumours of the pituitary have not been observed in patients with Addison's disease.

Cushing's syndrome clinically manifests its presence with obesity, hypertension, plethora, asthenia, moon facies, diabetes mellitus, osteoporosis, violaceous striae, virilism in the female, and feminism in the male. The plasma cortisol levels are elevated and the normal diurnal variation is absent. The urinary excretion of 17-ketosteroids is generally elevated.

Since Cushing's syndrome may have any of several aetiologies, its cause must be determined prior to any decision regarding treatment. It is particularly important to determine whether an adrenal tumour is present since this calls for a direct surgical approach. Benign adrenal adenomas are cured by surgical removal.

If, however, adrenal hyperplasia is present, due to excess production of pituitary ACTH, surgery, pituitary irradiation, or a combination of these modalities may be employed. Orth and Liddle (1971) have reported the results of primary radiation therapy in 51 such patients who received doses of 4,000–5,000 rads in a period of about one month; 10 patients appeared to be cured while an additional 13 improved sufficiently to require no further therapy except for aminoglutethimide given to some. The authors do not indicate whether or not pituitary adenomas were present in any of this group of patients. Levitt, Prather and Bogardus (1970) reviewed the results of treatment of primary pituitary tumours associated with Cushing's syndrome and found that only 3 of 23 patients treated with pituitary irradiation demonstrated a persistent symptomatic response. Those responding received doses in excess of 4,000 rads. Of 8 patients with proven chromophobe adenoma, only 1 responded but this patient was the only one to receive 4,000 rads. The authors conclude that the number of patients with reported treatment details is too small to draw definite conclusions about poor response to irradiation. Lawrence and colleagues (1971) indicate that heavy-particle therapy is effective in Cushing's disease. Since 1959, they have irradiated 25 patients with doses usually in excess of 10,000 rads and report 'dramatic benefits in their endocrine and metabolic status' in 19. They have also treated 6 patients following bilateral adrenalectomy who have developed pigmentation of the skin with or without enlarged sella and report stabilization or decrease in pigmentation and a fall in ACTH levels in the 2 patients on whom such measurements were made.

Another approach to treatment where no pituitary or adrenal tumour is demonstrated involves unilateral adrenalectomy and pituitary irradiation used in combination. Van Seters, Jenny and Querido (1965), reporting on the results of so treating 38 patients, found a 50 per cent complete remission rate with an additional 13 per cent requiring no further therapy.

CRANIOPHARYNGIOMA

While not actually a tumour of pituitary origin, the craniopharyngioma generally is found in close proximity to the sella turcica, is an important differential diagnosis for pituitary lesions, particularly in children, and is amenable to treatment by much the same radiotherapeutic techniques as pituitary adenomas. A number of other names have been applied to the craniopharyngioma, including Rathke's pouch tumour, epidermoid cyst, suprasellar cyst, hypophyseal duct cyst, and adamantinoma. The lesion is usually composed of multiple cystic cavities lined with squamous epithelium and filled with an oily fluid containing cholesterol crystals. Occasionally the tumour is solid. Its most common location is the suprasellar region but it may be intrasellar with or without suprasellar extension.

Craniopharyngioma is more commonly found in children than in adults. When seen in children, it may be accompanied by the adiposogenital syndrome. Impairment of vision is the most common presenting symptom but headache, growth disturbance and symptoms of panhypopituitarism are also noted. In the adult, the lesion may be difficult to distinguish from chromophobe adenoma on clinical grounds but the diagnosis can be established by transsphenoidal biopsy.

In the past, surgery has been regarded as the method of choice in treating craniopharyngioma. Since the lesion is histologically benign, complete removal should be tantamount to cure. Unfortunately it is often technically impossible to effect total removal due to the proximity to multiple delicate structures to which the lesion is often adherent including the hypothalamus, optic nerves and third ventricle.

Kramer, McKissock and Concannon in 1961 first reported a new approach to the treatment of this lesion by combined surgery and radiation therapy and more recently he has been given further follow-up of his original series of 10 patients and presented data on

16 additional cases (Kramer, Southard and Mansfield, 1968). The surgical aspect of treatment is confined to decompression of the cystic portion of the tumour and the establishment of a diagnosis. The trans-sphenoidal stereotaxic approach may be attempted but if unsuccessful a transcranial approach will be necessary. Radiation therapy is then administered to the lesion using megavoltage photons with an arc or rotation technique. Kramer has aimed for doses of 7,000 rads in seven weeks in adults and 5,500 rads in six weeks in children below 14 years of age. His results are quite impressive. All of the six children in the original series were alive and well 13–15 years after treatment. One adult was alive and well 15 years after treatment; the other three adults in the first series died of other causes without evidence of recurrence or brain damage at 2, 10 and 14 years. Of the 16 patients in the second series, 6 were referred after recurrence following surgical treatment but despite this 4 of 6 children and 7 of 10 adults were alive and well six months to eight years and ten months after treatment. It should be noted that Kramer emphasizes the need to avoid extensive surgical procedures to avoid compromising the blood supply of the brain as well as the need for precision radiation therapy with the irradiated volume kept to a minimum in order to avoid radiation complications with doses of this magnitude.

RADIATION TECHNIQUES

Prior to treatment planning it is essential that the extent of the tumour be determined as precisely as possible. The confidence one has in the tumour localization will determine the extent to which field size can be reduced since, with histologically benign tumours, margins need not take into account infiltration beyond the gross extent of the lesion. An exception to this is encountered with large chromophobe adenomas which may, indeed, be infiltrative. The pneumoencephalogram is the most useful study for tumour localization but additional information may be available with angiography particularly regarding the anterior extent of the lesion.

Absolute immobilization of the patient's head during treatment is another requisite to therapy with small fields. This requires a good head holder rigidly attached to the treatment chair or couch as well as a means of individualizing the head holder to the patient. Perspex or plaster masks may be used for this purpose but we have found Orthoplast to be simple to employ and yet highly effective. This orthopaedic plastic splinting material can be cut with scissors and when heated to 140°F is easily moulded to facial contours without discomfort to the patient. When cooled to room temperature, it hardens to retain the desired contours and when used with a suitable head holder gives the needed immobilization.

Beam direction is established by portal filming. It should be borne in mind that if an arc rotation is employed past pointing may be necessary. When satisfactory portal films are obtained, field localization marks should be tatooed on the skin. During the period of treatment, frequent checks of beam direction by repeat portal films is suggested.

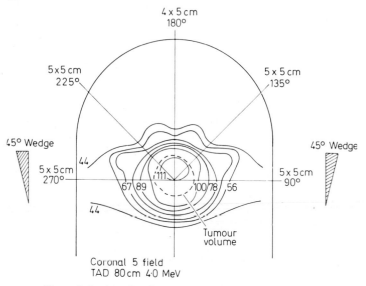

Figure 1. Isodose distribution using 5 fixed fields at 4 MeV

Treatment should be carried out using a well collimated megavoltage photon beam. The output of an x-ray generator such as a linear accelerator is preferable to cobalt-60 because of its sharper beam edges which produces a tighter isodose distribution in rotation techniques and reduces the dose to normal brain tissues.

In the past, radiation of the hypophyseal region has been largely by two portal technique, usually parallel opposed lateral portals. Chang and Pool (1967) found they could reduce the integral dose by almost one-half by changing their technique from two opposing 5 × 5 cm ports using cobalt-60 to 360 degree rotation of a 4 × 4 cm port using 6 MeV x-ray photons. Our preference is for treatment in the coronal plane since we believe that the area of greatest uncertainty as to tumour extent most often lies superiorly and the coronal rotation provides a less abrupt transition from the high dose region to the low dose region in this area than does rotation in a transverse plane. If rotation is not available a satisfactory plan may be achieved using five fields as shown in *Figure 1*. The lateral ports are wedged

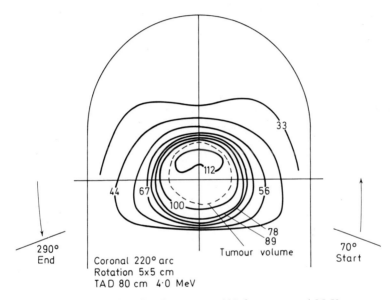

Figure 2. Isodose distribution using 220 degree arc at 4 MeV

and the ports are equally weighted. A somewhat improved distribution can be obtained using a 220 degree arc rotation in the coronal plane as advocated by Kramer, Southard and Mansfield (1968). The appearance of the isodose distribution for 4 MeV radiation using this technique is shown in *Figure 2*. For cases where there is a significant suprasellar component to the tumour without equal lateral extension, we favour the use of a double arc rotation with reversed wedges. This produces an upward elongation of the isodose contours as shown in *Figure 3* with a slow fall-off in dose which is desirable when there is uncertainty as to the superior extent of the lesion. By varying the degree of overlap of the two arcs the degree of elongation can be controlled.

Pituitary adenomas are treated at the rate of 200 rads/day with five treatments per week. This delivers a dose of 4,600 rads in about

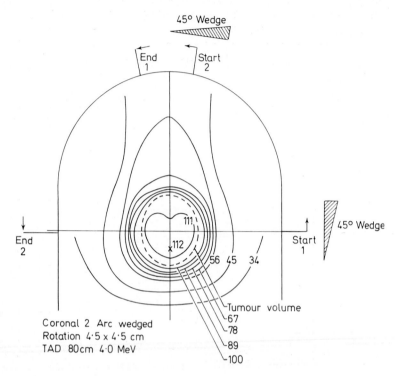

Figure 3. Isodose distribution using double arc rotation with reversed wedges at 4 MeV

$4\frac{1}{2}$ weeks. For large chromophobe adenomas the total dose is increased to 5,000 rads. Craniopharyngiomas are treated according to the plan presented by Kramer, Southard and Mansfield (1968) with 5,500 rads in six weeks for children under 14 and 7,000 rads in seven weeks for adults.

REFERENCES

Almquist, S., Dahlgren, S., Notter, G. and Sundbom, L. (1964). 'Brain necrosis after irradiation of the hypophysis in Cushing's disease.' *Acta radiol.*, **2**, 179.

Béclère, A. (1909). 'The radiotherapeutic treatment of tumors of the hypophysis, gigantism and acromegaly.' *Archs Roentgen Ray.*, **14**, 142.

Caplan, R. H. and Dobben G. D. (1969). 'Endocrine studies in patients with the "empty sella syndrome".' *Archs Intern. Med.*, **123**, 611.

Carlson, D. H. and Marsh, S. H. (1971). 'Cobalt-60 teletherapy of pituitary adenomas.' *Radiology*, **98**, 655.

Chang, C. H. and Pool, J. L. (1967). 'The radiotherapy of pituitary chromophobe adenomas.' *Radiology*, **89**, 1005.

Dawson, D. M. and Dingman, J. F. (1970). 'Hazards of proton-beam pituitary irradiation.' *New Engl. J. Med.*, **282**, 1434.

Gramegna, A. (1909). 'Un Cas d'Acromégalie Traité par la Radiothérapie.' *Rev. Neurologique*, **17**, 15.

Greenwood, F. C., Stewart, H. J., Forrest, A. P. M. and Wood, R. G. (1965). 'Plasma-growth-hormone levels in untreated acromegaly and after radioactive implants into the pituitary.' *Lancet*, **2**, 555.

Grundy, L., Goree, J. A. and Jimenez, J. P. (1970). 'Oxycephaly in the adult simulating pituitary tumor; clinical and roentgenologic manifestations.' *Am. J. Roentgenol.*, **108**, 762.

Hayes, T. P., Davis, R. A. and Raventos, A. (1971). 'The treatment of pituitary chromophobe adenomas.' *Radiology*, **98**, 149.

Henderson, W. R. (1939). 'Pituitary adenomata: a follow-up study of the surgical results in 338 cases.' *Br. J. Surg.*, **26**, 811.

Hirsch, O. (1910). 'Offizieles Protokoll der K.K. Gesellschaft der Aerzte in Wien.' *Wien. klin. Wochenschrift*, **23**, 563.

— (1921). 'Veber Radium behandlung der Hypophysentumoren.' *Arch. Laryngologie Rhinologie*, **21**, 133.

Horsley, V. (1906). 'Diseases of the pituitary gland.' *Br. med. J.*, **1**, 323.

Jadresic, A. V., Poblete, M., Reid, A., Riera, M., Matus, A. and Herroros, M. (1965). 'Therapeutic hypopituitarism induced by stereotaxic transfrontal implantation of yttrium-90 in patients with breast cancer.' *J. clin. Endocr.*, **25**, 686.

Kaufman, B. (1968). 'The "empty" sella-turcica—a manifestation of the intrasellar subarachnoid space.' *Radiology*, **90**, 931.

Kjellberg, R. N., Shintani, A., Frantz, A. G. and Kliman, B. (1968). 'Proton-beam therapy in acromegaly.' *New Engl. J. Med.*, **278**, 689.

— and Kliman, B. (1971). 'Proton-beam therapy.' *New Engl. J. Med.*, **284**, 333.

Kliman, B. and Kjellberg, R. N. (1971). 'Therapy of acromegaly.' *New Engl. J. Med.*, **284**, 673.

Kramer, S. (1968). 'The value of radiation therapy for pituitary and parapituitary tumors.' *Can. Med. Ass. J.*, **99**, 1120.

— McKissock, W. and Concannon, J. P. (1961). 'Craniopharyngiomas: treatment by combined surgery and radiation therapy.' *J. Neurosurg.*, **17**, 217.

— Southard, M. and Mansfield, C. M. (1968). 'Radiotherapy in the management of craniopharyngiomas.' *Am. J. Roentgenol.*, **103**, 44.

Lawrence, A. M., Pinsky, S. M. and Goldfine, I. D. (1971). 'Conventional radiation therapy in acromegaly.' *Archs Intern. Med.*, **128**, 369.

Lawrence, J. H., Born, J. L., Linfoot, J. A. and Chong, C. Y. (1970a). 'Heavy-particle radiation treatment of pituitary tumors.' *J. Am. Med. Ass.*, **214**, 2061.

— Tobias, C. A., Linfoot, J. A., Born, J. L., Lyman, J. T., Chong, C. Y., Manougian, E. and Wei, W. C. (1970). 'Successful treatment of acromegaly: metabolic and clinical studies in 145 patients.' *J. Clin. Endocr.*, **31**, 180.

— Okerlund, M. D., Linfoot, J. A. and Born, J. L. (1971). 'Heavy-particle treatment of Cushing's disease.' *New Engl. J. Med.*, **185**, 1263.

Levitt, S. H., Prather, C. A. and Bogardus, C. R. Jnr. (1970). 'Radiation therapy for primary pituitary tumors associated with Cushing's syndrome.' *Clin. Radiol.*, **21**, 47.

Lindholm, J., Rasmussen, P. and Korsgaard, O. (1969). 'Chromophobe adenomas of the pituitary gland in Cushing's disease.' *Acta endocr.*, **62**, 647.

McCombs, R. K. (1957). 'Proton irradiation of the pituitary and its metabolic effects.' *Radiology*, **68**, 797.

McCormick, W. F. and Halmi, N. S. (1971). 'Absence of chromophobe adenomas from a large series of pituitary tumors.' *Archs Path.*, **92**, 231.

McLachlan, M. B., Wright, A. D. and Doyle, F. H. (1970). 'Plain film and tomographic assessment of the pituitary fossa in 140 acromegalic patients.' *Br. J. Radiol.*, **43**, 360.

Miskin, M. M. (1970). 'Juxtasellar mass lesions.' *Sem. Roentgenol.*, **5**, 165.

Nelson, D. H., Meakin, J. W., Dealy, J. B. Jnr., Matson, D. D., Emerson, K. Jnr. and Thorn, G. W. (1958). 'ACTH-producing tumor of pituitary gland.' *New Engl. J. Med.*, **259**, 161.

— — and Thorn, G. W. (1960). 'ACTH-producing pituitary tumors following adrenalectomy for Cushing's syndrome.' *Ann. Intern. Med.*, **52**, 560.

Orth, D. N. and Liddle, G. W. (1971). 'Results of treatment of 108 patients with Cushing's syndrome.' *New Engl. J. Med.*, **285**, 243.

Peck, F. C. Jnr. and McGovern, E. R. (1966). 'Radionecrosis of the brain in acromegaly.' *J. Neurosurg.*, **25**, 536.

Quick, D. (1920). 'Radium and x-rays in tumors of the hypophysis.' *Archs Ophthal.*, **49**, 256.

Rasmussen, T., Harper, P. V. and Kennedy, T. (1953). 'Use of a beta ray point source for destruction of the hypophysis.' *Surg. Forum*, **4**, 681.

Richmond, J. J. (1958). 'Pituitary tumors: the role of radiotherapy.' *Proc. R. Soc. Med.*, **51**, 911.

Roth, J., Glick, S. M., Cuatrecasas, P. and Hollander, C. S. (1967). 'Acromegaly and other disorders of growth hormone secretion.' *Ann. intern. Med.*, **66**, 760.

— Gordon, P. and Kirkland, B. (1970). 'Efficacy of conventional pituitary irradiation in acromegaly.' *New Engl. J. Med.*, **282**, 1385.

Rothenberg, S. F., Jaffe, H. L., Putman, T. J. and Simkin, B. (1955) 'Hypophysectomy with radioactive chromic phosphate in treatment of cancer.' *Archs Neurol.*, **73**, 193.

Schloffer, H. (1906). 'Zur Frage der Operationen an der Hypophyse.' *Beitr. klin. Chir.*, **50**, 767.

REFERENCES

Sheline, G. E. (1971). 'Untreated and recurrent chromophobe adenomas of the pituitary.' *Am. J. Roentgenol.*, **112**, 768.

Sosman, M. C. (1949). 'Cushing's disease—pituitary basophilism.' *Am. J. Roentgenol.*, **62**, 1.

Stern, W. E. and Batzdorf, U. (1970). 'Intracranial removal of pituitary adenomas. An evaluation of varying degrees of excision from partial to total.' *J. Neurosurg.*, **33**, 564.

Talairach, J., Aboulker, J., Tournoux, P. and David, M. (1956). 'Technique stereotaxique de la chirurgie hypophysaire par voie nasale.' *Neuro-Chirurg.*, **2**, 3.

Tobias, C. A., Anger, H. O. and Lawrence, J. H. (1952). 'Radiological use of high energy deuterons and alpha particles.' *Am. J. Roentgenol.*, **67**, 1.

Van Seters, A. P., Jenny, M. and Querido, A. (1965). 'Unilateral adrenalectomy followed by pituitary irradiation in Cushing's disease; with observations on cortisol secretion after therapy.' *Acta endocrinol.*, **48**, 253.

Wilson, R. R. (1946). 'Radiological use of fast protons.' *Radiology*, **47**, 487.

Wolman, L. (1966). 'Symposium on pituitary tumours. 4. Unusual pathological features.' *Br. J. Radiol.*, **17**, 161.

Wright, A. D., McLachlan, M. S. F., Doyle, F. H. and Fraser, T. R. (1969). 'Serum growth hormone levels and size of pituitary tumour in untreated acromegaly.' *Br. Med. J.*, **4**, 582.

Zervas, N. T. (1969). 'Stereotaxic radiofrequency surgery of the normal and abnormal pituitary gland.' *New Engl. J. Med.*, **280**, 429.

Zulch, K. J. (1957). *Brain Tumors: Their Biology and Pathology.* New York; Springer.

12—Extradural Metastases of the Spinal Cord

Fazlur R. Khan

Compression of the spinal cord is a well recognized and troublesome complication of malignant disease caused by metastasis.

There are three main sources of epidural cord compression. By far the most common is vertebral metastasis; the second most common is soft tissue involvement around the vertebral body. The dura itself is quite resistant to tumour invasion but transmits the pressure of an epidural metastasis causing the signs and symptoms of cord compression.

INCIDENCE

Epidural cord compression can occur at any age. Most cases are reported in the 30 to 60 age group. The reason for this is that malignant diseases like breast, lymphoma and lung tumours are most common in these age groups.

Sex

There is no predominance of one sex over the other.

Site

Lower thoracic and upper lumbar regions are the most common sites. Cord compression can occur from first cervical to second lumbar vertebra. Sometimes pressure on the cauda equina can produce neurological defects. Khan and colleagues (1967) reported 82 patients of whom 62 had their thoracic region involved, 15 the lumbar and 5 the cervical.

SIGNS AND SYMPTOMS

Table 1 shows the most common signs and symptoms from the Khan series. This distribution agrees with that reported by other authors (Brice and McKissock, 1965; Posner, 1971; Rubin, Meyer and Porter, 1969).

TABLE 1
Frequency of Symptoms

Sign or symptom	Number/total	%
Pain	69/82	84
Motor loss	67/82	80
Sensory loss	46/82	56
Sphincter control loss	39/82	47

Pain

There is general agreement in the literature that pain is the predominant symptom; 80 to 90 per cent of patients have pain, which may be local backache only, with or without tenderness. Pain may also be radicular in nature or of a mixed variety. Most of the cases have the latter type.

Motor Loss

About 70 per cent of patients have some degree of motor weakness. Out of 82 patients in the series by Khan and colleagues, 15 had no motor deficit, 35 had weakness of varying degree and 32 were paraplegic.

Sensory Loss

About half the patients present with a sensory deficit identifying the level of obstruction, but on occasion it was above the level of obstruction of the spinal cord shown on the myelogram.

Sphincter Function

Sphincter loss commonly develops late in the course of the condition and is present in about 47 per cent of cases.

The above symptoms seem to occur in the same order in most patients and probably reflect an orderly process of cord compression starting anteriorly with motor loss, and pain later due to compression of the posteriorly sensory fibres, then complete interference of cord function with loss of sphincter control.

Most patients have a known primary malignant disease, but cord compression can be the primary manifestation of the neoplastic process as reported by Brice and McKissock (1965). The malignant diseases which most commonly give rise to epidural cord compression are shown in Table 2 from Khan and colleagues.

TABLE 2
Sites of Origin of Primary Tumours

Primary	Total No. of patients	%
Carcinoma of breast	22	27
Lymphosarcoma	15	19
Reticulum cell sarcoma	14	17
Hodgkin's disease	7	8
Unknown primary	4	5
Miscellaneous	20	24
Total	82	100

Reproduced from Khan and colleagues (1967) by courtesy of the Editor of *Radiology*.

The above series have a predominance of lymphomas (44 per cent) and of breast cancer. This may be because of large populations of patients in these two diseases treated at the Memorial Hospital. The miscellaneous category included myeloma, prostate and lung carcinoma. The relative lack of lung carcinoma in this series is puzzling, since patients with carcinoma of the lung were present in good supply at the Memorial Hospital. In Brice and McKissock's series the most common primary was lung.

PHILOSOPHY OF TREATMENT

Compression of the spinal cord with epidural cord disease is a grave situation. It requires a very urgent and realistic approach in the management of these patients as an emergency if a paraplegia is to be avoided. While cord compression is usually a manifestation of disseminating neoplasm where the overall prognosis commonly is limited, it is still true that paraplegics present a very difficult medical and socio-economic problem. It is the concensus that immediate therapy is necessary in these patients. A general review of the literature was made by Rubin (1969) and serves as the basis for most of Table 3. Surgical laminectomy followed by radiation therapy is the usual treatment. Surgery usually fails to remove the tumour completely. Symptomatic relief, when it occurs, is a consequence of the decompression.

TABLE 3

Review of Literature

Year	Author	No. of patients	Histology: Lymphoma, Hodgkin's disease, lymphosarcoma, leukaemia, myeloma	Carcinoma	Other
Surgery and Radiation:					
1945	Shenkin, Horn and Grant	33	10	9	14
1954	Love, Miller and Kernohan	39	39	0	0
1957	Mullan and Evans	50	15	20	15
1958	Rogers	22	All type	0	9
1958	Perese	30	7	15	8
1959	Williams and colleagues	118	118	—	—
1963	Wright	84	18	60	6
1963	Wild and Porter	45	7	32	6
1965	Smith	52	0	52	—
1965	Viets and Odom	78	0	58	20
1966	Mones, Dozier and Berrett	46	14	23	2
1970	Posner	31	6	25	—
Radiation Alone:					
1967	Khan and colleagues	82	36	22	24
1970	Rubin and colleagues	12	5	5	2
1970	Posner	75	25	Not known	—
Surgery Alone:					
1957	Torma	250	40	131	79
1967	Hardy and Dugger	39	14	23	2

Reproduced from Rubin (1969) by courtesy of the Editor of *Radiology*.

Looking at the above experience it is obvious that laminectomy followed by radiation has been the most common method of treatment. It has resulted in an ambulation rate varying from 38 to 45 per cent.

The large experience of Torma (1957) with surgery alone gave a poor response. Out of 199 patients only 18 had a good palliation, a rate of 9 per cent.

Radiation alone is a more recent method of treatment. Khan and colleagues (1967) showed good response in 34 out of 82 patients (41 per cent). Rubin, Meyer and Porter (1969) have shown a response rate of 9 out of 12 patients with radio-sensitive neoplasms. The treatment technique used by Rubin was based on his own experimental work. He used high daily doses initially. The report looks promising.

Treatment of spinal cord compression necessitates immediate measures to reduce pressure in an effort to reverse the process before the cord is damaged permanently. At present, according to the knowledge and information available, treatment may be classified as follows:

(1) Radiation therapy with high doses initially should be the treatment of choice for the following situations: (a) all radio-sensitive tumours (e.g. lymphomas, leukaemias, neuroblastoma) in all stages of cord compression; (b) all moderately radio-sensitive tumours, including breast and lung carcinomas, have a slow onset of compression.

(2) Laminectomy and radiation therapy: (a) patients who have developed symptoms and signs of cord compression suddenly, especially those with paraplegia; although these patients do not do well, they should still be treated with laminectomy and radiation; orthopaedic devices may be helpful; the prognosis of this group may alter, if massive dose therapy (doses of 1,000 to 1,200 rads in single treatment) proves to be beneficial; (b) patients with radio-resistant tumours like teratocarcinoma or prostatic cancer, should, I believe, have a laminectomy followed by radiation; here the rate of tumour regression is slow and damage may be averted by the surgical act; (c) I know of no evidence that chemotherapy aids prognosis; (d) patients with an unknown primary should have laminectomy for the operation will establish the diagnosis, which is imperative; (e) all laminectomies should be followed by radiation.

RADIOTHERAPEUTIC TECHNIQUES

Volume

An adequate, properly chosen volume is a most important factor in determining the results. Relevant x-rays, a neurological examination and detailed myelographic evidence should be obtained. Whenever a complete block is found, a cysternal cervical myelogram should be considered to establish the length of the block and to test the possibility that there is more than one site of cord compression. This is most likely to occur in patients with lymphomas. Neurological evidence of level or levels of involvement or evidence of the presence of nodes in paravertebral areas is also helpful, especially in the lymphomas. All the above information should be used to dictate the volume to be treated. Every effort should be made to include all the disease around the site of compression. On balance it is better to err on the side of too large a volume. Treatment of the contents of the spinal canal will give only very temporary results.

Time Dose

Rubin's technique (Rubin, Meyer and Porter, 1969) of 400 to 500 rads as the initial fraction, then reducing the dose to 200 rads per day, seems to be logical, and is based on his experimental data as well as his clinical experience. The total dose is determined on the basis of histology and of the general condition of the patient. 2,500 rads in ten fractions over two weeks to 3,500 rads and fifteen fractions in three weeks is his range.

In Khan's series (Khan and colleagues, 1967), doses of 200 rads per day given daily from Monday to Friday, varying from 2,500 rads tumour dose to 4,500 rads tumour dose, did not show any significant difference in response as a function of total dose.

Millburn, Hibbs and Hendrickson (1968) have done a few cases with massive doses of 1,000 rads in a single treatment. This is worth considering and might reduce the indications for laminectomy. Radiation-induced oedema is an event of very low probability, as was nicely shown by the experimental and clinical work of Rubin, Meyer and Porter (1969) and by Irvine and Robertson (1964). In case it does occur, steroids and high osmolarity solutions can be used. The post-laminectomy patient may be treated by equal daily doses or by a high initial dose technique.

Quality of Radiation

Supervoltage radiation is the treatment of choice. Analysing various plans of treatments with different modalities shows that a direct electron port of 20 to 30 MeV will commonly give an excellent distribution (*Figure 1*). Plans using two wedges at 45 degrees to the vertical give a very adequate volume distribution of energy (*Figure 2*). A single posterior port using cobalt-60, 60 cm FSD or 80 cm FSD is a common method of treatment; it is useful when electrons are not available and if the patient's condition (urgency of treatment) does not allow time to develop a wedge plan. However, it is not a satisfactory method, particularly if the patient remains or becomes paraplegic. The high skin and subcutaneous dose enhances the likelihood of subsequent ulceration in these patients. The dose should be specified at a depth usually of 5 to 6 cm, and a minimum dose to tumour

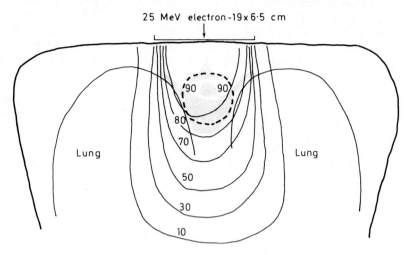

Figure 1. Direct electron beam for spinal cord compression, section at level of T7

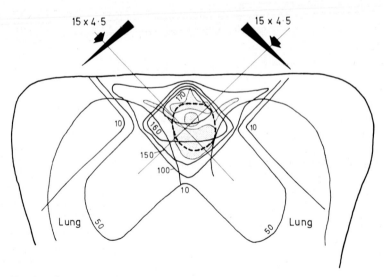

Figure 2. Six MeV, 100 SSD, 45 degree wedge—two posterior fields, section at level of T7

should be stipulated. The use of orthovoltage therapy should be discouraged but, if used, the maximum dose should be noted.

No real complication has occurred with the above methods of treatment, other than as noted for single posterior ports. Some reaction in oesophagus and pharynx might occur, but this is transient and negligible.

PROGNOSIS

Histology did not affect the prognosis appreciably in the Khan series (Khan and colleagues, 1967). No favourable difference was found in patients with lymphomas, 15 out of 36 patients with

TABLE 4

Spinal Cord Compression—Duration of Signs and Symptoms
and Response of Radiotherapy

Sign or symptom	Duration	Total No. of patients	Response			
			Excellent	Fair	Poor	Nil
Pain	1 day to 1 week	8	3	1	2	2
	1–4 weeks	9	1	1	5	2
	4–8 weeks	19	3	1	6	9
	Over 8 weeks	33	8	10	13	2
		69	15	13	26	15
No pain		13	4	2	4	3
Motor loss	1 day to 1 week	27	9	5	8	5
	1–4 weeks	19	4	6	5	4
	4–8 weeks	11	2	0	7	2
	Over 8 weeks	10	2	1	7	0
		67	17	12	27	11
No motor loss		15	2	3	3	7
Sensory loss	1 day to 1 week	20	3	2	10	5
	1–4 weeks	15	2	3	6	4
	4–8 weeks	6	1	1	1	3
	Over 8 weeks	5	2	1	1	1
		46	8	7	18	13
No sensory loss		36	11	8	12	5
Sphincter control loss	1 day to 1 week	22	4	4	9	5
	1–4 weeks	7	—	—	5	2
	4–8 weeks	7	—	1	3	3
	Over 8 weeks	3	—	—	1	2
		39	4	5	18	12
No sphincter control loss		43	15	10	12	6

lymphomas having a useful response with preservation or restoration of ambulation and complete or partial remission of symptoms. Recent experience at the Memorial Hospital (Posner, 1971) showed also that about half the patients had a useful response irrespective of the histology of the tumour.

The duration and severity of signs and symptoms before the onset of treatment is very important prognostically.

(1) Acute paraplegia without prodromal symptoms has a very poor prognosis. It seems that vascular damage associated with a very rapidly growing tumour or with abrupt vertebral collapse contributes to the rapid development of permanent damage of the cord.

(2) Loss of sphincter control lasting more than 24 hours is a very poor prognostic sign.

(3) Patients with complete paraplegia do very badly. Only 5 out of 32 patients had a useful response, whereas 29 out of 50 patients had a useful response without a paraplegia. A poor response in the paraplegic patient was also true in major surgical series (Torma, 1957). Rubin's new technique of high dose therapy has given some improvement in patients with radio-sensitive tumours who also had paraplegia.

Table 4 gives a good understanding of response, as it relates to signs and symptoms. Excellent and fair responses are those where rehabilitation was possible. A patient with a slowly developing cord compression will usually respond favourably.

SUMMARY

Epidural spinal cord compression is a common manifestation of metastatic cancer. It requires immediate treatment.

The key to therapeutic success is early recognition of the process and prompt relevant treatment. More emphasis should be placed on radiation therapy. Radiation alone may produce better results with the new regimen of high dose technique. This would eliminate surgical morbidity.

Results indicate that radiation alone produces as good a result as surgery and radiation in most cases.

ACKNOWLEDGEMENT

It is a pleasure to acknowledge the assistance given by Dr J. J. Nickson in the preparation of this paper.

REFERENCES

Baker, G. S. (1942). 'Lymphoblastoma of the spinal cord simulating other organic diseases: report of 2 cases.' *Proc. Staff Meet. Mayo Clin.*, **17**, 588.

Brice, J. and McKissock, W. (1965). 'Surgical treatment of malignant extradural spinal tumours.' *Br. Med. J.*, **1**, 1341.

Browder, J. and DeVeer, J. A. (1939). 'Lymphomatoid disease involving the spinal epidural space: pathologic and therapeutic consideration.' *Archs Neurol.*, **41**, 328.

Hardy, I. M. and Dugger, G. S. (1967). 'Myelopathy caused by metastatic spinal epidural neoplasms.' *Sth med. J.*, **60**, 72.

Irvine, R. A. and Robertson, W. B. (1964). 'Spinal cord compression in the malignant lymphomas.' *Br. med. J.*, **1**, 1354.

Khan, F. R., Glicksman, A. S., Chu, F. C. H. and Nickson, J. J. (1967). 'Treatment by radiotherapy of spinal cord compression due to extra-dural metastases.' *Radiotherapy*, **89**, 495.

Lawes, F. A. E. and Ham, H. J. (1953). 'A case of Hodgkin's disease with spinal cord involvement treated by nitrogen mustard.' *Med. J. Aust.*, **1**, 104.

Love, J. G., Miller, R. H. and Kernohan, J. W. (1954). 'Lymphomas of spinal epidural space.' *Archs Surg.*, **69**, 66.

Millburn, L., Hibbs, G. G. and Hendrickson, F. R. (1968). 'Treatment of spinal cord compression from metastatic carcinoma: review of the literature and presentation of a new method of treatment.' *Cancer*, **21**, 447.

Mones, R. J., Dozier, D. and Berrett, A. (1966). 'Analysis of medical treatment of malignant extradural spinal cord tumors.' *Cancer*, **19**, 1824.

Mullan, J. and Evans, J. P. (1957). 'Neoplastic disease of the spinal extra-dural space; a review of fifty cases.' *Archs Surg.*, **74**, 900.

Perese, D. M. (1958). 'Treatment of metastatic extradural spinal cord tumors; a series of 30 cases.' *Cancer*, **11**, 214.

Posner, J. B. (Ed.) (1971). 'Medical grand rounds.' *Clin. Bull. Memorial Sloan-Kettering Cancer Center*, **1**, 65.

Rogers, L. (1958). 'Malignant spinal tumours and the epidural space.' *Br. J. Surg.*, **45**, 416.

Rubin, P. (1969). 'Extradural cord compression by tumour. Part I. Experimental production and treatment trial.' *Radiology*, **93**, 1243.

— Meyer, E. and Porter, C. (1969). 'Extradural cord compression by tumour. Part II. High daily dose experience without laminectomy.' *Radiology*, **93**, 1248.

Smith, M. J. and Sternstrom, K. W. (1948). 'Compression of the spinal cord caused by Hodgkin's disease: case reports and treatment.' *Radiology*, **51**, 77.

Smith, R. (1965). 'An evaluation of surgical treatment for spinal cord compression due to metastatic carcinoma.' *J. Neurol. Neurosurg. Psychiat.*, **28**, 152.

Torma, T. (1957). 'Malignant tumours of the spine and the spinal extradural space: a study based on 250 histologically verified cases.' *Acta chir. scand.*, Suppl. **225**, 157.

Viets, H. R. and Hunter, F. T. (1933). 'Lymphoblastomatous involvement of the nervous system.' *Archs Neurol.*, **24**, 1246.

Wild, W. O. and Porter, R. W. (1963). 'Metastatic epidural tumor of the spine.' *Archs. Surg.*, **87**, 825.

Williams, H. M., Diamond, H. D., Craver, L. F. and Parsons H. (1959). *Neurological Complications in Lymphomas and Leukemias.* Springfield, Ill.; Thomas.

Wright, R. L. (1963). 'Malignant tumors in the spinal extradural space: results of surgical treatment.' *Ann. Surg.*, **157**, 227.

13—Cerebral Metastases

Thomas J. Deeley

INTRODUCTION

Estimates of the incidence of cerebral metastases have varied in the literature; this is probably due to the special interests of the hospitals concerned, the proportion of those patients having a post-morten and the care with which a search is made for deposits. Autopsy information is, of necessity, that obtained on a selected group of patients; those who are admitted die and have a necropsy investigation at that hospital; as such it gives only an indication of the true incidence of metastases. Aronson, Garcia and Aronson (1964) reported 397 intracranial metastases in 2,406 autopsies with extracranial malignancies, an incidence of 16·5 per cent; Richards and McKissock (1963) estimated that 10 per cent of intracranial neoplasms were metastatic.

The most common primary sites of the neoplasm are lung, breast, gastro-intestinal tract, kidney, skin (mainly melanomas), but occasional metastases have been found from most other sites. Aronson, Garcia and Aronson (1964) reported that 46 per cent of central nervous system metastases were from the bronchus, and Hindo and colleagues (1970) reported an incidence of 52 per cent. In patients with a primary carcinoma of the bronchus the incidence of cerebral metastases has varied from 8 per cent, reported by Engelman and McNamara (1954), to 61 per cent, reported by Chao, Phillips and Nickson (1954). Line and Deeley (1971) reported a 28 per cent incidence of brain metastases in cases of carcinoma of the bronchus. These authors also correlated this incidence with the histological type of the lung lesion; brain metastases were found in 42 per cent of oat cell lesions, 39 per cent of adenocarcinomas, 24 per cent of anaplastic tumours and 17 per cent of squamous tumours.

In Aronson's series the next most common primary site, carcinoma

253

of the breast, accounted for only 13 per cent of secondary central nervous system deposits; the gastro-intestinal tract accounted for 9 per cent, melanotic sarcoma and urinary tract each for 3 per cent. These authors reported a low incidence from cancer of the prostate, uterus and cervix.

It has been suggested that the frequency of cerebral metastases decreases with advancing age (Onuigbo, 1962). Aronson, Garcia and Aronson reported that the highest incidence of central nervous system metastases was found in patients dying during the first decade of life and that the rate diminished in succeeding decades. In bronchus and breast malignancies there were sufficient numbers of patients to allow an analysis of the age-associated rates to be calculated and these showed decreasing incidence with advancing age. Galuzzi and Payne (1955), who had noticed this with bronchial neoplasms, suggested that it may have been because the incidence of squamous cell lesions increases with advancing age and, also, that older patients may die before there is an opportunity to develop metastases. It is possible that there may sometimes be a less thorough examination of the brains of elderly patients who have obvious causes of death. We cannot therefore, be too certain about this association, especially when we consider the limitation of carrying out analyses on autopsy material.

NUMBER OF METASTASES

Deposits in the brain may be single or multiple—single has been used here to refer to a single mass of metastatic tumour with no macroscopic evidence of other deposits in the brain. Galuzzi and Payne (1956) reported that 36 per cent of brain metastases were single and 64 per cent multiple. Line and Deeley (1971) found 45 per cent of metastases were single and 55 per cent multiple—both these investigations were on secondary deposits from a primary carcinoma of the bronchus. Line and Deeley went further and associated the number of metastases with the histological type. In patients with a primary oat cell carcinoma single deposits were present in 44 per cent of those who had cerebral metastases, in anaplastic tumours 47 per cent, in squamous lesions 42 per cent and in adenocarcinoma 46 per cent; thus the histology does not affect the incidence of single or multiple metastases.

These findings were, of course, those found at necropsy; it is extremely difficult to make a correct diagnosis clinically. Sophisticated methods of localization, including arteriography, ventriculography, isotope investigations, and so on, fail to differentiate between single and multiple lesions; this is almost certainly because the larger lesion will always overshadow the smaller ones and also because the methods of diagnosis at present available fail to pick up very small lesions. This difficulty of differentiation dictates the subsequent treatment, as will be shown later.

LOCATION OF METASTASES

The deposits may be situated anywhere in the brain, but Rubin and Green (1968) suggested that about 60 per cent were found in the cerebrum, 30 per cent in the cerebellum, and 10 per cent in the brain stem, the incidence being roughly in proportion to the bulk of these structures. Galuzzi and Payne (1956), investigating the distribution of metastases from carcinoma of the bronchus, considered only the two sites; the cerebrum and cerebellum; they found that 38 per cent of lesions were located in the cerebellum. Line and Deeley (1971), also investigating the necropsy findings in carcinoma of the bronchus, reported that of all metastases in the brain the cerebrum was involved in 76 per cent of cases, the cerebellum in 23 per cent and the pituitary gland in 23 per cent. When the deposits in the brain were multiple the cerebrum only was involved in 60 per cent of cases, in 35 per cent there were also deposits in the cerebellum and in 5 per cent deposits were also present in the pituitary gland. Where there was only one single deposit in the brain this was found in the cerebrum in 47 per cent of cases, in the pituitary in 45 per cent and in the cerebellum in 8 per cent. The authors concluded that when the pituitary gland was involved the lesion was more likely to be single, and when the cerebellum was involved deposits were more likely to be multiple.

SOLITARY METASTASES

If a proportion of the brain metastases were solitary it would seem reasonable to give treatment aimed at ablating both the primary lesion and the metastasis in the brain. A metastasis can be defined as 'solitary' when it is the only one found in the body; there may, or may not, be a primary lesion present depending on whether this has been adequately dealt with by radical surgery or radiotherapy. Estimates of the incidence of solitary brain metastases vary tremendously. Richards and McKissock (1963) estimated that 16 per cent of brain metastases were solitary. Galuzzi and Payne (1956), reviewing brain metastases in lung cancer, found that 25 per cent were solitary. Flavell (1949) had reported an incidence of 10 per cent and Stern

(1954), in a small series of 14 patients, found no other metastases in 7. In cancer of the bronchus Deeley and Line (1969) found solitary metastases in 20 per cent of cerebral metastases, and showed that the incidence depended on the histological type of the tumour. In squamous lesions 27 per cent were solitary, in oat cell 19 per cent and in both anaplastic tumours and adenocarcinomas 14 per cent.

We have mentioned the difficulty of determining whether metastases in the brain are single; the same difficulty is experienced in detecting solitary metastases. Pack and Ariel (1959) and Lang and Slater (1964) reported that their original pre-operative diagnosis that metastases were solitary was often proved to be wrong at necropsy.

It appears, then, that quite a fair number of these metastases may be solitary, especially in cases of carcinoma of the bronchus. This may be because the metastasis results from the only tumour cell, or clump of cells, that have broken away from the primary tumour and entered the bloodstream; it may be that only one cell has survived, others being killed in the bloodstream; or that one cell only has been able to establish a good blood supply at the site of lodgement; or it may be that only one cell has established itself in a suitable soil where it can grow. It has been shown that tumours often give off several metastases which may be found in the circulating blood but that not all of these cells are viable and capable of forming metastatic deposits (Kuper and Bignall, 1966; Klassen, 1971). Is there any reason why the incidence of solitary metastases should be higher in the brain? Animal experiments have shown that a clump of malignant cells—about three, maybe more—are needed to form a metastasis; this may be because the outer cells are damaged in transport through the body or may be acted upon by certain body substances which destroy them or inhibit their growth either in the bloodstream or in the tissue in which they are lodged. The centre cell may thus be protected and enabled to start up a new growth. In its passage around the arch of the aorta this clump of cells will have a greater mass than the normal constituent cells of the blood and thus be acted on by a greater centripedal force pulling it out so that it enters the first large openings in the aorta—the carotid arteries.

CLINICAL FEATURES

Brain metastases may be found as the presenting symptom of a primary carcinoma elsewhere, at the same time as the primary lesion, during a course of treatment to the primary, or at some time after completion of treatment to the primary. In bronchus lesions Deeley and Rice-Edwards (1968) found that in half of the patients the metastasis was the presenting symptom or was found on examination before or during treatment to the primary. In those patients developing lesions after treatment half had symptoms within six months and 88 per cent within one year, but one patient did not have symptoms suggesting a metastasis until more than three years after successful treatment for a primary lesion. Lansberg (1968) reported cases occurring up to nine years after treatment for a primary lesion. Diagnosis is, of course, easier in the patient who is known to have a primary carcinoma. In the majority of cases the diagnosis of cerebral metastases is clinical. Biopsy is not usually indicated in the presence of a known carcinoma and may cause deterioration in the patient's general condition; Richards and McKissock (1963) reported that in a series of patients who had a biopsy 69 per cent survived no more than one month. The possibility of brain secondaries must always be thought of in a patient with a known carcinoma who develops central nervous system symptoms. However, the possibility of an independent primary cerebral tumour, a cerebrovascular accident, an intracranial abscess or other intracranial lesion must also be borne in mind. In addition care must be taken to exclude cases of metabolic encephalopathy due to the growth.

The most important feature in the differential diagnosis is the natural history: metastatic tumours usually have an ominously progressive course, whereas cardiovascular disorders often occur dramatically and then either cause rapid death, remain stationary or improve over a period of time. Mental deterioration and lapses of memory—most marked for recent events—are fairly common presenting symptoms of metastases. Neurological investigations may help in the location of the lesions but often do not give sufficient information on which to base a definite diagnosis. Brain scans may be particularly helpful in demonstrating supratentorial secondaries but not as helpful in posterior fossa lesions; they are more useful in diagnosing multiple deposits than any other investigation. We reported that cerebral secondaries were detected in 80 per cent of cases by brain scan (Deeley and Rice-Edwards, 1968). Not too much reliance should be placed on the finding of a single deposit on brain scan because we know, from autopsy examination, that multiple lesions may be present in half of the patients. Electroencephalograms are usually abnormal and may demonstrate the presence of multiple foci. Angiography may be of help in the diagnosis of cerebral metastases and it has been reported to show evidence in more than half of the cases (Deeley and Rice-Edwards, 1968). Zachrisson (1963) also thought that it was possible to give a fairly confident diagnosis.

These diagnostic procedures have all been discussed in previous chapters. It is important not to take too much time seeking a precise diagnosis before starting definitive treatment. A radioactive brain scan should be carried out in all cases; it is a relatively simple procedure which can be performed with very little upset to the patient. Where the brain scan is negative the decision to treat will depend on the clinical features, the history and the progression of the symptoms over the course of a few days.

Metastatic tumours may be mistaken for primary cerebral tumours and may be treated as such, the primary only becoming evident some time later. An interesting study by Kindt (1964) showed that a definite site of predilection for metastases was posterior to the Sylvian fissure near the junction of the temporal, parietal and occipital lobes, a site which receives its blood supply from the terminal branches of the middle cerebral artery; no such predilection was found for primary tumours.

TREATMENT

The treatment given may be surgery or radiation therapy. Complete cure is possible after excision of a solitary metastasis in the brain and indeed cures have been reported; Flavell (1949) reported a sixteen-year survivor and Simonescu (1960) a six-year survivor. Richards and McKissock (1963) carried out complete surgical excision in 70 patients and 14 of these survived for more than six months. Deeley and Rice-Edwards reviewed the literature in 1968 and reported that of 149 cases operated on for a secondary deposit from a carcinoma of the bronchus 8 (5 per cent) survived for more than one year. The authors pointed out that this represented survival only and was not synonymous with 'significant' palliation, which they defined as improvement which was sufficient to enable the patient to return home and live a relatively normal life after treatment. Bouchard (1966) considered that excision was justified and worth while especially in those cases where the metastasis manifested itself some time after the primary had been removed and the results were best in breast and kidney lesions. Lansberg (1968) reported that six out of ten patients operated on for a secondary hypernephroma survived for more than a year and one patient survived for ten years; one patient with a metastatic melanoma lived three years without symptoms. No patients with a carcinoma of the bronchus lived for more than a year; he reported that the survival in breast cancer was poor.

The operative morality may be high, 24 per cent reported by

Stortebecker (1954), 38 per cent by Simonescu (1960) and 37 per cent by Stoier (1965).

RADIOTHERAPY

There are now several reports in the literature of the results of irradiation of cerebral secondaries. It is proposed to describe our own experience in the treatment of secondaries from a bronchial carcinoma (Deeley and Rice-Edwards, 1968). as these are by far the most common lesions, and then to review the relevant literature.

We have already pointed out that metastases may be multiple throughout the brain and, as a result, the whole brain must be irradiated. Opposing fields of either 15 or 17 cm length by 10 or 12 cm width, necessary to cover the whole brain, are used on either side of the skull. To avoid any oedema of the cerebral tissues with the consequent exacerbation of symptoms small doses of 50 rads are given to each field initially; this is increased by 50 rads daily; it is aimed to give a tumour dose of 3,000 rads in 20 treatments in four weeks. If symptoms of increased intracranial pressure develop intravenous mannitol is given. Such a course of treatment was completed in 69 per cent of patients; the remaining patients deteriorated rapidly or died before the prescribed course was completed. Palliation was assessed as 'significant' or 'not significant'. 'Significant' implies that improvement was sufficient to enable the patient to return home and live a relatively normal and comfortable life for at least one month after treatment; some patients returned to their normal work. 'Not significant' implies that the patient showed no improvement and rarely had relief of troublesome symptoms; he was unable to return to his normal life or if he showed an apparent improvement it lasted for less than one month.

The palliation achieved was 'significant' in 47 per cent of patients and 'not significant' in 53 per cent. 'Significant' palliation was present in 30 per cent at three months, 15 per cent at six months, 7 per cent at one year, 5 per cent at two years and 3 per cent at three years. We could demonstrate no way of predicting whether a certain patient would have a good response to therapy. There was no correlation between the degree or length of response and the initial level of consciousness, the presence or absence of papilloedema, the duration of cerebral symptoms, or whether cerebral or lung lesion appeared first. However, squamous lesions appeared to show a greater improvement than other lesions.

Some patients who did not get full relief of symptoms and in whom the response was 'not significant' were nevertheless made more comfortable; instead of a gradual deterioration in condition there was often a period of relief lasting weeks or months followed by a short terminal illness. Several comatose patients recovered sufficiently to become co-operative and this greatly eased the nursing problem. A few comatose patients recovered sufficiently to return to their home and work.

In this series of 61 patients, who received at least 3,000 rads tumour dose, the one-year survival was 14 per cent, the two-year survival six per cent and the three-year survival 4 per cent.

Nisce, Hilaris and Chu (1971) treated 560 patients with cerebral metastases, and irradiated the whole brain. Of these patients, 39 per cent had a breast carcinoma, 25 per cent a bronchial carcinoma, 8 per cent a melanoma, and other sites accounted for 20 per cent. A total dose of between 3,000 and 4,000 rads was given in 3–4 weeks. They reported that 80 per cent improved as a result of treatment, the average duration of remission being six months for breast, five months for bronchus and three months for melanoma. They compared the results of treatment using either orthovoltage irradiation or supervoltage irradiation; except for less scalp reaction with supervoltage no statistical difference was noted. The use of adjuvant corticosteroid therapy often produced immediate improvement, making the administration of treatment easier but did not affect the overall results; 25 per cent of patients with a breast carcinoma, 15 per cent of the bronchial carcinoma and 10 per cent of melanomas survived for more than a year. The authors stressed the importance of treating the whole brain because of the frequency of multiple metastases.

Order and colleagues (1968) reported the results of whole brain irradiation in 108 patients; an improvement in functional status was achieved in 60 per cent, and 16 per cent of all cases survived for more than a year. These authors attempted to assess the response by defining four classes of function; they found the greatest improvement in those patients who had the least pre-treatment impairment.

Chao, Phillips and Nickson (1954) found a favourable response in 17 out of 26 patients treated; they recommended a dose of 3,000 to 4,000 rads in three to four weeks to the whole brain and found that doses of less than 2,000 rads were unlikely to be of much benefit.

Hindo and colleagues (1970) investigated the effect of a large single dose of radiation, giving a single midline tumour dose of 1,000 rads to the whole brain with a telecobalt machine: 54 patients were treated, 35 (65 per cent) showing a significant improvement; in 15 per cent of the patients this improvement lasted for one year, and 35 per cent of their patients survived for one year. These results are particularly encouraging. The treatment usually advocated has been of four weeks' duration, which has meant that the patient has to be in a reasonably good condition to start treatment and, in the series we reported, about one-quarter were unable to complete the prescribed dose. The short course of treatment has obvious advantages, more patients can be treated initially and the chance taken that the results may prove efficacious. This technique of treatment obviously needs more investigation.

Summary of Radiotherapy Treatment

From this brief survey some points have become apparent; the whole brain must be irradiated; doses of 3,000 to 4,000 rads in about four weeks will give a useful palliation and a chance of survival; breast and kidney tumours appear to have a slightly better prognosis than those from other sites; oedema as a result of treatment has not been a serious disadvantage and may be reduced either by giving the treatment slowly or by giving corticosteroids; large dose single treatments should be investigated further.

CORTICOSTEROIDS

There is little doubt that corticosteroids may help the patient who has symptoms due to cerebral oedema; they give sufficient temporary relief for the ill patient to be started on a course of radiotherapy. It has been suggested that all patients having radiotherapy should be given corticosteroids to prevent oedema but there is little evidence to suggest that this is necessary in all cases and steroids are probably best kept for those patients with signs of oedema. Hindo and colleagues (1970) suggested that oedema may, in fact, be due not to the irradiation but to haemorrhage or acute inflammation of the secondary mass. Horton and colleagues (1971) carried out a study on 48 patients to determine whether as much palliation can be achieved by prednisone alone; they concluded that a combination of prednisone and irradiation offered only a slight advantage over steroids alone. However, there was a suggestion that the remission and duration of survival produced by the combination of treatments were longer than those by prednisone alone. The continuation of prednisone, in those patients classified as responsive after combination therapy, did not prolong the remission; a subsequent relapse may be usefully treated by prednisone. These findings have not been verified by other workers. Nisce, Hilaris and Chu (1971) gave steroids to their patients, and found that, whilst there was a reduction in the radiation reaction permitting easier administration of the treatment, there was no influence on the overall response when compared to irradiation given without steroids.

Beresford (1969) thought that the results of treatment with corticosteroids and radiation were better than when radiation alone was given in the treatment of melanomas.

There is little evidence to suggest that useful palliation can be achieved by using any of the chemotherapeutic agents.

SUMMARY

The irradiation of intracranial metastases is worth while because about half of the patients obtain useful palliation. The whole brain should be irradiated, and further investigation is needed of the effect of treatment given in a single dose. The presence of cerebral metastases is usually associated in our minds with a hopeless prognosis; it is suggested that a more vigorous approach should be made to the treatment of these lesions and that the results may be quite encouraging.

REFERENCES

Aronson, S. M., Garcia, J. H. and Aronson, B. E. (1964). 'Metastatic neoplasms of the brain; their frequency in relation to age.' *Cancer*, **17**, 558.

Beresford, H. R. (1969). 'Melanoma of the nervous system.' *Neurology*, **19**, 59.

Bouchard, J. (1966). *Radiation Therapy of Tumours and Diseases of the Nervous System*. London; Kimpton.

Chao, J. H., Phillips, R. and Nickson, J. J. (1954). 'Roentgen-ray therapy of cerebral metastases ' *Cancer*, **7**, 682.

Deeley, T. J. and Rice-Edwards, J. M. (1968). 'Radiotherapy in the management of cerebral secondaries from bronchial carcinomas.' *Lancet*, **1**, 1209.

— and Line, D. H. (1969). 'Solitary metastases in carcinoma of the bronchus.' *Br. J. Chest*, **63**, 150.

Engelman, R. M. and McNamara, W. L. (1954). 'Bronchogenic carcinomas. Statistical review of 234 autopsies.' *J. thorac. Surg.*, **27**, 227.

Flavell, G. (1949). 'Solitary cerebral metastases from bronchial carcinomas Their incidence and a case of successful removal.' *Br. med. J.*, **2**, 736.

Galuzzi, S. and Payne, P. M. (1955). 'Bronchial carcinoma; statistical study of 741 necropsies with special reference to distribution of blood-borne metastases.' *Br. J. Cancer*, **9**, 511.

— — (1956). 'Brain metastases from primary bronchial carcinoma, a statistical study of 741 necropsies.' *Br. J. Cancer*, **10**, 408.

Hindo, W. A., DeTrana, F. A., Lee, M. S. and Hendrickson, F. R. (1970). 'Large dose increment irradiation in treatment of cerebral metastases.' *Cancer*, **26**, 138.

Horton, J., Baxter, D. H., Olson, K. B. and The Eastern Co-operative Oncology Group (1971). 'The management of metastases to the brain by irradiation and corticosteroids.' *Am. J. Roentgenol.*, **111**, 334.

Kindt, G. W. (1964). 'The pattern of location of cerebral metastatic tumours.' *J. Neurosurg.*, **21** 54.

Klassen, K. P. (1971). 'Blood cytology.' In *Modern Radiotherapy—Carcinoma of the Bronchus*, Ed. by T. J. Deeley. London; Butterworths.

Kuper, S. W. A. and Bignall, J. R. (1966). 'Survival after resection of bronchial carcinoma.' *Lancet*, **1**, 10.

Lang, E. F. and Slater, J. (1964). 'Metastatic brain tumours; results of surgical and non-surgical treatment.' *Surg. Clins N. Am.*, **44**, 865.

Lansberg, J. (1968). 'Operation for solitary intracranial metastases.' *Germ. Med.*, **13**, 93.

Line, D. H. and Deeley, T. J. (1971). 'The necropsy findings in carcinoma of the bronchus.' *Br. J. Chest Dis.*, **65**, 238.

Onuigbo, W. I. (1962). 'Lung cancer, metastasis and growing old.' *J. Gerontol.*, **17**, 163.

Nisce, L. Z., Hilaris, B. S. and Chu, F. C. H. (1971). 'A review of experience with irradiation of brain metastases.' *Am. J. Roentgenol.*, **111**, 329.

Order, S. E., Hellman, S., van Essen, C. F. and Kligerman, M. M. (1968). 'Improvement in quality of survival following whole-brain irradiation for brain metastases.' *Radiology*, **91**, 149.

Pack, G. T. and Ariel, I. M. (1959). *Treatment of Cancer and Allied Disorders*, 2nd Ed., Vol. 2: *Tumours of the Nervous System*, Chapter 15. New York; Harper and Row.

Richards, P. and McKissock, W. (1963). 'Intracranial metastases.' *Br. med. J.*, **1**, 15.

Rubin, P. and Green, J. (1968). *Solitary Metastases*. Springfield, Ill.; Thomas.

Simonescu, M. D. (1960). 'Metastatic tumours of the brain. 195 cases with neurosurgical consideration.' *J. Neurosurg.*, **17**, 361.

Stern, R. O. (1954). 'The morbid anatomy of carcinoma of the bronchus, an analysis of 87 cases with special reference to solitary cerebral metastases.' *Br. J. Cancer*, **8**, 412.

Stoier, M. (1965). 'Metastatic tumours of the brain.' *Acta neurol. scand.*, **41**, 262.

Stortebecker, T. P. (1954). 'Metastatic tumours of the brain from a neurosurgical point of view, F.U. study of 158 cases.' *J. Neurosurg.*, **11**, 84.

Zachrisson, L. (1963). 'Angiography of cerebral metastases.' *Acta radiol. diag.*, **1**, 521.

14—The Treatment of Recurrent Tumours

Thomas J. Deeley

INTRODUCTION

The patient who develops recurrent symptoms after a radical course of radiotherapy presents quite a difficult problem; there may be recurrence of the tumour, radio-necrosis in the irradiated area, or a mixture of both. Whilst a second course of radiation may be indicated for the recurrent tumour it is strongly contra-indicated for the necrotic lesion. The differential diagnosis between recurrence and necrosis is not easy; both cause irritation of the cerebral tissues with the appropriate neurological response for that site.

The patient's clinical history may give an indication—for example, signs developing within a few months of the irradiation may suggest a recurrence more than a necrotic lesion and symptoms developing some months, or even years, after treatment may suggest that the lesion is more likely to be radio-necrotic; but, some lesions of the brain are relatively slow-growing and not too much reliance can be placed on the time of recurrence of symptoms. The presence of signs of increased intracranial pressure would usually suggest the presence of a space-occupying lesion.

Special tests do little to elucidate the problem; electroencephalography will reveal a focus of irritation only and this may be due to either cause; the same is true of pneumoencephalography and cerebral angiography. Serial investigations, however, may show an increase in the size of the lesion, suggesting that it is growing. It is possible that radioisotope studies may be more helpful; necrotic tissue is unlikely to take up the isotope and actively-growing tissues are more likely to take it up, but it must be realized that considerable alterations in the surrounding cerebral tissues may have occurred due

264

to the previous irradiation or surgery. MacDonald, Green and Rubin (1968) carried out clinical and experimental studies; after lobectomy, in animals there was an increased activity of isotope concentration over the areas which gradually disappeared by the end of the third month. The application of liquid nitrogen to the dura in animals was followed by increased isotope uptake for one month and then a return to normal. In patients the irradiation of a brain tumour was followed by residual activity but the authors were undecided whether this was due to residual tumour or to an altered blood–brain barrier. They suggested that serial brain scans may reveal either a decrease or increase in activity.

It would appear that in cases of recurrence of symptoms soon after treatment there may be an increased isotope uptake even when the tumour is ablated, but that in these cases repeated investigations may show a decrease within the next few months—whereas with residual tumours there is often an increasing uptake. Where symptoms occur at a later period an uptake is suggestive of tumour activity and that suggestion may be further strengthened by the demonstration of a further increase in uptake on repeating the test one month later.

Unequivocal evidence of recurrent or residual tumour will only be obtained by histological examination, and Rubin and Casarett (1968) considered that the risk of re-treating the area by further irradiation was often greater than the risk of carrying out a craniotomy to determine the pathology.

RADIATION

When a decision has been made that the lesion is recurrent we have to decide whether or not further radiation is indicated. In radiotherapy practice is has become accepted that when a radical course of radiation is contemplated this must be an all-out attempt to cure, by a dose which cannot be repeated. If the tumour does not respond to this dose it is unlikely to respond to the same dose given again; thus a higher dose will be required and the effects on normal tissues will be further increased by the treatment and result in a high risk of radiation necrosis of the normal tissues. Re-treatments have thus been unfashionable.

Let us state an opposing point of view: when a patient is seen with a malignant lesion we, as radiotherapists, have three choices; either to treat radically aiming for a cure; to palliate if there are symptoms; or to do nothing if there are no symptoms or no chance of a cure. If a radical course of radiation has been given and the tumour recurs there is thus no chance of cure by radiotherapy so we must consider whether surgical treatment is possible—and in a few sites this may be possible. In the remaining patient with recurrence we have two possibilities; if the patient has no symptoms obviously further radiotherapy is contra-indicated, but if there are distressing symptoms which could be palliated by radiation this treatment should be given. It is possible to relieve distressing haemoptysis due to recurrence after radiotherapy to the lungs, and to relieve haematuria due to recurrence. Admittedly there is a greater risk of radiation damage to normal tissue but invariably the expectation of life is too short for this to develop and the relief of distressing symptoms in a dying patient far outweighs the possibility of late effects. This is a generalization and we must decide how we can adapt it to the problem of re-treatment of central nervous tumours. We can best do this in the way that we have discussed for the primary treatment in this book—that is, for whole central nervous system irradiation, for localized treatments and for secondary deposits.

WHOLE CENTRAL NERVOUS SYSTEM

Where the whole central nervous system has not been irradiated and growth occurs outside the treated area there is no problem with re-treatment and that new area can be treated to a radical tumour dose. The problems of re-treatment of medulloblastomas have been discussed in Chapter 7; Horns and Webber (1967) reported the results of re-treatment of four cases of medulloblastoma, who survived 4, 7, 25 and 29 months after re-treatment, two cases of ependymoma were re-treated, one died at 3 months and the other was alive at $3\frac{1}{2}$ years. Sheline, Phillips and Boldrey (1965) described the re-treatment of a patient who had received treatment for a medulloblastoma; he developed a spinal cord compression two years later which was re-treated and he died of a further recurrence at seven years.

Further palliative treatment in patients who have had the whole central nervous system irradiated should be limited to the site of the recurrence; however, because of the relative radio-sensitivity of these tumours and their propensity to spread, a fairly generous area should be irradiated and a relatively high dose can often be achieved because the previous dose given to the whole central nervous system was low.

LOCALIZED LESIONS

We have already pointed out the problems of the localization of a brain lesion (Chapter 6); the use of small fields creates the possibility of a 'geographical miss', and leads us to use fields of a larger size with a lower tumour dose. An increase in the activity of a tumour may bring about various signs and symptoms, which may be distressing to the patient and relatives, depending on the site of the primary tumour. Symptoms may be local or general or there may be an increased intracranial pressure or coma. If even short-term palliation can be achieved by re-treatment this would seem to warrant its use. The comatose patient is a problem of nursing care and re-treatment is justified if he can be brought to a co-operative state. Medical methods of reducing the increased pressure may be used but medication must be maintained and often becomes ineffective; radiotherapy may have a more lasting effect. Horns and Webber (1967) described the re-treatment of three astrocytomas; one lived 9 months, one 20 months and the third was alive at 3 years but with severe disability and blindness. The same authors reported two brain stem and one pontine tumour who survived respectively 3, $5\frac{1}{2}$ and 22 months after treatment. Bray, Carter and Taveras (1958) reported the result of re-treatment in 12 children with brain stem tumours—seven showed an improvement. Whyte, Colby and Layton (1969), discussing the treatment of 57 patients with brain stem tumours, reported that 15 patients (26 per cent) had a second course of therapy and 2 received a third course; 3 of these patients were still alive (time unspecified), 1 patient was alive six years later, having had three courses of therapy and having only slight residual disability. These authors recommended an aggressive approach to the treatment of brain stem tumours.

Shenkin (1965) reported four patients who had recurrence of symptoms from an oligodendroglioma at 24, 41, 68 and 20 months after irradiation, who were re-treated and subsequently had remission of symptoms for an additional 24, 24, 54 and 48 months respectively; it must be remembered that these are relatively slow-growing tumours but that there was remission of symptoms with re-treatment. Sheline, Phillips and Boldrey (1965), reporting the treatment of 16 oligodendrogliomas, gave re-treatment in 3 cases; 1 patient then had removal of a fluid-filled cyst which revealed no evidence of the original tumour.

SECONDARY DEPOSITS

The dose of radiation given to cerebral deposits is relatively low, the aim being to produce palliation; it is thus possible to repeat this treatment if it is necessary. Also because it is palliative treatment, given where the expectation of life is extremely poor, we do not have to consider the late effects of the irradiation. Re-treatment by radiotherapy is considered if the patient has distressing symptoms or is comatose. We reported a patient (Deeley and Rice-Edwards, 1968) who was comatose due to cerebral deposits; she was treated palliatively and returned to normal life for six months, the tumour recurred and she was again comatose. She was again treated, improved for a further three months after which she deteriorated and died within three weeks. Order and colleagues (1968) reported re-treatment in 16 patients whose general condition was good even though they had recurrence of neurological symptoms; 7 of these patients again showed improvement after treatment.

CONCLUSION

The fear of the consequences of the re-treatment of central nervous system tumours often dissuades radiotherapists, but the majority of the patients who are being treated will not live long enough to develop symptoms of radiation damage. If there is definite recurrence of a tumour and distressing symptoms occur the patient should be re-treated with the idea of palliating these symptoms. It is suggested that we should re-appraise our approach to the question of further palliative treatment. The literature contains very few references to its use. As a first step it would be useful to collect retrospective information on these patients who have been re-treated; if a sufficient number could be obtained it might be possible to correlate the response with other parameters, such as tumour type, site of lesion, dose given initially and in re-treatment, and to assess the morbidity, palliation and even, perhaps, survival as a result of re-treatment.

There is very little information on the effect of chemotherapeutic agents in the treatment of recurrent lesions; again we need to collect information about those patients who have had this therapy and to analyse the results.

REFERENCES

Bray, P. F., Carter, S. and Taveras, J. M. (1958). 'Brainstem tumours in children.' *Neurology*, **8**, 1.
Deeley, T. J. and Rice-Edwards, J. M. (1968). 'Radiotherapy in the management of cerebral secondaries from bronchial carcinoma.' *Lancet*, **1**, 1209.
Horns, J. and Webber, M. M. (1967). 'Retreatment of brain tumours.' *Radiology*, **88**, 322.

MacDonald, J., Green, J. P. and Rubin, P. (1968). 'Serial scanning of brain following irradiation; experimental observation.' In *Clinical Radiation Pathology*, Ed. by P. Rubin and G. W. Casarett. Philadelphia; Saunders.

Order, S. E., Hellman, S., Von Essen, C. F. and Kligerman, M. M. (1968). 'Improvement in quality of survival following whole-brain irradiation for brain metastases.' *Radiology*, **91**, 149.

Rubin, P. and Casarett, G. W. (Eds.) (1968). *Clinical Radiation Pathology*. Philadelphia; Saunders.

Sheline, G. E., Phillips, T. L. and Boldrey, E. (1965). 'The therapy of unbiopsied brain tumours.' *Am. J. Roentgenol.*, **93**, 664.

Shenkin, H. A. (1965). 'The effect of roentgen-ray therapy on oligodendrogliomas of the brain.' *J. Neurosurg.*, **22**, 57.

Whyte, T. R., Colby, M. Y. and Layton, D. D. (1969). 'Radiation therapy of brain-stem tumours.' *Radiology*, **93**, 413, 421.

15—Chemotherapy

William R. Shapiro

INTRODUCTION

In 1969 the clinical and experimental aspects of the chemotherapy of brain tumours were reviewed by Shapiro and Ausman. It was pointed out that while the most hopeful advances in the treatment of patients with brain tumours lay in the field of chemotherapy, no 'break-through' had yet been achieved. Since then, considerable progress has been made in both the laboratory and the clinic, towards the goal of effective chemotherapy in patients with brain tumours. At the recent meeting of the American Association for Cancer Research, Walker and Gehan (1972) gave a preliminary report of the use of 1.3-bis(2-chloroethyl)-1-nitrosourea (BCNU) both with and without radiation therapy in the treatment of glioblastoma multiforme. For the first time, a controlled clinical study demonstrated significant increased survival of patients with glioblastoma multiforme who received chemotherapy and radiotherapy. Whether this constitutes a 'breakthrough' remains to be determined, but the results suggest that we are entering into an era in which chemotherapy of brain tumours may be expected to play an increasingly significant role in the overall treatment of such patients.

In this chapter, the experimental studies based on the murine ependymoblastoma model, as used at both the National Cancer Institute and the Sloan-Kettering Institute, will be reviewed, following which some of the preliminary results in the clinical studies at the Memorial Hospital for Cancer and Allied Diseases will be presented. The relationship of this work to that of others in this field should provide the reader with an 'over-view' of current experimental and clinical research.

Reference will be made to a number of chemotherapeutic drugs as they have been used in experimental and clinical studies. Except for the brief comment which follows, no attempt will be made to des-

270

cribe in any detail the previous work with these agents, their pharmacology or toxicity. The reader is referred to several excellent recent monographs on the various agents (Livingston and Carter, 1970).

All chemotherapeutic agents kill cells, frequently in an indiscriminate manner, i.e. both tumour cells and normal cells can be affected. The mechanisms by which such agents are lethal to cells may be defined in two broad categories: the first consists of agents whose mechanism of action may be operative at any time during the cell's life cycle; the second category consists of agents whose effect occurs principally during those portions of the cell cycle in which cell division takes place. The latter group is defined as 'cell cycle specific' agents. In the first category of non-cell cycle specific agents is found the alkylating agents, of which nitrogen mustard is the prototype. Other agents of this type include cyclophosphamide and probably also the nitrosoureas BCNU, 1-(2-chloroethyl)-3-cyclohexyl-nitrosourea (CCNU) and other related nitrosoureas. Examples of cell cycle specific agents include the anti-metabolites methotrexate (MTX), arabinosyl cytosine (ara-C) and 5-fluorouracil (5-FU). These agents interfere directly with DNA synthesis and therefore directly alter cell division. There are also compounds whose mechanism of action is unknown; in brain tumour chemotherapy the principal example is vincristine. Finally, corticosteroid hormones may be considered as chemotherapeutic agents and are of major usefulness in patients with brain tumours.

EXPERIMENTAL STUDIES

In the past, the poor clinical results in the chemotherapy of brain tumours were due in part to the absence of a proved animal model which could predict clinical therapeutic outcome. The initial purpose of the laboratory studies was to establish such a model and to test its ability to screen for chemotherapeutic agents. The ependymoblastoma mouse model uses a readily transplantable tumour, small animals, and has the ability to reproduce brain tumours in large numbers of animals for statistically valid testing; it has now been in use for five years (Ausman, Shapiro and Rall, 1970; Shapiro, Ausman and Rall, 1970). In those years, the aims of the laboratory investigation have been sharpened and include, first, the testing of chemotherapeutic agents by survival of tumour-bearing animals; secondly, the testing of chemotherapeutic agents for the effect on intracellular metabolism and entry of drugs into brain tumours; and thirdly, the testing of corticosteroid hormones and their effect both on the surrounding cerebral oedema and on tumour growth.

271

Four chemically induced tumour lines of murine glioma have been used. The first is the ependymoblastoma of Zimmerman and Arnold (1941); the second is glioma 261, induced by Seligman and Shear (1939); the third is glioma 26, induced by Sugiura (1969); and the fourth is ependymoblastoma A, a mutant subline of the original Zimmerman and Arnold ependymoblastoma. Histologically, all tumours are ependymoblastomas consisting of small uniform poly-gonal cells with oval, darkly-staining nuclear chromatin and scanty cytoplasm. The cells are arranged in sheets with little connective tissue stoma. Pseudo-rosettes are present and occasionally central canal-like formations can be seen. Mitotic figures are prominent, especially at the periphery of the tumours.

TABLE 1

Biological Characteristics of Intracerebral Implanted Gliomas

Tumour	*Approximate tumour generation time (hours)*	*Average median survival time* $\pm$ SD (days)*	*No-take rate (%)**
Ependymoblastoma	69	29 $\pm$ 3	1·0
Glioma 261	57	25 $\pm$ 2	2·0
Glioma 26	55	25 $\pm$ 3	2·0
Ependymoblastoma A	45	20 $\pm$ 2	2·0

* Mice with intracerebrally implanted tumours.

The tumours are maintained subcutaneously through bi-weekly transplantation. For intracerebral experiments, they are inoculated into the brains of lightly anaesthetized mice by a needle inserted directly through the scalp and skull into the right cerebral hemi-sphere. The needle was especially designed to carry a small fragment, approximately 1×1 mm, to a constant depth. By this method, 75 to 100 mice can be inoculated in one hour. The tumours grow intra-cerebrally and prove fatal in a predictable period of time. There is some difference in the biological behaviour of the four tumour lines, primarily in terms of their rate of growth. Table 1 depicts the approxi-mate generation time, the median survival time of animals bearing intracerebral tumours, and the rate of no-takes for each of the tumours. In general, there is a rough correlation between the generation time of the cells of the tumour and the average median survival time of animals bearing intracerebral tumours. The no-take rate, based on animal deaths within 60 days of implantation, is 2 per cent or less. Thus, treated animals surviving longer than 60 days can be considered 'long-term survivors' and yield an additional measure for evaluation. Of the original four tumours, only glioma 261, glioma 26 and ependymoblastoma A have been used in recent years.

Survival Studies

In each chemotherapy experiment, non-treated animals serve as tumour controls and corresponding tumour and non-tumour bearing groups receive five different doses of the experimental drug. Drugs are given at doses which span the toxicity range from LD_0 to LD_{100} (the LD, or lethal dose, means the dose of drug which yields a given percentage of dead animals). Animals are observed and the day of death for each is recorded. Results are evaluated using three measures: first, the median survival time of the treated groups is compared with the median survival time of the control group, and the treatment/control ratio is determined. Secondly, the days of death of all animals are ranked in a modification of the Wilcoxon rank sum test (Gehan, 1965) to determine statistically significant prolongation of lifespan afforded by the drug. Lastly, the long-term survivors are tabulated at 60 days after implantation, when 98 per cent of non-treated animals have died of their brain tumours.

Table 2 depicts the overall results of testing a variety of chemo-therapeutic agents. As can be seen, the most effective drug so far tested is CCNU. BCNU was not quite as effective, and of the other agents, only cyclophosphamide showed significant increase in survival. So far, none of the cell cycle specific agents has been more than minimally effective; only ara-C yielded some increase in survival.

In the initial studies, CCNU was tested as a suspension adminis-tered intraperitoneally (Shapiro, 1971). The drug is lipid soluble and almost entirely insoluble in aqueous media. In a repeat series, the CCNU was dissolved in sesame oil and administered intramuscularly (Table 2) (Shapiro, 1972 c). The combination is highly effective. As yet the oil method is not available for clinical use, but parenteral administration may prove more useful than the available orally administered agent.

Survival studies have also been used for drug combinations. Previous studies (Schabel, 1969) suggested that a combination of a cell cycle non-specific agent followed by a cell cycle specific agent might be more effective than either type of drug given alone. One combination tested in our laboratory was BCNU and vincristine. The combination failed to demonstrate any usefulness of the vin-cristine over that already afforded by BCNU. Other combination

273

TABLE 2

Chemotherapeutic Agents versus Intracerebral Murine Gliomas. (Maximum increased life span as percentage of control at the approximate LD_{10} for each drug. All drugs given intraperitoneally except where noted)

Drug	Dose (mg/kg)	Schedule	Tumour			
			Ependymoblastoma	Glioma 261	Glioma 26	EpA
CCNU	50	Single day 2		>400*	235	>400*
	50	Single day 7		300		
	50	Single day 14		300		
CCNU in oil IM	50	Single day 2		>400*	>400*	>400*
	50	Single day 7		256	273	>400*
	50	Single day 14		213	214	238
BCNU	30	Single day 2	194	235	135	224
Cyclo-phosphamide	200	Single day 2	124	150	138	
Arabinosyl cytosine	300†	E2d x10‡		137	109	
VM–26	7·5	E4d x4‖		122	98	
Mithramycin	1·0	D3–8¶	98	96		
Methotrexate	32	E4d x4‖	100	104	102	
Vincristine	0·375	E4d x4‖		98	102	105
5–FU	30	E4d x4‖		102	93	103

* Calculated at four times the control median survival time.   † LD_{10} not reached, maximum dose used 300 mg/kg.
‡ E2d x10 = every two days for ten doses.   ‖ E4d x4 = every four days for four doses.   ¶ D3–8 = every day, days 3 to 8.

studies are in progress. Survival studies permit testing of various schedules based on kinetic growth characteristics of the tumours. We are currently investigating CCNU given in low doses in multiple dose schedules in an effort to match the clinical studies more closely (Hansen and colleagues, 1971; Walker and colleagues, 1971). Further schedules of drugs based on the growth kinetics of the tumours are also under investigation.

The results in these studies were similar to those reported with other models and raised some question about the requirement for an intracerebral tumour to test for chemotherapeutic agents. To define more clearly the value of the intracerebral model, a comparative drug study was accomplished. VM26 is a semi-synthetic podophyllotoxin derivative which was tested in the usual survival studies and found to be essentially ineffective in prolonging survival of intracerebral brain tumour-bearing animals (Table 2). A subcutaneous implantation was done with the same tumour, and the same schedule of VM26 was administered; the drug afforded a major reduction in tumour size (Shapiro, 1972 a). The difference between the poor showing in the intracerebral tumour and the excellent results obtained with subcutaneous tumour was similar to that which occurred with the drug mithramycin. Other investigators had reported tumour inhibition when mithramycin was administered to subcutaneous tumour-bearing animals (Kennedy and colleagues, 1968) but we had failed to demonstrate any increased survival of treated intracerebral tumour-bearing animals (Table 2). As noted below, mithramycin also failed to increase the survival of patients with brain tumours. These data suggest that survival time in intracerebral test systems may be a better measure of drug effectiveness than tumour growth inhibition in subcutaneous tumours.

DNA Precursor Studies

Besides the survival time model, an additional system was established (*a*) for preliminary testing of chemotherapeutic agents in experimental brain tumour chemotherapy, (*b*) to examine possible mechanisms of drug action, and (*c*) to measure the ability of drugs to enter tumour cells within the substance of the brain (Shapiro, 1972 d). Experiments consisted of administration of deoxyribonucleic acid (DNA) precursors, tritiated thymidine (TdR-3H) or labelled uridine (UdR-14C), and evaluation of the uptake and incorporation of the precursor into the DNA of the tumour tissues and frequently normal tissues in treated and control animals. Tumour-bearing mice were given one dose of a drug at various intervals prior to the injection of labelled precursor. Two hours after the thymidine, the animals were

275

sacrificed and the brains, tumours, and frequently other tissues, were removed, analysed for DNA and counted for radioactivity. The incorporation was expressed as DPM of labelled precursor per microgram of DNA.

Drugs were selected for the initial set of experiments based on their usefulness in the survival studies and the question of their mechanism of action and/or their possible entry into tumour cells. BCNU was found to retard markedly the incorporation of tritiated thymidine into the tumours ependymoblastoma A, glioma 261 and glioma 26. Retardation varied from 25 to 50 per cent of control values. BCNU was found to be most effective 24 hours after its administration, confirming earlier work (Mizuno and Humphrey, 1969). CCNU was administered in oil to define the time course of action of the drug. It produced marked retardation in uptake of tritiated thymidine; the maximum effect occurred about 12 hours after its administration and lasted at least 72 hours. The results with BCNU and CCNU suggested either an indirect effect on DNA synthesis or a delayed effect related to the requirements for metabolism of the drug to an active form. Since these agents had been found to be non-cell cycle specific, the latter mechanism appears to be most likely.

As noted above, ara-C had demonstrated a mild effect on survival of tumour-bearing animals when administered every two days for ten doses (Table 2). The effect of ara-C on uptake of tritiated thymidine, however, was considerably more impressive. A dose of 40 mg/kg administered once reduced the uptake of tritiated thymidine by over 90 per cent. Ten times that dose retarded the uptake of tritiated thymidine to zero in tumour, bone marrow and lymph nodes. The differences between the survival and the uptake results are probably related to the finding that ara-C must be administered frequently to be most effective, e.g. every three hours for L1210 leukaemia (Skipper, Schabel and Wilcox, 1967). In this case, the uptake studies suggested a way by which a drug could be checked for preliminary effectiveness, following which more detailed survival studies could then be undertaken. It also demonstrated that ara-C entered brain tumour cells, confirming the previous demonstration that the drug enters spinal fluid in low concentrations (Dixon and Adamson, 1965).

The initial poor survival results with methotrexate (Table 2) and its known inability to cross the blood–brain barrier suggested that its failure to gain entry into the tumour made it ineffective. However, Ausman and Levin (1969) and Levin, Clancy and Ausman (1969) demonstrated that MTX occupied approximately the same space within the murine ependymoblastoma as did inulin, a space close to 27 per cent and considerable larger than the 1–2 per cent space found in normal brain. Recently, Tator (1971) demonstrated autoradio-graphically the presence of MTX within experimental brain tumours but not normal brain. To measure possible intracellular entry of MTX, the effect of the drug on the uptake and incorporation of DNA precursors was studied in our laboratory. MTX blocks the methyla-tion of deoxyuridine monophosphate to deoxythymidine mono-phosphate. Under such circumstances, deoxyuridine uptake is de-pressed and thymidine uptake might be expected to be increased. Indeed, such results were found in the brain tumour model. MTX increased the uptake of tritiated thymidine to 140 per cent of control while retarding the uptake of 14C-uridine to 23 per cent of control. These results clearly demonstrated that MTX does enter brain tumours, at least in the experimental murine ependymoblastoma model, and excludes the blood–brain barrier as the sole factor in its poor chemotherapeutic showing.

Cerebral Oedema and Corticosteroid Hormones

Brain tumours produce their symptoms in two ways: first, the size of the tumour itself displaces and infiltrates into brain tissue. Secondly, the tumour is associated with cerebral oedema, an increase in fluid content of the brain around the tumour, which produces neurological deficit. The value of corticosteroid hormones in re-ducing the signs and symptoms of patients with brain tumour has been ascribed to reduction in surrounding cerebral oedema, but attempts to confirm this in an experimental animal model have been contradictory. Although some reduction in the surrounding oedema was demonstrated, a more impressive result was inhibition of tumour growth. Cortisone was found to inhibit the growth of subcutaneously transplanted ependymomas in mice as early as 1951 (Brzustowicz and colleagues, 1951). Kotsilimbas and colleagues (1967) examined the effect of dexamethasone intraperitoneally in mice bearing intra-cerebrally implanted melanoma. A 25 per cent increase in mean survival time was afforded by the drug. The water content of tumour, adjacent brain and distant brain was reduced by steroids and the sodium–potassium (Na/K) ratios were decreased in the brain tissue. However, a more striking finding was marked reduction in both wet and dry weight of brain tumour in steroid treated animals. In an-other subcutaneous model, Wright, Shaumba and Keller (1969) reported tumour growth inhibition by methyl prednisolone and depo-methyl prednisolone in mice with subcutaneous ependymomas and rats with subcutaneous gliomas. Gurcay and colleagues (1971) reported that methyl prednisolone increased survival in transplant-able intracerebral rat gliomas and afforded a reduction in both surrounding cerebral oedema and the wet weight of treated tumours. Mealey, Chen and Schanz (1971) demonstrated transient inhibition of tumour growth by steroids in human glioblastomas carried in tissue culture. Methyl prednisolone was more injurious than dexamethasone but resistance occurred within one day.

In an effort to evaluate the effect of corticosteroid hormones, a series of experiments was performed in our laboratory utilizing such hormones and the ependymoblastoma model (Shapiro, 1972 b). The first series of experiments consisted of testing corticosteroids on survival of mice bearing intracerebral ependymoblastoma A. Both dexamethasone and depo-methyl prednisolone were used in a variety of doses and starting days. The drugs were administered daily. As shown in Table 3, dexamethasone at a dose of 40 mg/kg significantly

TABLE 3

Effect of Corticosteroids on Survival of Mice Bearing
Intracerebral Ependymoblastoma A

Drug	Dose (mg/kg)	Starting day	Median survival % control
Dexamethasone	1	2, 14	95–105
	10	2	118
		14	113
	40	1	124
		12	95
Depo-methyl prednisolone	0·4–2·8	12, 17	90–97

Drugs were administered intraperitoneally daily beginning on the starting day shown.

increased survival of tumour-bearing mice but only to 24 per cent greater than controls. In parallel experiments, animals were sacrificed 18 days after the implantation of the tumour and the animals treated with dexamethasone. The brains and tumours of the animals were removed and weighed, dried and re-weighed, and electrolytes determined on the dried specimens. Early treatment with dexamethasone, 1 mg/kg, reduced the water content of adjacent brain from 81·5 to 79·6 per cent, a significant reduction, as well as reducing the Na/K ratio from 0·891 to 0·738. No change in water content of distant brain occurred and no change occurred with treatment delayed to day 14. With dexamethasone at 10 mg/kg, the water content was reduced from 82·1 to 79·9 per cent, again a significant reduction, and the Na/K ratio fell from 0·897 to 0·686, also significant. These studies showed a modest effect of the corticosteroid drugs both on survival of animals bearing intracerebral tumours and on the water content and Na/K ratio of the adjacent brain in such animals. A more impressive result was found when the weights of the tumours were compared with those of the controls (*Figure 1*); a significant reduction in both wet and dry weight occurred, suggesting a direct growth

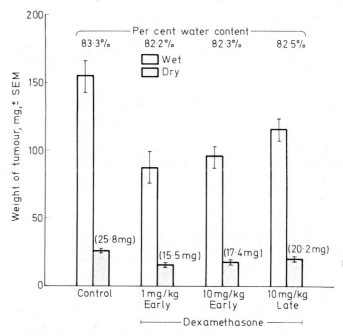

Figure 1. *The effect of dexamethasone on the weight of intracerebral ependymoblastoma A. The drug was given daily intraperitoneally starting early (day 2 after implantation) or late (day 14 after implantation). The reduction in wet and dry weight of brain tumour was significantly different from control with all three schedules. No significant change in water content occurred*

inhibiting effect of steroids on the tumours. In an effort to define more clearly the effect of the dexamethasone on brain tumour growth, a tritiated thymidine uptake experiment was performed. Dexamethasone was given in a dose of 40 mg/kg at times 0, 4 hours, 12 hours and 24 hours prior to the administration of 40 microcuries per animal of tritiated thymidine. *Figure 2* shows the results as percentages of control. Lymph node uptake was markedly depressed, as would be expected from the lympholytic effect of corticosteroids.

Bone marrow was unchanged. Uptake in the tumour was significantly retarded, the maximum depression occurring after four hours.

These studies confirmed that tumour growth inhibition by corticosteroid drugs does occur in experimental brain tumours as well as reduction in surrounding cerebral oedema. They further demonstrated that uptake and incorporation of DNA precursors can be altered

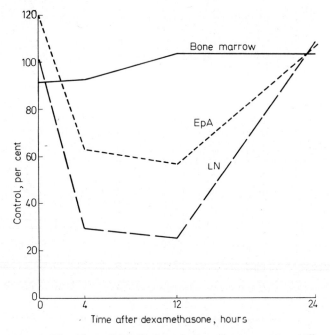

Figure 2. The effect of dexamethasone 40 mg/kg intraperitoneally on uptake and incorporation of TdR-3H by intracerebral ependymoblastoma A, lymph node and bone marrow. Note time course of retarded uptake of TdR-3H

by large doses of corticosteroids, although the exact mechanism by which such uptake is altered is still unknown. The relationship between such growth inhibiting functions of corticosteroids and their clinical usefulness in patients with brain tumour is also unknown, although the possibility is raised of a tumour growth inhibiting function. Studies on corticosteroid mechanism of action continue.

Comment

The relevance of the survival studies in the experimental animal model to patients with brain tumours constitutes one possible definition of a 'screen' for chemotherapeutic agents. Whether or not a given model will predict human response to the drugs tested depends on the kind of clinical studies undertaken. Three randomized studies utilizing chemotherapy in patients with primary brain tumours have been reported. The first of these used mithramycin *versus* radiation therapy; the mithramycin was ineffective in prolonging survival (Leventhal and Walker, 1969). The second compared 5-FU with radiation therapy and chemotherapy in combination (Edland, Javrid and Ainsfield, 1971), and again the 5-FU was ineffective. Finally, BCNU has been used in combination and alone in patients with primary brain tumours (Walker and Gehan, 1972) (*see below*) and was found to be effective. The murine screening data noted above showed both mithramycin and 5-FU unable to increase survival time of tumour-bearing mice, whereas BCNU was highly effective. This limited comparative experience suggests that the experimental tumour system does indeed predict for human brain tumour response. Whether it does so in a more precise way than other available models remains to be seen.

The data derived from the uptake experiments tend to confirm that the blood–brain barrier is not a significant impediment to entry of chemotherapeutic agents into the midst of brain tumours. Thus, MTX clearly alters the uptake and incorporation of DNA precursors in an experimental brain tumour—an intracellular process. It would appear that the blood vessels within the centre of a brain tumour resemble vessels found outside the brain and are quite porous. It is therefore necessary to explain why drugs like the nitrosoureas, which enter both brain tumour and surrounding brain, appear to be more effective than water soluble agents whose entry is restricted to the tumour centre. One possibility may be that the drug must find entry to that portion of the tumour carrying the most sensitive cells. It has been demonstrated (Kirsch, Schulz and Leitner, 1967) that while most of the cells in a brain tumour are located in the central regions, the actively proliferating cells are found along the edge. In the latter site, there is a low inulin space, implying a relatively tight blood–brain barrier (Ausman and Levin, 1969). It is in such a site that the water soluble anti-metabolites (methotrexate) have restricted entry, while the lipid soluble nitrosoureas may easily enter (Levin and colleagues, 1970). Theoretically, then, the nitrosoureas are more effective because they can affect cells both in the centre and at the periphery, while the water soluble drugs can affect only that small fraction of actively dividing cells found in the centre. The blood–brain barrier appears to be most important at the edge of the tumour.

Experimental work now being carried out in our own and other laboratories promises further to expand the study of experimental brain tumours. The new trend in such work involves the concept of non-transplantable tumours, i.e. those arising within the brain and therefore avoiding some of the problems related to transplantation. Tumours may be induced in the brain by insertion of viral particles directly (Vick, Bigner and Kredar, 1971) or by the intravenous administration of nitrosoureas (Swenberg, Koestner and Wechsler, 1972; Schmidek and colleagues, 1971). Such models, although more difficult to work with, are one step closer to the clinical situation.

CLINICAL STUDIES

A major problem for the physician who would treat patients with brain tumours by the administration of chemotherapeutic agents is to determine a standardized system for evaluating the results of such studies. Such evaluation presents specific problems not present in patients with systemic disease. Thus, a lung nodule that can be seen on x-ray examination, lymph nodes and skin tumours than can be palpated and measured, and bone marrow that can be examined, all permit a direct measure of response. In patients with brain tumours, there is no acceptable method to determine the response of intra-cranial neoplasms to chemotherapy. The various radiographic procedures, brain scans and echograms, do not measure the size of the tumour itself but also include the surrounding oedema. This is especially true in primary brain tumours, where survival time of patients is the only quantitative means available for determining precise end-points in chemotherapy. In carcinoma metastatic to the brain, patients may die of systemic metastases or of the primary tumour, excluding survival as a means of evaluating chemotherapy.

Despite such problems, several treatment centres now have active programmes in chemotherapy, using primarily the nitrosoureas. The following review will be in the nature of a preliminary report on such studies.

Glioblastoma Multiforme

Several years ago, Jelsma and Bucy (1969) reported their results on the surgical and radiation therapy of patients with glioblastoma multiforme. They divided their patients into three groups: those with extensive surgery, those with partial resection, and patients who only had biopsies. The survival time of patients with extensive surgery and radiation therapy was similar to that reported by Frankel and German (1958) and that at The New York Hospital. The survival curve of such patients has two components. The first is a straight exponential curve from the time of operation to approximately two years following operation, when 10–13 per cent of patients are still alive. A flatter curve then commences until five years is reached. The median survival time of the first 90 per cent of the patients (the straight curve) is between 5 and 7·5 months. The second group of patients has a considerably longer survival time, with approximately 3 per cent of the original group of patients still alive at five years. The existence of this second, tail group of patients means that the longer a patient survives following operation, the greater his chance of falling into this long-term survival group. Evaluation of chemotherapy in such patients thus becomes very difficult since they may already be 'long-term survivors'. In recognition of this fact, most centres today begin chemotherapy shortly after the initial resection. The Brain Tumor Study Group, sponsored by the National Cancer Institute, has utilized Phase III type studies with randomization of patients in drug therapy, drug therapy plus radiation therapy, radiation therapy alone, and control groups. At Memorial Hospital, we have randomized into drug therapy and drug therapy plus radiation groups. Such randomization protocols are of relatively recent origin, however, and prior to approximately five years ago most studies on brain tumour patients were of the Phase II type in which all patients, no matter how long their survival from operation, were entered into the same treatment schedule. It was left to the individual investigators to determine the method for evaluating such patients, and comparing the many studies was difficult at best. Such a comparison was done by Shapiro and Ausman (1969) for the first 15 years of chemotherapy in brain tumours. On the whole, results were not particularly impressive. Although occasional patients achieved significant palliation, no discernible positive effect could be seen in the majority.

The first major effort at quantitative evaluation of chemotherapy in glioblastoma was accomplished by the Brain Tumor Study Group in their study of mithramycin (Leventhal and Walker, 1969). The drug was ineffective but the study demonstrated the possibility of co-operative trials among several centres in controlled clinical studies. BCNU had been tried in Phase II type trials by Walker and Hurwitz (1970) and by Wilson, Boldrey and Enot (1970) and found to be effective in improving the clinical status of patients with recurrent glioblastoma multiforme. These data, along with the animal data noted above, made this drug ideal to try for the second drug in the Brain Tumor Study Group's chemotherapy trials. Walker and Gehan (1972) have recently reported the preliminary results of the BCNU study undertaken by the Group. BCNU was administered as 80 mg/ sq m/day for three days every six to eight weeks. Radiation consisted of 6,000 rads of whole brain in six to eight weeks, 4,500 rads of whole head plus 1,500 rads to the involved hemisphere. Preliminary analysis of the first 180 patients randomized for the study indicated divergence of the survival curves. The median survival times from randomization were: control 17 weeks, BCNU alone 20 weeks, radiation 28 weeks (significantly different from control), and BCNU plus radiation 41 weeks (significantly different from control). The study continues but even the preliminary results clearly indicate that the combination of BCNU and radiation therapy offers a significant chance for increased survival in patients with glioblastoma.

As noted above, we have elected to randomize patients into two groups: those who received chemotherapy alone and those who received a combination of chemotherapy and radiation therapy. We have relied on the Brain Tumor Study Group protocol to supply data on patients who receive only radiation therapy and those who receive no additional primary therapy following the operation (controls). Our protocols also differ in that we have added vincristine to the regimen of BCNU. Vincristine had been initially reported by Lassman, Pearce and Gang (1965) to be effective in patients with primary brain tumours, although their subsequent studies had failed to confirm the initial impression. All of the patients received BCNU 80 mg/sq m/day for three days and vincristine 1·4 mg/sq m on days 1 and 8 of each course. The course is repeated at about six-week intervals. In addition, half of the patients receive 6,000 rads of whole brain radiation therapy. The study is too early to draw any firm conclusions, although no major difference is discernible yet between the two groups of patients.

We also see patients who are operated on elsewhere and who come to us with symptoms of recurrent growth of their brain tumours. Such patients have been treated by two protocols; the first is the same chemotherapy protocol as used in the randomized group, i.e. BCNU and vincristine; the second utilizes CCNU (Hansen and colleagues, 1971; Walker and colleagues, 1971). Such patients have already survived varying intervals of time since their initial operation, and survival cannot be used to evaluate chemotherapy results. Instead, we have had to rely on qualitative estimates of response in which patients are evaluated neurologically and brain scans and appropriate contrast studies are performed. Corticosteroids are used because of their obvious effectiveness in relieving symptoms of such patients. Soon after chemotherapy is started, however, the corticosteroids are reduced and the subsequent clinical course is used as one measure of chemotherapy response. We have treated six patients with a combination of BCNU and vincristine and three of these responded with improvement in the signs and symptoms lasting at least three months. Four patients so far treated with oral CCNU did not show significant improvement at doses ranging from 80 to 130 mg/sq m repeated at six-week intervals. Subsequent patients have been treated at doses of 150 mg/sq m at six week intervals or at lower doses at two- or three-week intervals. Several patients appear to have responded to new schedules.

Metastatic Brain Tumours

When a patient with primary systemic cancer presents with metastatis to the brain, evaluation of chemotherapy is even more difficult than with primary brain tumours. Metastases may occur late or early in the course, for example, breast cancer and melanoma tend to occur toward the end of the general course of the patient's disease but in carcinoma of the lung about 7–10 per cent of patients present with brain tumour. Evaluation of chemotherapy in patients with metastatic brain tumour may be especially difficult in that the patient may die either from his brain tumour or his systemic disease. Survival time, a good method of evaluating primary brain tumours, is of almost no value in evaluating chemotherapy of metastatic brain tumours; it is necessary to utilize the patient's neurological signs and symptoms to measure response. Patients are usually treated with corticosteroids to reduce oedema, and differentiating the effects of the steroids from those of the chemotherapeutic agents may be difficult. Patients with metastatic brain tumours may show improvement in neurological signs and symptoms but may have progression of their systemic disease. Patients with metastatic brain tumours are usually treated with radiation therapy first and residual neurological signs and symptoms make it difficult to evaluate changes from chemotherapy. Metabolic problems can frequently produce neurological abnormalities and systemic cancer is notorious for producing metabolic encephalopathy, further complicating evaluation. Thus, evaluating the results of chemotherapy in patients with metastatic brain tumours requires careful documentation of changes in signs and symptoms as well as critical evaluation of the results of autopsy should the patient expire.

We have used both BCNU and CCNU to treat patients with metastatic brain tumours. The results have been disappointing. Of seven patients with malignant melanoma metastatic to the brain treated with intravenous BCNU, there was improvement in two patients, one lasting four months and the other three months. Of three patients with melanoma in the brain treated with oral CCNU on the initial lower dose, none demonstrated improvement. Two patients treated recently with high doses of CCNU both demonstrated reduction of neurological signs and symptoms and requirement for corticosteroid hormones, each lasting about five months. Of seven patients with bronchogenic carcinoma treated with BCNU, only one improved and remained symptom free for five months; the remaining patients had progressive central nervous system dysfunction and died one to three months following the start of chemotherapy. Bronchogenic carcinoma treated with CCNU has not fared much better. Four patients died between three and five months after starting therapy, all with progressive disease and all with little evidence of improvement. Too few patients with breast carcinoma have been treated with chemotherapeutic agents to permit evaluation. These results are not dissimilar to those obtained using these newer agents in systemic disease (Walker and Hurwitz, 1970; Wilson, Boldrey and Enot, 1970; Hansen and colleagues, 1971).

Medulloblastoma

Patients with recurrent medulloblastoma who have received full dosage of radiation therapy in the past have been treated with several different combinations of drug therapy. Several years ago the drugs used were BCNU and intrathecal MTX, the MTX being delivered by Ommaya reservoir (Ratcheson and Ommaya, 1968). Our initial enthusiasm for this method was dampened by one patient who, after initial improvement, subsequently developed bilateral decerebrate rigidity, mutism, and died. Two other patients developed a similar syndrome. The combination of surgical intervention in one case and autopsy results in the others demonstrated periventricular necrosis secondary to the intrathecal MTX (Shapiro, Chernik and Posner, 1973). The common denominator in these patients was the presence of ventricular obstruction, which apparently permitted the MTX to penetrate in relatively high concentrations into the periventricular white matter with resulting necrosis and demyelination. Intraventricular MTX is no longer used if ventricular obstruction is present. CCNU has proved to be effective in two medulloblastoma patients, one of whom survived six months following the initiation of treatment and another is alive seven months after beginning CCNU.

Meningeal Carcinomatosis

We see approximately 20 patients per year with diffuse meningeal involvement from metastatic brain tumour. In the past, the prognosis for such patients was quite poor. We have made an effort to utilize Ommaya reservoirs and intrathecal medication to treat these patients. Treatment with MTX and ara-C for malignant melanoma metastatic to the meninges was unsuccessful with no evidence of response. More recently, we have treated three patients with breast carcinoma metastatic to the meninges with MTX delivered in an Ommaya reservoir. An excellent response was obtained with improvement in neurological signs and symptoms as well as a return toward normal of the cerebrospinal fluid abnormalities. In one patient, whole brain radiation therapy was included because of signs of a cerebral metastasis.

Drug Toxicity

Except for the problem noted above with intrathecal MTX, the drugs have been fairly well tolerated. The nitrosoureas produce primarily bone marrow toxicity with thrombocytopenia and, to a lesser extent, leukopenia. The bone marrow depression is unusual in that it tends to occur in a delayed fashion; evidence of thrombocytopenia rarely begins before the 21st day following BCNU, reaching its nadir about the 30th day. There is gradual recovery so that at about 40 days the peripheral platelet counts are usually normal. Leukopenia follows the thrombocytopenia by about five days, both in its fall and subsequent recovery. Some patients treated with chemotherapy who have survived long intervals have had mild, permanent bone marrow damage with gradually progressive delays in recovery of both platelet counts and white counts, and subsequent development of anaemia. Additional toxicity problems include mild elevations in the serum glutamic oxaloacetic transaminase and, to a lesser degree, serum alkaline phosphatase. With oral CCNU, fairly marked but reversible elevations in liver-derived enzymes have been seen as well as the delayed bone marrow depression. A problem of note in medulloblastoma is the fact that these children have usually had total spine irradiation in the past. As a result, their bone marrow reserves are lower than usual and they have an increased risk of serious bone marrow toxicity from chemotherapeutic agents.

Summary

In total, at Memorial Hospital we have treated some 80 patients with a variety of primary brain tumours and secondary metastatic brain tumours with BCNU, vincristine, CCNU and intrathecal medication. A 30–40 per cent overall response rate was found with BCNU and vincristine in primary tumours. Treatment of metastatic carcinoma, however, remains poor and the nitrosoureas have not contributed in any major way to improvement. CCNU is a new drug whose primary difficulty relates to irregular absorption from the gastrointestinal tract, as manifested by difficulty in controlling dose and toxicity. Parenteral preparations in animals have been designed (Shapiro, 1972c) but are not yet available for human use. Methyl-CCNU, another member of the nitrosourea family, is now being evaluated at Memorial and at other centres.

CONCLUSIONS

In 1952, French and colleagues reported on the use of intracarotid nitrogen mustard in patients with brain tumours. The drug and route of administration proved to be very toxic; the authors concluded that nitrogen mustard was toxic to normal brain tissue and that chemotherapy by intracarotid injection was contra-indicated. However, in 1959 Woodhall and colleagues began using several alkylating agents to treat patients with brain tumours. For the next 10 years a number of investigators, utilizing different routes of administration and different drugs, attempted to treat their patients with brain tumours using a variety of chemotherapeutic agents. It was not until the advent of the nitrosoureas, however, that any major inroads have been made in this complicated task. The survival time of patients with glioblastoma has now been doubled by the use of nitrosoureas in combination with radiotherapy, but much work obviously remains to be done. Continued screening for new drugs and both experimental and clinical studies on drug combinations are currently under way. The problem of the kinetics of drug entry, the problem of the kinetics of brain tumour growth, and the relationship between steroids, oedema and chemotherapeutic drugs remain as fields of investigation. Perhaps the single most important advancement made in the last five years in the chemotherapy of patients with brain tumours has been the recognition that neurosurgeons and neurologists must lead the way in both the experimental study of chemotherapy in brain tumours and the clinical application of methods derived from the laboratory.

REFERENCES

Ausman, J. I. and Levin, V. A. (1969). 'Intra- and extravascular distribution of standard drug molecules in brain tumor and brain.' In *Fourth International Congress of Neurological Surgery*, p. 41, Ed. by C. G. Drake and R. Duvoisin. New York; Excerpta Medica.
— Shapiro, W. R. and Rall, D. P. (1970). 'Studies on the chemotherapy of experimental brain tumors: development of an experimental model.' *Cancer Res.*, **30**, 2394.
Brzuntowicz, R. J., Svien, H. J., Bennett, W. A. and Higgins, G. M. (1951).

'The effect of cortisone on the growth of transplanted ependymomas in mice.' *Proc. Staff Meet. Mayo Clin.*, **26**, 121.

Dixon, R. L. and Adamson, R. H. (1965). 'Antitumor activity and pharmacologic disposition of cytosine arabinoside (NSC 63878).' *Cancer Chemother. Rep.*, **48**, 11.

Edland, R. W., Javrid, M. and Ainsfield, F. J. (1971). 'Glioblastoma multiforme. An analysis of the result of postoperative radiotherapy alone vs radiotherapy and concomitant 5-fluorouracil.' *Am. J. Roentgenol.*, **111**, 337.

Frankel, S. A. and German, W. J. (1958). 'Glioblastoma multiforme. Review of 219 cases with regard to natural history, pathology, diagnostic methods and treatment.' *J. Neurosurg.*, **15**, 498.

French, J. D., West, P. M., von Amerongen, F. K. and Magoun, H. W. (1952). 'Effects of intracarotid administration of nitrogen mustard on normal brain and brain tumors.' *J. Neurosurg.*, **9**, 378.

Gehan, E. A. (1965). 'A generalized Wilcoxon test for comparing arbitrarily singly censored samples.' *Biometrika.*, **52**, 203.

Gurcay, O., Wilson, C., Barker, M. and Eliason, J. (1971). 'Corticosteroid effect on transplantable rat glioma.' *Archs Neurol.*, **24**, 266.

Hansen, H. H., Selawry, O. S., Muggia, F. M. and Walker, M. D. (1971). 'Clinical studies with 1-(2-chloroethyl)-3-cyclohexyl-1-nitrosourea.' *Cancer Res.*, **31**, 223.

Jelsma, R. and Bucy, P. C. (1969). 'Glioblastoma multiforme: Its treatment and some factors affecting survival.' *Archs Neurol.*, **20**, 161.

Kennedy, B. J., Yarbro, J. W., Kickertz, V. and Sandberg-Wollheim, M. (1968). 'Effect of mithramycin on a mouse glioma.' *Cancer Res.*, **28**, 91.

Kirsch, W. M., Schulz, D. and Leitner, J. W. (1967). 'The effect of prolonged ischemia upon regional energy reserves in the experimental glioblastoma.' *Cancer Res.*, **27**, 2212.

Kotsilimbas, D. G., Meyer, L., Berson, M., Taylor, J. M. and Scheinberg, L. C. (1967). 'Corticosteroid effect on intracerebral melanomata and associated cerebral edema.' *Neurology*, **17**, 223.

Lassman, L. P., Pearce, G. W. and Gang, J. (1965). 'Sensitivity of intracranial gliomas to vincristine sulfate.' *Lancet*, **1**, 296.

Leventhal, C. M. and Walker, M. D. (1969). 'Chemotherapy of malignant glioma: A collaborative study.' In *Fourth International Congress of Neurological Surgery*, p. 33, Ed. by C. G. Drake and R. Duvoisin. New York; Excerpta Medica.

Levin, V. A., Clancy, T. P. and Ausman, J. I. (1969). 'Methotrexate permeability and steady-state distribution in the murine ependymoblastoma.' *Trans. Am. Neurol. Ass.*, **94**, 294.

— Shapiro, W. R., Clancy, T. P. and Oliverio, V. T. (1970). 'The uptake, distribution and antitumor activity of 1-(2-chloroethyl)-3-cyclohexyl-1-nitrosourea in the murine glioma.' *Cancer Res.*, **30**, 2451.

Livingston, R. B. and Carter, S. K. (1970). *Single Agents in Cancer Chemotherapy*. New York; IFI/Plenum.

Mealey, J. Jnr., Chen, T. T. and Schanz, G. P. (1971). 'Effects of dexamethasone and methylprednisolone on cell cultures of human glioblastoma.' *J. Neurosurg.*, **34**, 324.

Mizuno, N. S. and Humphrey, E. W. (1969). 'Effect of combined therapy with cytosine arabinoside (NSC 63878) and 1,3-bis(2-chloroethyl)-1-nitrosourea (NSC 409962) on Sarcoma 180 and L1210 in vivo.' *Cancer Chemother. Rep.*, **53**, 215.

Ratcheson, R. A. and Ommaya, A. K. (1968). 'Experience with the subcutaneous cerebrospinal fluid reservoir. Preliminary report of 60 cases.' *New Engl. J. Med.*, **279**, 1025.

Schabel, F. M. Jnr. (1969). 'The use of tumor growth kinetics in planning "curative" chemotherapy of advanced solid tumors.' *Cancer Res.*, **29**, 2384.

Schmidek, H. H., Nielsen, S. L., Schiller, A. L. and Messer, J. (1971). 'Morphological studies of rat brain tumors, induced by N-nitrosomethylurea.' *J. Neurosurg.*, **34**, 335.

Seligman, A. M. and Shear, M. J. (1939). 'Studies in carcinogenesis. VIII. Experimental production of brain tumors in mice with methylcholanthrene.' *Am. J. Cancer*, **37**, 364.

Shapiro W. R. (1971). 'Studies on the chemotherapy of experimental brain tumors: Evaluation of 1-(2-chloroethyl)-3-cyclohexyl-1-nitrosourea, vincristine and 5-fluorouracil.' *J. natn. Cancer Inst.*, **46**, 359.

— (1972a). 'A comparative study of intracerebral vs subcutaneous implantation of murine glioma: Differential sensitivity to VM26.' *Proc. Am. Ass. Cancer Res.*, **13**, 122.

— (1972b). 'Corticosteroid hormones in an experimental mouse brain tumor.' *Neurology*, **22**, 401.

— (1972c). 'Effect of 1-(2-chloroethyl)-3-cyclohexyl-1-nitrosourea (CCNU, NSC 79037) in sesame oil intramuscularly on experimental brain tumors.' *Cancer Chemother. Rep.*, **56**, 457.

— (1972d). 'The effect of chemotherapeutic agents on incorporation of DNA precursors by experimental brain tumors.' *Cancer Res.*, **32**, 2178.

— and Ausman, J. I. (1969). 'The chemotherapy of brain tumors: A clinical and experimental review.' In *Recent Advances in Neurology*, pp. 149–235, Ed. by F. Plum. Philadelphia; Davis.

— — and Rall, D. P. (1970). 'Studies on the chemotherapy of experimental brain tumors: Evaluation of 1,3-bis(2-chloroethyl)-1-nitrosourea, cyclophosphamide, mithramycin and methotrexate.' *Cancer Res.*, **30**, 2401.

— Chernik, N. L. and Posner, J. B. (1973). 'Necrotizing encephalopathy following intraventricular instillation of methotrexate.' *Archs Neurol.*, **28**, 96.

Skipper, H. E., Schabel, F. M. Jnr. and Wilcox, W. S. (1967). 'Experimental evaluation of potential anticancer agents. XXI. Scheduling of arabinosylcytosine to take advantage of its S-phase specificity against leukemic cells.' *Cancer Chemother. Rep.*, **51**, 125.

Sugiura, K. (1969). 'Tumor transplantation.' In *Methods of Animal Experi-*

mentation, Ed. by W. I. Gay, Vol. 2, pp. 171–222. New York; Academic Press.

Swenberg, J. A., Koestner, A. and Wechsler, W. (1972). 'The induction of tumors of the nervous system with intravenous methylnitrosourea.' *Lab. Invest.*, **26**, 74.

Tator, C. H. (1971). 'The uptake of tritiated methotrexate by an experimental glioma.' *Cancer Res.*, **31**, 1600.

Vick, N. A., Bigner, D. D. and Kvedar, J. P. (1971). 'The fine structure of canine gliomas and intracranial sarcomas induced by the Schmidt–Ruppin strain of the Rous sarcoma virus.' *J. Neuropath. expl. Neurol.*, **30**, 354.

Walker, M. D. and Gehan, E. A. (1972). 'An evaluation of 1,3-bis(2-chloroethyl)-1-nitrosourea (BCNU) and irradiation alone and in combination for the treatment of malignant glioma.' *Proc. Am. Ass. Cancer Res.*, **13**, 67.

— and Hurwitz, B. S. (1970). 'BCNU (1,3-bis(2-chloroethyl)-1-nitrosourea; NSC 409962) in the treatment of malignant brain tumor—a preliminary report.' *Cancer Chemother. Rep.*, **54**, 263.

— Rosenblum, M. L., Smith, K. A. and Reynolds, A. F. Jnr. (1971). 'The treatment of brain tumor with 1-(2-chloroethyl)-3-cyclohexyl-1-nitrosourea (CCNU).' *Proc. Am. Ass. Cancer Res.*, **12**, 51.

Wilson, C. B., Boldrey, E. B. and Enot, K. J. (1970). '1,3-bis(2-chloroethyl)-1-nitrosourea (NSC 409962) in the treatment of brain tumors.' *Cancer Chemother. Rep.*, **54**, 273.

Woodhall, B., Hall, K., Mahaley, S. and Jackson, J. (1959). 'Chemotherapy of brain cancer. Experimental and clinical studies in localized hypothermic cerebral perfusion.' *Ann. Surg.*, **150**, 640.

Wright, R. L., Shaumba, B. and Keller, J. (1969). 'The effect of glucocorticoids on growth and metabolism of experimental glial tumors.' *J. Neurosurg.*, **30**, 140.

Zimmerman, H. M. and Arnold, H. (1941). 'Experimental brain tumors. I. Tumors produced with methylcholanthrene.' *Cancer Res.*, **1**, 919.

16—Scanning After Irradiation

Antero Voutilainen

INTRODUCTION

For correct irradiation dosage in cases of intracranial neoplasm the position and the extent of the tumour must be determined. In attempting this, one usually has at one's disposal the results of neuro-radiological examination and frequently, in addition, data provided by neurosurgical operations. Nevertheless, the overall picture often remains obscure, particularly regarding the extent of the growth in different directions into the brain tissue. In some cases an earlier examination no longer provides an up-to-date picture by the time radiotherapy is planned.

That intracranial neoplasm belongs to a group of diseases in which it is exceedingly difficult to give a prognosis does not remove the need to assess the situation as accurately as possible when irradiation is planned. It is, moreover, also necessary to devise means of checking, by comparable methods, the effect of the treatment at different stages of the disease.

Neurological methods of examination, valuable though they are in themselves, have certain disadvantages and limitations. Not only are they difficult to carry out but most of them also involve pain, risks, expense and, particularly if repeated, opposition and fear on the part of the patient.

Either scintigraphy or gamma-encephalography of the brain would seem a valuable method of determining the condition after irradiation. The advantages are that they are easy to carry out on non-hospital-ized patients and are painless and convenient for the patient being examined. This is important when the condition of a patient must be continuously observed. In patients with a poor prognosis—when, for

292

example, malignant tumours are being treated by irradiation or cytostatic drugs—it has seemed especially unreasonable to subject them repeatedly to frightening or painful examinations for the sake of objective observation of their condition, although this may for several reasons be advisable and necessary.

In the light of studies made and experience gained over about 15 years it seems possible that since radioactive isotopes seek, and are retained in, pathological intracranial tissue formations—especially tumours—the need for less painful methods of examination can be met, at least in part, by isotope scanning of the brain.

Gamma-encephalography is based on the following physiological and patho-physiological factors:

(1) The large quantity of blood circulating in the intracranial structure.

(2) The changes produced by pathological processes in the barrier of cerebral blood vessels, with radioactive isotopes very actively seeking the brain tumour and subjecting it to chemical influence as well.

In supratentorial brain tumours positive findings in 80–90 per cent of patients can be achieved when using the scanner or the gamma camera. In infratentorial tumours we obtained only 30–40 per cent positive findings. When the tumour is located near the base of the cranium, the third or fourth ventricle or in the region of the mid-brain, the scanning does not always show it—this results from the increased uptake in these regions which is present normally, for example, from the tongue and the great blood vessels such as the transverse sinus (*Figure 1*).

Another factor which produces negative results is the small size of the tumours. A review of the literature shows that supratentorial tumours or metastases larger than 1 cm and infratentorial tumours or metastases larger than $1\frac{1}{2}$–2 cm cannot possibly be verified by the scanning method.

What then can be found by scanning after irradiation of the brain tumours? This matter has not been investigated thoroughly because the patients often go to other hospitals for follow-up examinations after the treatment. In this case we have to try to clear up certain problems:

(1) The importance of repeated scanning in the patient's follow-up period after irradiation.

(2) Does the examination verify possible brain tumours or their position after the treatment?

(3) Whether it is possible to verify by scanning a residual or recurrent tumour after irradiation.

(4) Whether there is a correlation between the clinical picture and the scanning findings.

A study of this kind was made in 1965 in the Department of Radiotherapy, University Central Hospital and Hesperia Hospital, Helsinki, and one or more radioisotope scannings were carried out on a total of 48 patients after radical irradiation.

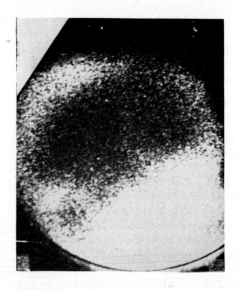

Figure 1. The lateral brain scan in the normal person. The uptake of radioisotope is in the base of the skull and the sagittal and transverse sinuses (gamma camera)

SCANNING

Scintigraphies were carried out by means of a commercial scanner (Nuclear Chicago Model 1700) using the photographic recorder. The dimensions of the scintillation crystal was 2 × 2 inches. In most cases a collimator of $7\frac{1}{2}$ cm length, tapered towards the radiation source, was used. The diameter of the hole varied from 2·5 to 1 cm. In some cases a 19-hole focusing collimator was used.

The radioactive isotope used was ^{203}Hg-neohydrin in intravenous doses of 700 μCi and the scanning was made five hours later, in sagittal and lateral directions.

Histological verification was obtained in 35 tumours; in three of these, isotope scanning before the irradiation revealed no uptake. In 17 patients both a clinical and neuro-roentgenological definition of the brain tumour was obtained—only 3 of them gave a negative finding on isotope scanning. Metastases were diagnosed clinically and neuroradiologically in 6 patients and scanning gave a positive result in 4 of these. All these patients had received the usual tumour dose of telecobalt irradiation which we employ—that is, a tumour dose of 5,000 rads.

After irradiation, isotope scanning was repeated in all the cases at least once and in 17 cases twice at about three-monthly intervals. The

TABLE 1

Results of Brain Scanning and its Correlation with the Clinical Picture

	Total	Before irradiation Positive	After irradiation		Correlation Good
			Positive	Negative	
Histologically proved tumour	35	32	21	14	28 (80%)
Clinically diagnosed tumour	7	4	1	6	3
Clinically diagnosed metastases	6	4	3	3	4
Total	48	40	25	23	35 (73%)

scanning was accompanied by a careful clinical and neurological examination, and the findings compared with the clinical picture to see whether they could be correlated. Post-irradiation scanning gave positive findings in 21 cases and negative in 14 cases in the group, verified by histopathological diagnosis (Table 1). In the group of probable brain tumours, the results were positive in 1 case and negative in 6 cases. In the 6 patients with metastases, the results were positive in 3 and negative in 3 cases. Isotope scanning and the

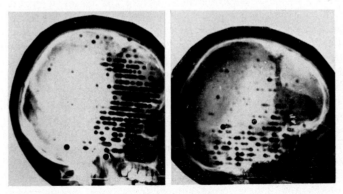

Figure 2. A lateral scan of an oligodendroglioma of the frontal region before and after irradiation (scanner)

295

patient's clinical picture were correlated in 28 of the verified cases, 3 of the unverified cases and in 4 cases in the metastatic group; that is, a total of 35 positives out of 48 (73 per cent). It is shown that the patient's clinical picture and isotope scanning were compatible and correlated in 80 per cent of the histologically proved cases. We could see very good uptake in the scanning before radiation; after the radiation, however, uptake was very small; gamma-encephalography findings correlated with the clinical picture in the same way as scintigraphy (*Figure 2*).

It is recommended that isotope scanning of the brain is made a part of the routine follow-up examination, because it can be performed on non-hospitalized patients and the more complicated pneumo-encephalographic and arteriographic examinations can be avoided.

GAMMA CAMERA

In isotope scannings the gamma camera has been used in recent years in clinical practice because it will give rapid results. In the Department of Radiotherapy of University Central Hospital, Turku, brain tumour examinations after irradiation have been performed since 1968, when the clinic had the Nuclear Chicago PHO/Gamma III-camera. The radioactive isotope tracer used is technetium as pertechnetate (^{99m} Tc) which rapidly reaches the brain blood flow and the tumour. Its physical half life is only six hours; 10 mCi of isotope is injected into a cubital vein and then travels unmixed to the superior vena cava, the right heart, the lungs, left heart and through the carotid artery to the cerebral blood vessels. The isotope thus reaches the assumed brain tumour immediately and the scanning can start immediately after injection. Before the tracer injection the patient is given calcium perchlorate to prevent, or at least to reduce, the tracer uptake in the salivary and thyroid glands (*Figure 1*).

The gamma camera has in its head a so-called technetium collimator with about 7,000 holes and a crystal of 11 inches in diameter. The equipment's recorder registers the pulses and after 200 kilopulses have been registered we obtain pictures on the oscilloscope from the brain's frontal, dorsal and lateral directions, and sometimes in addition from the vertex projection, which are permanently recorded by a Polaroid camera.

Twenty-nine patients with brain tumours were examined and, of these, 20 had been histopathologically verified; 7 cases were clinically diagnosed as brain tumours by neuroradiological examination methods, and 2 cases were clinically diagnosed brain metastases (Table 2). The histological pattern of the 20 patients with proved

TABLE 2

Results of Gamma-encephalography and its Correlation with the Clinical Picture in Histopathological Cases

	Total	Before irradiation		After irradiation		Correlation		Residual tumour	Operation or post-mortem
		Positive	Negative	Positive	Negative	Good	Poor		
Histologically proved tumours	20	15	5	14	6	17	3	16	6
						(85%)			
Clinically diagnosed tumours	7	4	3	3	4	4	3	2	
Clinically diagnosed metastases	2	2			2	2		2	
Total	29	21	8	17	12	23	6	20	
						(78%)			

297

lesions are shown in Table 3: the majority were astrocytomas and gliomas.

All these patients have had a brain scan before irradiation. Seven patients had had a partial tumour operation. A further scanning was performed at two to three months, six months, nine months and a year later and in some cases also two years after irradiation. In addition to the brain scan the patient also had an accurate neurological examination. Thus we can make a good clinical assessment of the condition of the tumour. In six patients with residual or recurrent tumours the finding was again verified histologically, four had a repeat surgical operation and in two the tumour was found at post mortem.

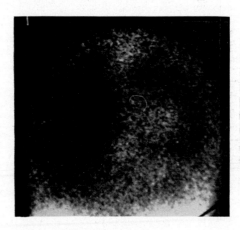

Figure 3. The frontal gamma-encephalography of a metastasis from a breast cancer before radiotherapy

Fifteen (75 per cent) patients whose tumour was verified histologically had a positive uptake shown by the brain scan and in five patients (25 per cent) there was no uptake before irradiation. In two astrocytomas a negative uptake was found after operation, in one medulloblastoma, in one spongioblastoma and in one ependymoma. The correlation between the clinical and the gamma camera findings was good in 17 cases and poor in 3 cases. Thus, 85 per cent of this group had good correlation and the scan and the clinical picture were compatible. Of 6 patients with negative findings after treatment, 3 cases showed no evidence of tumour either clinically or on the scan, while 3 patients were shown to have a residual tumour on the clinical finding and other neuroradiological examinations. Definite positive recurrences were proved in all 16 patients in this group; 4 were verified by operation and 2 at post mortem (Tables 2 and 3).

TABLE 3

Results of Gamma-encephalography and its Correlation with the Clinical Picture in Histopathological Cases

	Total	Before irradiation		After irradiation		Correlation		Residual tumour positive	Operation or post-mortem
		Positive	Negative	Positive	Negative	Good	Poor		
Astrocytoma	10	8	2	7	3	10	0	7	2
Glioma	4	4	0	4	0	4	0	4	1
Pinealoma	1	1	0	0	1	1	0		1
Medulloblastoma	2	1	1	2	0	1	1	1	
Spongioblastoma	1	0	1	0	1	0	1		
Ependymoma	2	1	1	1	1	1	1	2	2
Total	20	15	5	14	6	17	3	14	6

In the group of clinically diagnosed tumours the scan was positive in four and negative in three cases. The tumours of this group were located near the cranial surface or infratentorially; thus, the scan and the clinical picture correlated well in four (57 per cent) and poorly in three cases. One metastatic carcinoma of the breast gave a positive finding before irradiation and negative after it and the correlation with the clinical examination was, in this case, good (*Figures 3* and *4*).

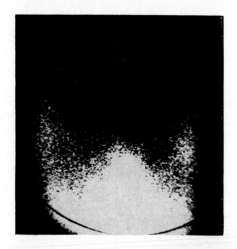

Figure 4. The same case as in Figure 3 after radiotherapy

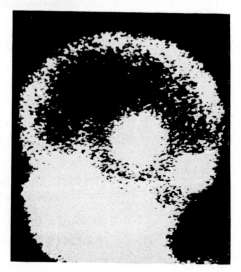

Figure 5. The uptake of a pinealoma in the lateral projection

When all the cases are added together (Table 3), the clinical picture and the gamma scan agreed in 23 out of 29 cases (78 per cent). As an example of good correlation and to demonstrate the scanning finding, we can give the findings in a two-year-old boy who had brain compression symptoms and hydrocephalus internus. Ultrasound examinations revealed a brain tumour (*see Figure 5*). To improve the cerebrospinal fluid circulation a Spitz-Holter valve was inserted and, at the same time, an inoperable tumour of 4 centimetres in diameter was found which was proved histologically to be a

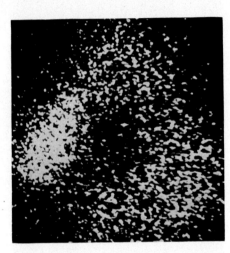

Figure 6. ^{131}I-human serum albumin in first and second ventricles

pinealoma. After operation 10 μCi ^{131}I were injected into the first ventricle and a brain scan was performed immediately. The uptake of the radioactive iodine was regular in the first and second ventricles (*Figure 6*) and the tumour revealed a defect. Eighteen hours later a new scan was performed and we could see that the isotope was normal in the ventricular system (*Figure 7*). This examination revealed that the Spitz–Holter valve was functioning. Later the patient had a course of radiation to a tumour dose of 4,800 rads and cytotoxic treatment. Six months later no uptake was shown at the tumour site (*Figure 8*); in addition a repeat ^{131}I examination revealed that the cerebrospinal fluid was flowing normally and that the valve was patent. Six months later the Spitz–Holter was removed and the hydrocephalus has not recurred and the patient remains in good condition.

The infratentorial tumours are revealed only with difficulty by scanning. For example, we will quote the negative scans in a two-year-old boy who had a medulloblastoma in the fourth ventricle.

The tumour was surgically removed and then irradiated to a 5,000-rad tumour dose by a cobalt machine. After radiation the patient had renewed brain compression symptoms and the clinical findings suggested a residual tumour. Repeat gamma camera scanning was

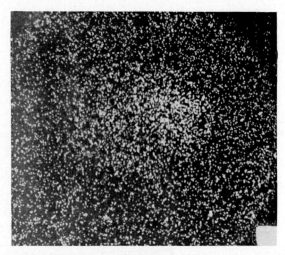

Figure 7. The same case as in Figure 6, 18 hours later. The isotope has disappeared

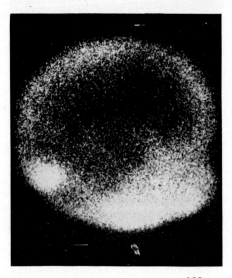

Figure 8. Scintigraphy of the same case as in Figure 5 after radiotherapy

performed and an extremely heavy uptake was shown in the frontal lobe (*Figure 9*). Despite further irradiation the patient died and post mortem revealed infratentorial and frontal tumour tissue (*Figure 10*).

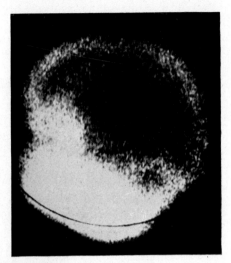

Figure 9. Medulloblastoma; a lateral brain scan of the frontal region. Infratentorially there is no uptake despite the presence of the tumour

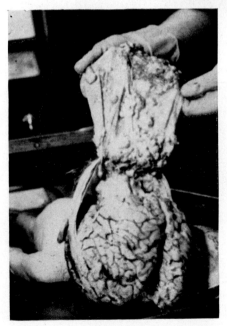

Figure 10. At post-mortem tumour tissue can be seen in the frontal and occipital region. The same case as in Figure 9

Astrocytomas, glioblastoma multiformes and oligodendrogliomas are not easily removed by radical surgery. This can be shown by radioactive scanning after operation (*Figure 11*). After radical irradiation the scan showed a completely negative uptake and no uptake could be seen in the irradiated area (*Figure 12*), suggesting that the irradiation had abated the growth. Possible recurrence can at first be verified by a neurological examination, electroencephalogram,

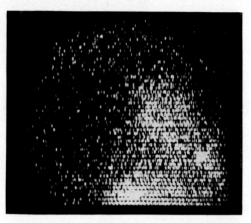

Figure 11. Gamma-encephalography in which a heavy uptake in an astrocytoma can be seen in the temporal region

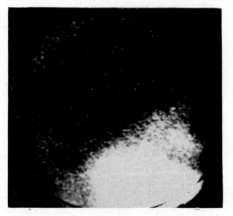

Figure 12. The same case as in Figure 11 after radiotherapy. No uptake and the patient is clinically very well

arteriography or pneumoencephalogram. Isotope brain scanning should also be performed and the recurrent area can be seen as a heavy uptake, limited and obviously located (*Figure 13*).

Glioblastoma multiforme has a very heavy uptake and the tumour limits are well defined (*Figure 14*). In spite of what appears to be a macroscopically complete removal of the tumour, it may still be

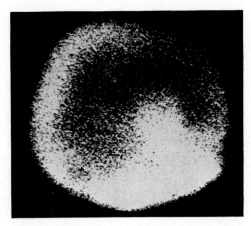

Figure 13. The same case as in Figures 11 and 12, 3½ years after irradiation. The uptake results from a recurrence

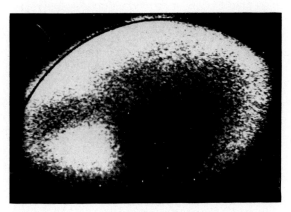

Figure 14. Glioblastoma multiforme in the frontal region which has a very heavy uptake of radioisotope

shown that there is an uptake at the site three to four weeks later (*Figure 15*). At about two months after irradiation, when the tumour has been destroyed, the finding on scanning is shown to be negative (*Figure 16*). Repeated examinations are necessary at three-monthly intervals because of probable recurrences. The clinical symptoms do not cause the patient much trouble and recurrence may not be suspected. Neurological examinations do not always show recurrences

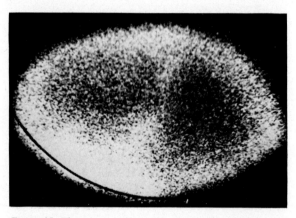

Figure 15. The same case as in Figure 14 after radical operation. A little uptake of isotope can be seen in the area of the operation

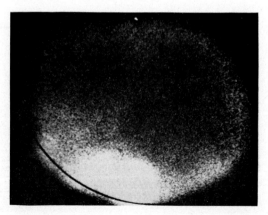

Figure 16. The same case as in Figures 14 and 15 two months after radiotherapy. No uptake and the patient is very well

but the scan may suggest recurrence, as can be seen in *Figure 17* taken ten months after irradiation. This patient was examined 13 months after the original irradiation and an obvious radioactive uptake in the frontotemporal region was found; the patient did not have any clinical symptoms but a neurological examination showed an obvious recurrence. Surgery revealed recurrence (*Figure 18*).

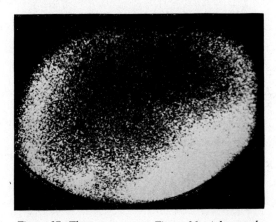

Figure 17. The same case as Figure 16; eight months later the radioactive uptake is in the same area as the original tumour but the patient is well

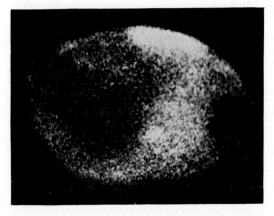

Figure 18. Same case as in Figure 17; the uptake is very clear in the scan 13 months after irradiation. Recurrence was verified at operation

The uptake in scanning is very small when the brain tumour is necrotic or badly vascularized (*Figure 19*); at operation necrotic material is frequently found and can be removed by suction. In the patient a recurrence was shown on repeat scanning four months later (*Figure 20*).

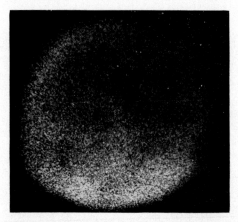

Figure 19. Gamma-encephalography in lateral projection before treatment. The uptake is very poor. At operation the tumour was very necrotic

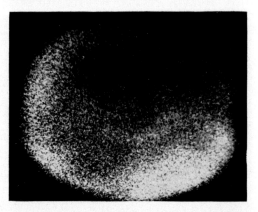

Figure 20. The same case as in Figure 19; four months after treatment by surgery and radiotherapy, the uptake is clearer and the clinical picture showed the recurrence

DISCUSSION

Brain scan after a course of radiotherapy justifies its place as a method of examination to complement the neuroradiological, neurological and clinical examinations. In these studies a good correlation was achieved between clinical findings and isotope scanning in 80–85 per cent of the histologically verified cases. When the clinically diagnosed and metastatic tumours were taken into account, there was good correlation between the clinical findings and the scan in 73–78 per cent.

In few cases the scan has played a significant part in deciding the subsequent treatment to be given. For example, in a patient with a pinealoma it was possible to determine that the Spitz–Holter valve could be removed; this was done with improvement in the patient's condition. In another patient it was possible to arrange for an operation on the second recurrence in time.

Gamma-encephalography may be recommended in follow-up examinations especially because the examination can easily be performed on non-hospitalized patients without any risk and the much more troublesome pneumoencephalographic or arteriographic examinations can thereby be avoided. In addition isotope scanning is easy to perform on a patient who is in poor general condition and can even be repeated frequently. Scanning provides a clear idea of the location and size of a tumour recurrence.

The examination can thus be performed when the patient comes for a follow-up examination. The first examination should be carried out at about two to three months after treatment and then routine control examinations every three months for two to three years because recurrences may appear later despite successful irradiation. A good clinical picture, a tumour that has been surgically removed and no suspicious findings at follow-up examination may suggest less frequent scanning examinations—say at about six-monthly intervals.

SUMMARY

In this paper the importance of regular brain scans after treatment by irradiation has been shown. In this study a commercial scanner and gamma camera have been used, using as the radioactive isotope tracer either [203]Hg-Neohydrin or ^{99m}Tc as pertechnetate. Scanning has been performed two to three months, six months, nine months and a year after radiotherapy to the brain tumour and it justifies its place as a method of post-irradiation control to complement neuro-radiological, neurological and clinical examinations. A good correlation was achieved between clinical findings and isotope scanning in 80–85 per cent of the histologically verified cases and in 78 per cent of all cases if clinically diagnosed; and metastatic tumours are included.

REFERENCES

Blau, M. and Bender, M. A. (1962). 'Radiomercury (Hg^{203}) labeled neo-hydrin: a new agent of brain tumor localization.' *J. nucl. Med.*, **3**, 83.

Brenner, M., Pihkanen, T. A. and Voutilainen, A. (1964). 'Radioisotopic diagnosis of brain tumors.' *Annls Med. exp. Fenn.*, **42**, 145.

— — — (1964). 'Aivo-scanning—uusi kallonsisäisten sairauksien tut-kimiskeino.' *Duodecim*, **80**, 915.

Dugger, G. S. and Pepper, F. D. (1963). 'The reliability of radioisotopic encephalography.' *Neurology*, **13**, 1042.

Quimby, E. H. and Feitelberg, S. (1963). *Radioactive Isotopes in Medicine and Biology*. Philadelphia; Lea & Febiger.

Voutilainen, A. and Pihkanen, T. (1965). 'Gammaencephalography as a method of checking on irradiation of brain tumours.' *Annls Med. int. Fenn.*, **54**, 143.

Index

Acoustic neuroma, surgery of, 103
Acromegaly, 12, 101, 224, 226, 227, 230 (*see also* Pituitary tumours)
Adamantinoma, 234
Adrenal cortex, tumours of, 232
Adrenalectomy, 233
Age, affecting radiation effect, 133
Anaesthesia, raised intracranial pressure and, 126
Anaplasia, 23
Angiography, 35
  spinal, 47
Angiomas, calcification, 34
Anosmia, 117
Aqueduct stenosis, 43
Arabinosyl cytosine, 271
  DNA precursor studies, 276
  experimental studies, 274
  meningeal carcinomatosis, in, 286
Arteriography, radio-isotope, 66
Astrocytomas,
  calcification, 34
  cerebral hemisphere, 94
  cerebral scanning, 62, 299, 304
  classification, 18
  localization of, 138
  malignancy of, 93
  optic nerve, 95
  pathology, 19
  pontine, electroencephalography in, 81
  posterior fossa, 99
  prognosis, 96
  radiology of, 47
  radiosensitivity of, 136
  radio-sensitization of, 176

radiotherapy, 132, 142, 148
  field size, 138
  post-operative, 143
recurrence, 267
reversion of, 5
spinal, 106
surgery of, 94, 99, 142, 148
survival rates, 142
treatment, general principles, 5

Basilar artery, involvement of, 92, 103
Basophil adenoma of pituitary, 12
Benign intracranial hypertension, 110
  lumbar puncture in, 122
  papilloedema in, 112
Biopsy of tissue, 137
1,3-Bis(2-Chloroethyl)-1-nitroso-urea (BCNU), 270
  cerebral metastases, in, 285
  DNA precursor studies, 276
  effectiveness of, 281
  experimental studies, 273, 274
  glioblastoma multiforme, in, 270, 283
  recurrent medulloblastoma, in, 286
  toxicity, 287
Bitemporal hemianopsia, 117, 226, 231
Blindness following radiotherapy, 11
Blood brain barrier, chemothera-peutic agents passing, 281

INDEX

Indium-113, cerebral scanning with, 58
Infratentorial tumours,
  cerebral scanning, 301
  electroencephalography in, 78
  herniation in, 113
  survival rate, 98
Interstitial implantation therapy, 225
Intracranial pressure, raised (*see* Raised intracranial pressure)
5-Iodo-2-deoxycytidine, 172
Ipsilateral hemiplegia, 116
Isotope studies in diagnosis (*see* Cerebral scanning)

Jugular canal, chemodectoma, 51

Kernohan classification, 18
17-Ketosteroids, 233
Kidney, metastases from, 105, 253, 258

Laminectomy for spinal cord metastases, 244, 246
Lateral rectus palsies, 116
Leukaemia, meningeal deposits in (*see* Meningeal leukaemia)
Location of tumours,
  calcification in, 32
  cardinal radiological signs, 28
  echo-encephalography, by, 71
  electro-encephalography, by, 78–87
  erosion, 29
  expansion, 31
  false signs, 116
  hyperostosis, 31
  need for accuracy, 139, 235
  pressure, 28
  radiotherapy and, 137, 147
Lumbar puncture, measurement of intracranial pressure by, 121

Lung cancer,
  cerebral metastases from, 82, 100, 253, 255, 256
    treatment, 258, 259, 260, 286
  spinal metastases, 105
Lung metastases,
  chordoma from, 197
Lymphoma,
  spinal cord involvement, 104
  radiotherapy, 107
Lymphosarcoma, spinal metastases from, 244

Malignancy, changing order of, 4
Mannitol in cerebral oedema, 125, 126
Medulloblastoma, 24, 153–9
  cerebral scanning in, 298, 299
    following radiation, 298, 301, 303
  chemotherapy of, 159
  classification, 18
  growth and spread, 24, 26
  incidence, 153
  pathology, 25, 153
  prognosis, 157
    factors influencing, 158
  radiosensitivity, 4, 135, 136
  radio-sensitization of, 176
  radiotherapy, 7, 155
    complications, 164
    fields used, 156
    fractionation, 156
    palliative, 158
    supervoltage, 156
    technique, 155
    whole central nervous system, 155
  recurrence, 158
    chemotherapy, 286
    treatment, 266
  surgical biopsy in, 155
  surgery of, 7, 99, 154
  survival rate, 7, 157
  treatment, 7, 154

317